T0205790

Informatik aktuell

Reihe herausgegeben von

Gesellschaft für Informatik e.V. (GI), Bonn, Deutschland

Ziel der Reihe ist die möglichst schnelle und weite Verbreitung neuer Forschungs- und Entwicklungsergebnisse, zusammenfassender Übersichtsberichte über den Stand eines Gebietes und von Materialien und Texten zur Weiterbildung. In erster Linie werden Tagungsberichte von Fachtagungen der Gesellschaft für Informatik veröffentlicht, die regelmäßig, oft in Zusammenarbeit mit anderen wissenschaftlichen Gesellschaften, von den Fachausschüssen der Gesellschaft für Informatik veranstaltet werden. Die Auswahl der Vorträge erfolgt im allgemeinen durch international zusammengesetzte Programmkomitees.

Weitere Bände in der Reihe https://link.springer.com/bookseries/2872

Klaus Maier-Hein · Thomas M. Deserno ·
Heinz Handels · Andreas Maier ·
Christoph Palm · Thomas Tolxdorff
(Hrsg.)

Bildverarbeitung für die Medizin 2022

Proceedings, German Workshop on
Medical Image Computing,
Heidelberg, June 26–28, 2022

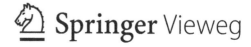

Hrsg.

Klaus Maier-Hein
Medical Image Computing, E230
Deutsches Krebsforschungszentrum
(DKFZ)
Heidelberg, Deutschland

Heinz Handels
Institut für Medizinische Informatik
Universität zu Lübeck
Lübeck, Deutschland

Christoph Palm
Fakultät für Informatik und Mathematik
Ostbayerische Technische Hochschule
Regensburg
Regensburg, Deutschland

Thomas M. Deserno
Peter L. Reichertz Institut für Medizinische
Informatik der TU Braunschweig und der
Medizinischen Hochschule Hannover
Braunschweig, Deutschland

Andreas Maier (ID)
Lehrstuhl für Mustererkennung
Friedrich-Alexander-Universität
Erlangen, Deutschland

Thomas Tolxdorff
Institut für Medizinische Informatik
Charité – Universitätsmedizin Berlin
Berlin, Deutschland

ISSN 1431-472X
Informatik aktuell
ISBN 978-3-658-36931-6   ISBN 978-3-658-36932-3   (eBook)
https://doi.org/10.1007/978-3-658-36932-3

Die Deutsche Nationalbibliothek verzeichnet diese Publikation in der Deutschen Nationalbibliografie; detaillierte bibliografische Daten sind im Internet über http://dnb.d-nb.de abrufbar.

Planung: Petra Steinmüller
Springer Vieweg ist ein Imprint der eingetragenen Gesellschaft Springer Fachmedien Wiesbaden GmbH und ist ein Teil von Springer Nature.
Die Anschrift der Gesellschaft ist: Abraham-Lincoln-Str. 46, 65189 Wiesbaden, Germany

Bildverarbeitung für die Medizin 2022

Veranstalter

MIC   Medical Image Computing
                   Deutsches Krebsforschungszentrum (DKFZ)
                   Heidelberg

Unterstützende Fachgesellschaften

BVMI	Berufsverband Medizinischer Informatiker
CURAC	Computer- und Roboterassistierte Chirurgie
DAGM	Deutsche Arbeitsgemeinschaft für Mustererkennung
DGBMT	Fachgruppe Medizinische Informatik der Deutschen Gesellschaft für Biomedizinische Technik im Verband Deutscher Elektrotechniker
GI	Gesellschaft für Informatik – Fachbereich Informatik in den Lebenswissenschaften
GMDS	Gesellschaft für Medizinische Informatik, Biometrie und Epidemiologie
IEEE	Joint Chapter Engineering in Medicine and Biology, German Section

Tagungsvorsitz

Prof. Dr. Klaus H. Maier-Hein
Medical Image Computing (MIC)
Deutsches Krebsforschungszentrum (DKFZ), Heidelberg

Tagungssekretariat

Stefanie Strzysch, Theresa Klocke und Michaela Gelz
Medical Image Computing (MIC), DKFZ

Anschrift:	Im Neuenheimer Feld 223, 69120 Heidelberg
Email:	orga-2022@bvm-workshop.org
Web:	https://bvm-workshop.org

Lokale BVM-Organisation

Prof. Dr. Klaus Maier-Hein, Jasmin Metzger, Dr. Peter Neher, Dr. Beatrix Tettmann, Dr. Daniel Walther, Dimitrios Bounias, Dr. Kathrin Brunk, Maximilian Fischer, Philipp Schader, Shuhan Xiao, Silvia Dias Almeida, u.v.m.

Verteilte BVM-Organisation

Begutachtung	Heinz Handels und Jan-Hinrich Wrage – Institut für Medizinische Informatik, Universität zu Lübeck
Mailingliste	Klaus Maier-Hein – Medical Image Computing, Deutsches Krebsforschungszentrum (DKFZ) Heidelberg
Special Issue	Andreas Maier – Lehrstuhl für Mustererkennung, Friedrich-Alexander Universität Erlangen-Nürnberg
Sponsoring	Thomas Tolxdorff und Thorsten Schaaf – Institut für Medizinische Informatik, Charité-Universitätsmedizin Berlin
Tagungsband	Thomas M. Deserno, Michael Völcker, Nick Igelbrink und Nico Stautmeister – Peter L. Reichertz Institut für Medizinische Informatik (PLRI), Technische Universität Braunschweig und Medizinische Hochschule Hannover
Web & News	Christoph Palm, Leonard Klausmann, Alexander Leis und Sümeyye R. Yildiran – Regensburg Medical Image Computing (ReMIC), Ostbayerische Technische Hochschule Regensburg

BVM-Komitee

Prof. Dr. Thomas M. Deserno, Peter L. Reichertz Institut für Medizinische Informatik (PLRI), Technische Universität Braunschweig und Medizinische Hochschule Hannover

Prof. Dr. Heinz Handels, Institut für Medizinische Informatik, Universität zu Lübeck

Prof. Dr. Andreas Maier, Lehrstuhl für Mustererkennung, Friedrich-Alexander-Universität Erlangen-Nürnberg

Prof. Dr. Klaus Maier-Hein, Medical Image Computing, Deutsches Krebsforschungszentrum Heidelberg

Prof. Dr. Christoph Palm, Regensburg Medical Image Computing (ReMIC), Ostbayerische Technische Hochschule Regensburg

Prof. Dr. Thomas Tolxdorff, Institut für Medizinische Informatik, Charité–Universitätsmedizin Berlin

Programmkomitee

Jürgen Braun, Charité-Universitätsmedizin Berlin
Thomas M. Deserno, TU Braunschweig
Jan Ehrhardt, Universität zu Lübeck
Sandy Engelhardt, Universitätsklinik Heidelberg
Ralf Floca, DKFZ Heidelberg
Nils Forkert, University of Calgary, Canada
Michael Götz, Universitätsklinikum Ulm
Horst Hahn, Fraunhofer MEVIS, Bremen
Heinz Handels, Universität zu Lübeck
Tobias Heimann, Siemens Healthcare, Erlangen
Mattias Heinrich, Universität zu Lübeck
Anja Hennemuth, Charité-Universitätsmedizin Berlin
Alexander Horsch, The Arctic University of Norway, Tromsø, Norwegen
Dagmar Kainmüller, MDC Berlin
Ron Kikinis, Harvard Medical School, Boston, USA
Dagmar Krefting, Universität Göttingen
Andreas Maier, Universität Erlangen-Nürnberg
Klaus Maier-Hein, DKFZ Heidelberg
Lena Maier-Hein, DKFZ Heidelberg
Andre Mastmeyer, Hochschule Aalen
Dorit Merhof, RWTH Aachen
Jan Modersitzki, Fraunhofer MEVIS, Lübeck
Heinrich Müller, TU Dortmund
Nassir Navab, TU München
Marco Nolden, DKFZ Heidelberg
Christoph Palm, OTH Regensburg
Bernhard Preim, Universität Magdeburg
Stefanie Remmele, HAW Landshut
Petra Ritter, BIH Berlin
Karl Rohr, Universität Heidelberg
Daniel Rückert, TU München
Sylvia Saalfeld, Universität Magdeburg
Dennis Säring, FH Wedel
Julia Schnabel, TU München/Helmholtz Zentrum München
Ingrid Scholl, FH Aachen
Stefanie Speidel, HZDR (NCT Dresden)
Thomas Tolxdorff, Charité-Universitätsmedizin Berlin
Klaus Tönnies, Universität Magdeburg
Gudrun Wagenknecht, Forschungszentrum Jülich
René Werner, UKE Hamburg
Thomas Wittenberg, Fraunhofer IIS Erlangen
Ivo Wolf, Hochschule Mannheim

Preisträger der BVM 2021 in Regensburg

Beste wissenschaftliche Arbeiten

1. **Tristan M. Gottschalk**
   (Lehrstuhl für Mustererkennung, Friedrich-Alexander Universität Erlangen-Nürnberg)
   Gottschalk TM, Maier A, Kordon F, Kreher BW
   Learning-Based Patch-Wise Metal Segmentation with Consistency Check

1. **Jan Macdonald**
   (Institut für Mathematik, Technische Universität Berlin)
   Macdonald J, März M, Oala L, Samek W
   Interval Neural Networks as Instability Detectors for Image Reconstructions

3. **Alexander Bigalke**
   (Institut für Medizinische Informatik, Universität zu Lübeck)
   Bigalke A, Hansen L, Heinrich MP
   End-to-end learning of body weight prediction from point clouds with basis point sets

Bester Vortrag

Katharina Breininger
(Lehrstuhl für Mustererkennung, Friedrich-Alexander-Universität Erlangen-Nürnberg)
Breininger K, Pfister M, Kowarschik M, Maier A
Move Over There: One-click Deformation Correction for Image Fusion During Endovascular Aortic Repair

Bestes Poster

Carina Tschigor
(Frauenhofer MEVIS, Bremen)
Tschigor C, Chlebus G, Schumann C
Deep Learning-basierte Oberflächenrekonstruktion aus Binärmasken

Vorwort

Die Tagung *Bildverarbeitung für die Medizin (BVM)* wird seit weit mehr als 20 Jahren an wechselnden Orten Deutschlands veranstaltet. Inhaltlich fokussiert sich die BVM dabei auf die computergestützte Analyse medizinischer Bilddaten mit vielfältigen Anwendungsgebieten, z.B. im Bereich der Bildgebung, der Diagnostik, der Operationsplanung, der computerunterstützten Intervention und der Visualisierung.

In dieser Zeit hat es bemerkenswerte methodische Weiterentwicklungen und Umbrüche gegeben, wie zum Beispiel im Bereich des maschinellen Lernens, an denen die BVM-Community intensiv mitgearbeitet hat. In der Folge dominieren inzwischen Arbeiten im Zusammenhang mit *Deep Learning* die BVM. Auch diese Entwicklungen haben dazu beigetragen, dass die Medizinische Bildverarbeitung an der Schnittstelle zwischen Informatik und Medizin als eine der Schlüsseltechnologien zur Digitalisierung des Gesundheitswesens etabliert ist.

Zentraler Aspekt der BVM ist neben der Darstellung aktueller Forschungsergebnisse schwerpunktmäßig aus der vielfältigen deutschlandweiten BVM-Community insbesondere die Förderung des wissenschaftlichen Nachwuchses. Die Tagung dient vor allem Doktorand*innen und Postdoktorand*innen, aber auch Studierenden mit hervorragenden Bachelor- und Masterarbeiten als Plattform, um ihre Arbeiten zu präsentieren, dabei in den fachlichen Diskurs mit der Community zu treten und Netzwerke mit Fachkolleg*innen zu knüpfen. Trotz der vielen Tagungen und Kongresse, die auch für die Medizinische Bildverarbeitung relevant sind, hat die BVM deshalb nichts von ihrer Bedeutung und Anziehungskraft eingebüßt.

Inhaltlich kann auch bei der BVM 2022 wieder ein attraktives und hochklassiges Programm geboten werden. Es wurden aus 88 Einreichungen über ein anonymisiertes Reviewing-Verfahren mit jeweils drei Reviews 24 Vorträge, 33 Posterbeiträge und eine Softwaredemonstration angenommen. Da aufgrund der strengen Covid Hygiene- und Abstandsregeln leider nur sehr wenige klassische Posterbeiträge zugelassen wurden, wird dieses Jahr erstmalig ein neues Format umgesetzt. Hierfür wurden 13 weitere Beiträge als e-Poster angenommen. Die besten Arbeiten werden auch in diesem Jahr mit Preisen ausgezeichnet. Die Webseite des Workshops findet sich unter https://www.bvm-workshop.org.

Das Programm wird durch drei eingeladene Vorträge ergänzt:

- **Prof. Dr. Ullrich Köthe**, Visual Learning Lab, Universität Heidelberg

- **Prof. Mihaela van der Schaar**, University of Cambridge, UK

- **Prof. Dr. Stefanie Speidel**, Translational Surgical Oncology, NCT Dresden

Des Weiteren werden im Vorfeld der BVM drei Tutorials angeboten:

- **Known Operator Learning and Hybrid Machine Learning in Medical Imaging The Past, the Present and the Future** (FAU Erlangen-Nürnberg)

- **Advanced Deep Learning** (DKFZ Heidelberg)

- **Hands-On Medical Image Registration** (Universität zu Lübeck)

An dieser Stelle möchten wir allen, die bei den umfangreichen Vorbereitungen zum Gelingen des Workshops beigetragen haben, unseren herzlichen Dank für ihr Engagement aussprechen: den Referent*innen der Gastvorträge, den Autor*innen der Beiträge, den Referent*innen der Tutorien, den Industrierepräsentant*innen, dem Programmkomitee, den Fachgesellschaften, den Mitgliedern des BVM-Organisationsteams und allen Mitarbeitenden der Abteilung Medical Image Computing des Deutschen Krebsforschungszentrums.

Wir wünschen allen Teilnehmer*innen des Workshops BVM 2022 spannende neue Kontakte und inspirierende Eindrücke aus der Welt der medizinischen Bildverarbeitung.

Januar 2022

Klaus Maier-Hein (Heidelberg)
Thomas M. Deserno (Braunschweig)
Heinz Handels (Lübeck)
Andreas Maier (Erlangen)
Christoph Palm (Regensburg)
Thomas Tolxdorff (Berlin)

Inhaltsverzeichnis

Die fortlaufende Nummer am linken Seitenrand entspricht den Beitragsnummern, wie sie im endgültigen Programm des Workshops zu finden sind. Dabei steht V für Vortrag, P für Poster, E für ePoster und S für Softwaredemonstration.

Session 2: Segmentation II

Session 3: Detection

Session 4: Registration / Detection

Session 5: Surgical Data Science / Virtual Reality

Session 6: Surgical Data Science / Simulation / Data Sets

Postersession 1

Postersession 2

Postersession 3

Software Demonstration

ePostersession

Unsupervised Segmentation of Wounds in Optical Coherence Tomography Images Using Invariant Information Clustering

Julia Andresen[1], Timo Kepp[1], Michael Wang-Evers[2], Jan Ehrhardt[1,3],
Dieter Manstein[2], Heinz Handels[1,3]

[1]Institute of Medical Informatics, University of Lübeck
[2]Cutaneous Biology Research Center, Department of Dermatology, Massachusetts General
Hospital, Harvard Medical School
[3]German Research Center for Artificial Intelligence, Lübeck
j.andresen@uni-luebeck.de

Abstract. Monitoring wound healing with optical coherence tomography (OCT) imaging is a promising research field. So far, however, few data and even less manual annotations of OCT wound images are available. To address this problem, a fully unsupervised clustering method based on convolutional neural networks (CNNs) is presented. The CNN takes image patches as input and assigns them to either wound or healthy skin clusters. Network training is based on a new combination of loss functions that require information invariance and locality preservation. No expensive expert annotations are needed. Locality preservation is applied to different levels of the network and shown to improve the segmentation. Promising results are achieved with an average Dice score of 0.809 and an average rand index of 0.871 for the best performing network version.

1 Introduction

The segmentation of anatomical or pathological structures is a crucial step in medical image processing that eases subsequent tasks such as disease monitoring or image registration. Manual segmentation however is time-consuming, error-prone and requires expert knowledge. Automatic segmentation methods such as convolutional neural networks (CNNs) speed up and harmonize medical image segmentation. Still, supervised training of CNNs depends on huge amounts of labelled data which are often not available. In contrast, clustering-based segmentation methods enable the delineation of structures without given labels by grouping similar and separating differing voxels.

In this paper, we present a clustering CNN for the segmentation of wounds in optical coherence tomography (OCT) images of the skin. The network receives image patches as input and assigns them to either wound or healthy skin clusters. Training is based on maximizing the mutual information between network outputs for pairs of original and randomly augmented image patches. This invariant information clustering [1] is combined with a locality-preserving (LP) loss. The LP loss favours similar encodings for close patches which leads to better clustering results. The resulting segmentations are compared to manual delineations of the wound area. Furthermore, we analyze the effect of applying the LP loss at different stages of the network on its clustering abilities.

2   Methods

In this section we first delineate the OCT data acquisition and preprocessing procedures. Subsequently, the network architecture and the training scheme for unsupervised wound segmentation are described.

2.1   Data acquisition

We used 12 human skin equivalents (EFT-400, MatTek, Ashland, MA, USA) and induced two circular wounds in the epidermis by a 1.5-mm biopsy punch. The skin equivalents were cultured in medium (EFT-400-ASY, MatTek), and the medium was exchanged daily for one week. An OCT scanner (TEL220C1, Thorlabs) with a central wavelength of 1300 nm was used to acquire volumetric images with an axial resolution of 4.2 μm, a lateral resolution of 13 μm (LSM03, Thorlabs), and a dimension of $3 \times 3 \times 3.5$ mm^3 (spatial FOV: $461 \times 461 \times 1024$ voxels). OCT images were taken on day 0, 1, 2, 3, 4 and 7 after the epidermal injury for each wound separately leading to 144 images in total.

2.2   Preprocessing

Due to poor contrast and large image size we perform average-smoothing on each horizontal slice and reduce the resolution to $64 \times 128 \times 284$ voxels. In a second step a flattening of the upper skin border is performed as shown in Figure 1. To do so, we 1) calculate the image gradient magnitude, 2) A-scan-wise extract the maximum gradient and enter its position into a height map, 3) mask the central area of the height map, 4) smooth the height map, 5) fill the masked area using bilinear interpolation and 6) translate each A-scan according to the height map so that the maximum gradient position is shifted to a fixed slice. The rectangular-shaped mask used in step 3) is selected by manual inspection and covers all wounds entirely. Like this, the translation of A-scans is based only on the position of the intact skin. Finally, the images are cropped to the upper $64 \times 128 \times 92$ voxels.

2.3   Clustering network

The architecture of the network is depicted in Figure 2. It consists of a convolutional backbone and two clustering heads each composed of three fully-connected (FC) layers

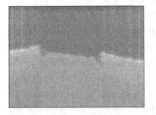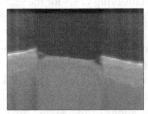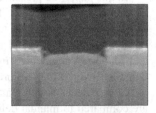

Fig. 1. Preprocessing steps taken before clustering. Left: original, middle: smoothing and downsampling, right: flattening.

and a final softmax activation. Input to our clustering network are 3D patches of size $11 \times 11 \times 92$ voxels. The output of the convolutional backbone is flattened and concatenated with a vector indicating the patch position in the image volume. The enlarged feature vector then serves as input to the first FC layers of main and overclustering head. The main head outputs a two-entry vector that contains the probabilities of the patch belonging to the wound and healthy skin clusters while the overclustering head produces ten instead of two clusters. Both heads are trained simultaneously with the same loss function allowing the overclustering head to discriminate patches inside the same cluster while maintaining the skin and wound predictions of the main head. This may help to increase expressivity in the learned features [1, 2].

2.4   Loss functions

The network $\Phi(\theta)$ with its corresponding parameters θ is trained using a two-component loss function based on invariant information clustering (IIC) and locality preservation. The objective of IIC is to maintain similarities between paired inputs and to discard instance-specific details. This is achieved by maximizing the mutual information between the soft clustering outputs of the paired inputs [1]. To use IIC for wound segmentation we apply this principle on pairs of image patches. Each pair consists of one original image patch x and a randomly augmented version x' of this patch. Augmentation includes the addition of random noise and random intensity transformations. The IIC part of the loss function is then given by

$$\mathcal{L}_{\text{IIC}}(\theta; x, x') = -\text{MI}\big(\Phi(\theta; x),\ \Phi(\theta; x')\big) \tag{1}$$

which has the effect of discarding differences between augmented and original patch and of making the network outputs the same for both patch versions.

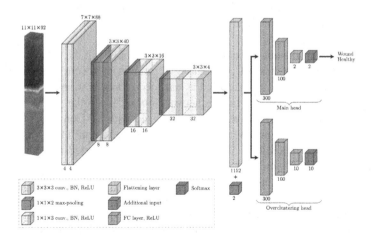

Fig. 2. Architecture of the patch-wise clustering network for wound segmentation. A convolutional backbone is followed by three FC layers. No padding is performed in the convolutional layers. Numbers below the convolutional layers indicate number of feature maps while the numbers above give the size of the outputs of the last convolutional layer.

To prevent inhomogeneous clusters, we add a second term to the loss function. The LP loss takes two patches x_i and x_j of the same image volume as input and favours similar encoded representations z_i and z_j for close patches. Inspired by [3, 4] we define

$$\mathcal{L}_{LP}(\theta; x_i, x_j) = \omega(\|l_i - l_j\|_2) \cdot s(x_i, x_j) \cdot \|z_i - z_j\|_2^2 \qquad (2)$$

Here, l_i is the location of patch x_i, s is an image similarity measure and ω a weighting function assigning small distances a large weight and setting large distances to zero. Like this, spatially close patches are pushed to similar encodings while distant patches may be clustered independently. The final loss function is calculated for all consecutive patch pairs in a batch and defined by

$$\mathcal{L}(\theta; x_i, x_j) = \mathcal{L}_{IIC}(x_i, x_i') + \mathcal{L}_{IIC}(x_j, x_j') + \mathcal{L}_{LP}(x_i, x_j) + \mathcal{L}_{LP}(x_i', x_j') \qquad (3)$$

The network is trained for 200 epochs, with Adam optimization and an initial learning rate of $1e^{-6}$. For each epoch, 150 pairs of patches per volume are drawn at random using a uniform distribution and passed through the network. During inference only original image patches (rather than pairs of patches) are input to the network and the overclustering head is ignored. The main head's clustering result is kept for the patch's central A-scan that is assigned the cluster with highest probability to achieve an A-scan-wise segmentation result.

3   Results

For evaluation, a six-fold cross-validation is performed, training the network on 120 images of 10 skin equivalents and testing it on the remaining 24 images. For each test set one of the four included wounds is manually segmented over all time points. The clustering ability of the networks is checked quantitatively comparing results to the manual segmentations and qualitatively using t-distributed stochastic neighbor embedding (t-SNE) for visualization [5].

We train several versions of our clustering method applying the LP loss on different levels of the network. Successively, the feature vectors output by convolutional backbone, first, second and third FC layer are used as encoded representations z in equation (3). Note that applying the LP loss on the network output is similar to the local spatial invariance used in [1]. Network versions are denoted with LP-Conv, LP-FC1, LP-FC2 and LP-FC3, respectively, and we report average DSC and rand index (RI) compared to the manual labels in Table 1. Additionally, results are reported for training without applying the LP loss (IIC only).

Results show that the clustering network learns to well distinguish between patches lying inside or outside of the wound. The LP loss greatly improves performance compared to the network trained on IIC alone leading to an average DSC of 0.809 for LP-Conv. For this best performing network version exemplar segmentation results are displayed in Figure 3 which shows that even the segmentation of the image with lowest DSC is still close to the actual wound area. Although the flattening does not work for this image because of the partially detached epidermis, the CNN still produces useful results.

Tab. 1. Results of the clustering network trained by applying LP on different levels. Average DSC and RI are reported. In brackets the minimal and maximal values are given and best results are presented in bold font.

Method	DSC	RI
IIC only	0.464 (0.339, 0.655)	0.479 (0.254, 0.743)
LP-Conv	**0.809** (0.678, 0.960)	**0.871** (0.768, 0.981)
LP-FC1	0.761 (0.596, 0.892)	0.832 (0.676, 0.939)
LP-FC2	0.777 (0.648, 0.914)	0.845 (0.743, 0.955)
LP-FC3	0.494 (0.312, 0.649)	0.607 (0.347, 0.779)

To further analyze the effect of the LP loss on the clustering abilities of the network, principle component analysis is used to reduce the high-dimensional feature vectors of convolutional backbone, first and second FC layer to a size of 50. Afterwards t-SNE plots are generated to visualize features in two dimensions (perplexity set to 50, further experiments with different values led to similar results). Plots are generated with 850 randomly selected patches per skin equivalent in the first test set. Representative results in Figure 4 show that especially for LP-FC1 and LP-FC2 the separability of clusters is increased in the feature space the LP loss is applied in. Also it can be seen that using the LP loss leads to clusters aligning well with wound and healthy skin whereas IIC only generates more intertwined clusters. This reflects the quantitive results showing how the LP loss helps to generate better segmentation results compared to training with IIC only.

4 Discussion

In this paper, a method for unsupervised segmentation of OCT wound images is presented. Without using any labelled data, the clustering network learns to distinguish

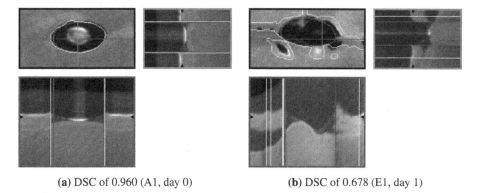

(a) DSC of 0.960 (A1, day 0)　　　　　　(b) DSC of 0.678 (E1, day 1)

Fig. 3. Segmentation results on best (a) and worst (b) performing test images compared to manual ground truth. Predicted and ground-truth segmentation contours are shown in green and red, respectively. Black triangles, blue and orange lines mark the position of the other depicted image slices.

Fig. 4. T-SNE plots displaying the feature vectors of convolutional backbone (1st and 4th columns), first (2nd and 5th columns) and second FC layer (3rd and 6th columns) in two dimensions for IIC only (a, b, c), LP-Conv (d, e, f), LP-FC1 (g, h, i) and LP-FC2 (j, k, l).

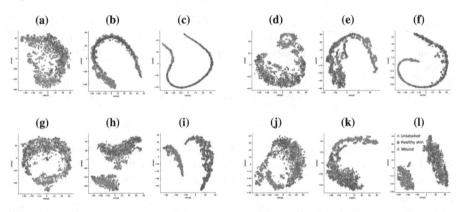

patches lying outside or inside of the wound. T-SNE plots show that the LP loss helps to form better separable clusters in the feature space leading to good segmentation results. Best results are achieved using the outputs of the convolutional backbone to calculate the LP loss with a mean Dice score of 0.809 compared to manually segmented images.

Still, further investigations on the best choice of hyperparameters and a more sophisticated quantitative evaluation of the method need to be done. We plan to analyze the effect of different patch sizes. The network tends to oversegment the wound area which we assign to the relatively large patch size. Smaller patch sizes down to A-scans might help prevent this problem. Moreover, we intend to test the clustering network for unsupervised segmentation of retinal OCT images.

All in all, our clustering network is a promising method for unsupervised detection and segmentation of pathologies in medical images. It is not limited to OCT images and may also be used to segment anatomical structures. Since no manual labels are required for network training the method is applicable to a wide range of datasets.

References

1. Ji X, Henriques JF, Vedaldi A. Invariant information clustering for unsupervised image classification and segmentation. Proc IEEE ICCV. 2019:9865–74.
2. Do K, Tran T, Venkatesh S. Clustering by maximizing mutual information across views. Proc IEEE ICCV. 2021:9928–38.
3. Aljalbout E, Golkov V, Siddiqui Y, Strobel M, Cremers D. Clustering with deep learning: taxonomy and new methods. arXiv preprint. 2018;arXiv:1801.07648.
4. Huang P, Huang Y, Wang W, Wang L. Deep embedding network for clustering. Proc IEEE ICRR. 2014:1532–7.
5. Van der Maaten L, Hinton G. Visualizing data using t-SNE. J Mach Learn Res. 2008;9(11):2579–605.

Iterative 3D CNN Based Segmentation of Vascular Trees in Liver CT

Mona Schumacher[1,2], Ragnar Bade[2], Andreas Genz[2], Mattias Heinrich[1]

[1]Institute of Medical Informatics, Lübeck University
[2]MeVis Medical Solutions AG, Bremen
mona.schumacher@mevis.de

Abstract. The segmentation of vascular systems is a challenging task since their sizes and structures vary greatly so that the spatial context becomes highly important. For further clinical analysis of the vascular system it is important to create a connected vascular tree starting from the main trunk, following the tree structure up to small branches. To address these issues, we propose a new iterative segmentation model that recursively evolves a segmentation of a vasculature by following its tree structure. Our iterative CNN alternates between three steps: First, a 3D segmentation of a sub-region is performed. Second, branches that are not part of the currently analyzed branch are removed and third, subsequent sub-regions are detected. These steps are repeated until the entire vascular system is segmented. We trained, validated and tested our model on 82 CT images. We showed that, in comparison to state of the art methods, our new model generates a more accurate segmentation, resulting in an improvement of the Dice score of 7 % and a reduction of the Hausdorff distance of approximately 20 %.

1 Introduction

Different clinical workflows require a precise segmentation of the vessels in the liver, e.g. for tumor resections. For these clinical applications, the correct detection of both small and large vessel structures is as important as the vessel tree connectivity and topology [1]. However, due to the low contrast between the vessels and surrounding liver parenchyma as well as the high complexity of the branching structures of the vessel systems, the segmentation is known to be a challenging task. In addition, the contrast between vessels and liver parenchyma can vary across CT scans since the timing of the acquisition is very important.

Deep learning methods for segmentation are less dependent and more robust against gray values and image quality. Popular architectures for the segmentation of structures are the U-Net [2] or variants of it [3, 4]. However, due to the size of the contrast enhanced CT input scan, the images often need to be downsampled or trained with a patch-based approach, because they cannot be processed at once due to the limited GPU memory. In the area of vascular segmentation this means, that small veins could possibly not be detected anymore because they would be removed during downsampling. Furthermore,

© Der/die Autor(en), exklusiv lizenziert durch
Springer Fachmedien Wiesbaden GmbH, ein Teil von Springer Nature 2022
K. Maier-Hein et al. (Hrsg.), *Bildverarbeitung für die Medizin 2022*,
Informatik aktuell, https://doi.org/10.1007/978-3-658-36932-3_2

the available 3D deep learning approaches also do not detect the tree topology correctly, which results in a segmentation with several unconnected components.

Due to the importance of parameter optimization, preprocessing, and data augmentation of the images that have a great influence on the performance of the network, the nnU-Net, introduced by Isensee et al. [5], has gained significant impact since its publication in 2019 and can currently be regarded as the state of the art method for medical image segmentation. However, even this approach does not generate a vessel segmentation with a continuous, connected tree structure that is important to analyze the blood flow and the supply of the remaining liver tissue.

1.1 Contributions

This paper presents a new iterative patch-based method to segment vessel trees from medical imaging data. Our proposed method overcomes the issues of currently available segmentation methods, and detect a continuous tree including small branches, and is able to cover the complex tree structure of the vessels. Starting from a manually selected seed, our method subsequently segments vascular trees in a 3D sub-region and detects the next regions of interest (ROI) depending on the course of the vessel and the number of branches in the segmented region until the entire vascular system is segmented.

2 Materials and methods

For training and evaluation of our method, a dataset of 82 contrast enhanced liver CT images of the venous phase from different centers and scanners with an image extend in a range of $313 \times 22 \times 86$ to $510 \times 421 \times 413$ voxels with voxel sizes of $0.39 \times 0.39 \times 0.97$ to $0.97 \times 0.97 \times 3.0$ mm are used.

Images are either acquired to plan a living liver donation (healthy patients) or a tumor resection. The dataset thus includes both images of healthy and diseased patients.

When acquiring contrast enhanced CT images, the timing is not always ideal in respect to the contrast enhancement of the vascular system to the surrounding structures. Our dataset shows a variety of contrasts in or outside of the portal vein, so that images with well contrasted (high gray values) as well as poorly contrasted portals veins (lower gray values, more similar to liver parenchyma) are included, which results in high variety of gray values of the portal vein.

For all of these images, ground truth labels are available. The data has been manually segmented and reviewed by three experienced radiologic technicians. The remarkable aspect of these annotations is that very small vessels are also included in the segmentation. Moreover, the resulting vascular tree is one connected component that can be used to analyze the blood supply of the liver parenchyma which is important to plan a liver surgery.

We clamped the image value range from 0 to 700 HU. The normalization of the images is done by subtracting the mean (170.81 HU) followed by a division by the standard deviation (36.70 HU) of the HU values within the portal vein of our training images and scale the image values from 0 to 1 afterwards. We do not resample our input data to a uniform voxel size to emphasize that vessel branches can be of different sizes.

Finally, we split the data for all experiments in a training, validation and testing set of 40, 10 and 32 image pairs, respectively.

To solve the issues described above, our model iteratively segments the vessels by following its tree structure. Starting from a manually selected seed point, the portal vein is segmented in a given sub-region with a 3D U-Net. Based on the segmentation in the sub-region, the next sub-region(s) are identified to follow the course of the vessels in consideration of the branching structure. The iterative segmentation stops if no new sub-regions are identified. An overview of the segmentation pipeline is shown in Figure 1. We start with a CT scan and an vessel tree result image in iteration step $i = 0$. The result image is accumulated with values at each iteration step to get the final segmentation. The queue is processed according to the FIFO (first-in-first-out) principle.

To demonstrate the beneficial effect of the removal of components from other vessel branches, we additionally evaluate our described iterative approach without the removal of these components (WithoutRemoval).

In addition, we train the 3D full resolution nnU-Net (3DnnU-Net), as described in [5] and a standard sliding window approach with a patch size of $128 \times 128 \times 64$ and an overlap of 50 %. To get a connected vascular tree, we perform a connected component analysis and keep the largest component to get the final segmentation result.

In the following, our method is described in more detail.

2.1 Segmentation of sub-regions

The segmentation of the sub-regions is done with a 3D U-Net. We train our model with two different patch sizes: $64 \times 64 \times 64$ (OursSmall) and $128 \times 128 \times 64$ (OursLarge).

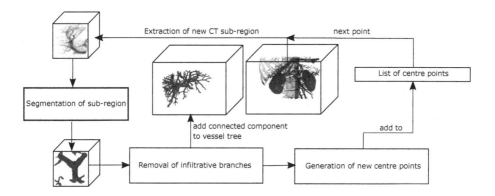

Fig. 1. Pipeline of proposed vessel segmentation method: Starting from a selected seed point, a 3D sub-region around the seed point is segmented with a U-Net. To contiguously track the vascular tree, connected branches in the segmented sub region are kept (components from other branches are removed) and new seed points for further tracking are detected. Such new seed points will be generated at the faces of the current cubical sub-region depending on the current tracking path and the number of tree branches in the segmented sub-region. Thus, iteratively the vascular tree is built up further until no new seed points are detected.

The networks contain an encoding and a decoding part that consists of two or three downsampling and upsampling parts respectively. The initial number of channels is 32 and the number is doubled for each downsampling step. We use batch normalization and leakyReLU with a slope of 0.1. We only use a central crop of approximately half dimensions of the segmented sub-region for further processing to overcome problematic issues induced by padded convolutions and other boundary conditions.

Because the sub-region is always located on a face of $i - 1$ (Sec. 2.3), except for the first iteration, the patches always overlap at least by quarter of the region size. Due to the iterative patch-based design of the proposed method, only patches containing portal vein can be used as training patches. As a result, the network can be trained more specifically for portal vein segmentation.

To train the network, we use a combined cross entropy and Dice loss function ($\epsilon = 0.0001$). The cross entropy loss function was weighted 0.3 and 1.0 for non-vessel and vessel voxel to address the imbalance between the classes. An Adam optimizer was used with a initial learning rate of 0.01. The learning rate was adapted using a learning rate scheduler that reduces the learning rate on a plateau by a factor of 0.1 with a threshold of zero. We use a new patch of each training sample in each epoch. Additionally, we augment the training data using small random affine transformations and random horizontal and vertical flips. If the midpoint of the sub-region is too close to the border of CT scan, we use zero padding. The training was done in 1500 epochs with a batch size of 2 which was the limitation of our used GPU (12 GB).

2.2   Removal of components from other paths

To ensure the tracking of the individual branches so that each path is considered separately and one after the other, branches that are currently not analyzed in the sub-region are removed and we only track branches connected to the current seed point (Fig. 2a-b). For this reason, we first generate a binary segmentation mask (Fig. 2a). Next, a connected component analysis (CCA) is done and all components not connected to the centre point are removed. This results in a segmentation mask only containing the currently analyzed path (Fig. 2b). In the next step, the probabilities for voxels identified as portal vein in step i are averaged with the probabilities of the steps before.

2.3   Detection of next sub-regions

Depending on the number of branches and the course of the vessel in the segmented region, the next regions are selected. For this reason, all parts of the sub-region that were segmented in iteration steps before are removed to ensure that it does not go backwards (Fig. 2c). The new centre points of the next sub-regions are determined by analysing a small region at all six faces. For all faces, a connected component analysis is done and each identified component represents a new region for the next iteration steps. By calculating the centre of mass of all connected components, the next centre points are determined (Fig. 2c-f).

Tab. 1. Resulting mean values and standard deviations of number of components, Dice scores (with and without CCA) and Hausdorff distances in mm (with and without CCA) of segmentation methods.

	OursSmall	OursLarge	Without Removal	Sliding Window	3D nnU-Net
Components	1 ± 0	1 ± 0	233 ± 133	329 ± 188	43 ± 34
Dice	**0.74 ± 0.08**	**0.74 ± 0.07**	0.66 ± 0.10	0.60 ± 0.07	0.71 ± 0.14
Dice (CCA)			0.66 ± 0.09	0.61 ± 0.09	0.69 ± 0.17
HD	54.06 ± 27.43	**42.88 ± 14.52**	93.79 ± 33.54	155.41 ± 35.50	43.95 ± 34.03
HD (CCA)			55.99 ± 25.04	54.01 ± 25.04	54.60 ± 43.08

3 Results

We compared the model outputs to the ground truth segmentation for our 32 test images and calculated the Dice scores and Hausdorff distances of the resulting masks. An overview of the mean Dice scores and mean Hausdorff distances are listed in Table 1. An example of one ground truth and the corresponding vessel segmentations predicted by the trained models are displayed in Figure 3.

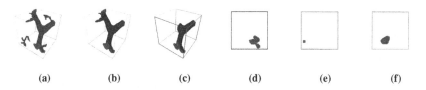

(a)   (b)   (c)   (d)   (e)   (f)

Fig. 2. Detection of new sub-regions: (a) U-Net segmentation result, (b) Connected component analysis to remove all vessels in the sub-regions that do not belong to current branch, (c) Parts of the sub-region that were segmented in an iteration step before are removed, (d)-(f) Analysis of the faces to find the next centre point for the next sub-regions. Only the non-empty slices are displayed. In this example, three new sub-regions are detected.

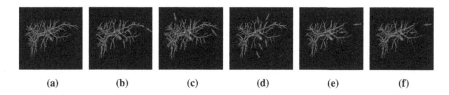

(a)   (b)   (c)   (d)   (e)   (f)

Fig. 3. Example of resulting vascular trees: (a) Ground Truth, (b) OursSmall, (c) OursLarge, (d) IterativeWithoutRemoval with CCA, (e) SlidingWindow with CCA, (f) 3DnnU-Net with CCA. The red arrows in the resulting images of the methods highlight example regions with a difference to the ground truth.

4 Discussion

The presented method creates a continuous vascular tree with one component and reaches a Dice score of 0.74, which is an improvement of up to 7 % in comparison to the state of the art method, the nnU-Net. Additionally, the presented iterative method shows a smaller Hausdorff distance, which can be seen as a proxy measure of the correctness of the tree topology. A paired Wilcoxon ranksum test show a statistical significance of the improvement of our proposed method ($p < 0.05$). Overall, it can be stated, that the presented iterative 3D patch-based segmentation approach is a great improvement in comparison to current state of the art techniques.

A limitation of the presented method is that the iterative approach can cause segmentation to stop too early and entire parts of the vessel system are not segmented. We observed this behavior in one of the 32 test cases. This behavior results in a high Hausdorff distance, in this case of 166.77 mm. In case of practical implementation, however, this could be improved quickly as the user can set additional seed points within missing parts, which would result in a mean Dice score of 0.75 and a mean Hausdorff distance of 39.21 mm for our method.

In future work, we will focus on the detection of new sub-regions and the combined segmentation to overcome the remaining limitation of stopping the segmentation too early as well as the inclusion of graph-based learning methods in our approach.

References

1. Selle D, Preim B, Schenk A, Peitgen HO. Analysis of vasculature for liver surgical planning. IEEE Trans Med Imaging. 2002;21(11):1344–57.
2. Ronneberger O, Fischer P, Brox T. U-Net: convolutional networks for biomedical image segmentation. International Conference on Medical image computing and computer-assisted intervention. Springer. 2015:234–41.
3. Livne M, Rieger J, Aydin OU, Taha AA, Akay EM, Kossen T et al. A U-Net deep learning framework for high performance vessel segmentation in patients with cerebrovascular disease. Front Neurosci. 2019;13.
4. Kitrungrotsakul T, Han XH, Iwamoto Y, Lin L, Foruzan AH, Xiong W et al. VesselNet: a deep convolutional neural network with multi pathways for robust hepatic vessel segmentation. Comput Med Imaging Graph. 2019;75:74–83.
5. Isensee F, Jaeger PF, Kohl SA, Petersen J, Maier-Hein KH. nnU-Net: a self-configuring method for deep learning-based biomedical image segmentation. Nat Methods. 2021;18(2): 203–211.

Robust Liver Segmentation with Deep Learning Across DCE-MRI Contrast Phases

Annika Hänsch[1], Felix Thielke[1], Hans Meine[1], Shereen Rennebaum[2],
Matthias F. Froelich[2], Lena S. Becker[3], Jan B. Hinrichs[3], Andrea Schenk[1]

[1]Fraunhofer MEVIS, Bremen
[2]Universitätsklinikum Mannheim
[3]Medizinische Hochschule Hannover
annika.haensch@mevis.fraunhofer.de

Abstract. Fully automatic liver segmentation is important for the planning of liver interventions and decision support. In patients with HCC, dynamic-contrast enhanced MRI is particularly relevant. Previous work has focused on liver segmentation in the late hepatobiliary contrast phase, which may not always be available in heterogeneous data from clinical routine. In this contribution, we demonstrate the training of a convolutional neural network across contrast phases of DCE-MRI, that is on par with a specialized late-phase network (mean Dice score 0.96) but in addition is more robust to other contrast phase images compared with the specialized network.

1 Introduction

Liver segmentation is a valuable pre-processing step for the planning of liver interventions and may be relevant for clinical treatment decision support. It is also a prerequisite for image analysis techniques such as Radiomics and may be useful during AI training, e.g. of liver tumor detection. In recent years, several algorithms based on Deep Learning (DL) techniques and convolutional neural networks have been proposed for fully automatic liver segmentation, in particular for CT image data [1]. For the diagnosis of hepatocellular carcinoma (HCC), dynamic contrast-enhanced MRI (DCE-MRI) has shown to lead to a higher sensitivity and higher diagnostic confidence in the diagnosis in patients with cirrhosis [2]. Therefore, this imaging technique is frequently used for HCC diagnosis and therapy planning. However, the automatic segmentation of MRI data is typically considered more difficult compared with the segmentation of CT data because the image appearance is highly dependent on various factors, such as the imaging device, the acquisition sequence and the contrast agent.

The late phase of hepatobiliary contrast agents such as Primovist® (Bayer Healthcare, Germany) is particularly suitable for DCE-MRI liver segmentation, due to the very high contrast between liver parenchyma and surrounding tissue. As a result, recent studies rely on the availability of this phase for automatic liver segmentation [3, 4]. This approach may be feasible and is indeed the best choice in study settings, where the imaging protocol is standardized and that contrast phase is always available. However, in a real-word setting where data acquired using highly heterogeneous MR protocols

Springer Fachmedien Wiesbaden GmbH, ein Teil von Springer Nature 2022
K. Maier-Hein et al. (Hrsg.), *Bildverarbeitung für die Medizin 2022*,
Informatik aktuell, https://doi.org/10.1007/978-3-658-36932-3_3

from multiple clinical sites and clinical routine need to be segmented, the late phase may not always be available or or not easy to recognise automatically, and other contrast agents may be used. Furthermore, the dynamic properties of DCE-MRI, i.e. arterial hyperenhancement and venous washout, are required for a correct diagnosis, therefore the direct segmentation of the corresponding images may be required.

In this contribution, we propose to train a convolutional neural network (CNN) for liver segmentation across the various contrast phases of DCE-MRI. The aim is to obtain a "generalist" neural network that can be applied to image data from clinical routine without requiring the availability or selection of a particular contrast phase. For comparison, we also train a specialized late-phase CNN optimized for late hepatobiliary phase images.

2 Materials and methods

2.1 Image and reference data

DCE-MRI data of 126 patients from two clinical sites was available for this study after ethical approval. The dataset was split into 80 cases for training, 6 cases for validation, and 40 cases for testing. For each patient, the liver was manually segmented by a technical radiologist assistant with more than 10 years of experience, using the DICOM series with the best tumor visibility. The resulting stratified split into training/validation/test sets with respect to contrast phases was as follows: arterial phase (9/1/6), portalvenous phase (15/1/9), venous phase (11/1/5), late (hepatobiliary) phase (41/3/20), or a different phase, e.g. the native image (4/0/0). For all non-late images, the corresponding late image was determined and registered to the annotated image, using a deformable registration algorithm optimized for DCE-MRI of the liver [5]. Overall, the data was acquired on 8 different MRI scanner models, with in-plane pixel resolution of 0.82–1.95 mm, and slice thicknesses of 1.8–6 mm.

The images were pre-processed by unifying the resolution to $1 \times 1 \times 3$ mm^3. The gray values were normalized by mapping the first and 99th gray value percentile to a fixed interval. For data augmentation, random scaling (standard deviation 5% of the original voxel size) and small rotations (standard deviation 5°) were performed on-the-fly in the axial plane.

2.2 Neural network and training

The neural network architecture was an anisotropic variant of the 2D U-Net [6], which introduces additional 3D convolutions in the network's lower three resolution levels [7]. As a result, the receptive field in the axial plane is equivalent to the 2D U-Net, but multiple slices are used for the prediction. This technique is supposed to mimic the way that radiologists annotate volumetric data, by scrolling up and down a few slices for determining the organ boundaries. Standard techniques for regularization such as batch normalization and dropout were integrated into the architecture. The architecture and training were implemented in Keras [8].

The neural network was trained on batches of two patches of size $52 \times 52 \times 32$ voxels with $92 \times 92 \times 20$ voxels symmetrical padding, to account for the decrease in patch size due to unpadded convolutions in the architecture. The Dice loss function was used for training, with ADAM optimizer and an initial learning rate of 10^{-4}. Every 500 iterations, the Jaccard coefficient was determined on the validation data. After 10 validation steps without improvement, the learning rate was halved. This procedure was applied until the 6th learning rate decay was reached, then the training was stopped. The network state with the highest Jaccard coefficient on the validation data was chosen for evaluation on the test data.

The training process was performed in two different manners: (1) on the annotated images, independent of the contrast phase, and (2) on the late-phase image for each patient, with reference segmentations directly annotated or registered as described above. We refer to these two trained network as (1) the "generalist CNN" and (2) the "specialized late-phase CNN".

During the inference step, we used the argmax of the networks' softmax output as voxel-wise binary classification result and performed a selection of the largest connected 3D component as simple post-processing.

2.3 Evaluation

We used three commonly employed metrics for the quantitative evaluation: Dice score, mean surface distance (MSD) and Hausdorff distance (HD). In addition, we calculated the Contour Dice (CDice) score with a tolerance of 5 mm [9]. The value of this score corresponds to the percentage of the predicted liver contour, that lies within the pre-defined tolerance to the reference contour. It can be seen as a surrogate for the correction effort. Statistical significance was determined using the Wilcoxon signed-rank test ($\alpha = 0.05$), with Benjamini-Hochberg correction to account for multiple testing (false discovery rate 0.05).

In addition, the liver contours predicted on the late-phase test cases (N=20) were rated by two clinical experts with respect to the required correction effort on a scale from 1 (unsuitable for correction/discard) to 5 (no corrections required).

3 Results

The quantitative evaluation is performed on three different test case subsets: all cases (N=40), all late-phase test cases (N=20), and all remaining test cases with different contrast phases (N=20) (Fig. 1, Tab. 1). On the late-phase test subset, both CNNs yield similar results with a mean Dice score of 0.955, mean MSD 1.83 mm vs. 1.91 mm, and mean HD 30.3 mm vs. 33.3 mm, without significant differences. Only the Contour Dice score with mean 0.915 vs. 0.902 is significantly higher for the generalist CNN. On the test cases from all other contrast phases, the generalist CNN significantly outperforms the specialized late-phase CNN w.r.t. all metrics, as expected. This also applies to the comparison on the full test set. Moreover, the performance of the generalist CNN is similar on both test subsets for late vs. non-late test images (mean Dice score 0.955 vs. 0.954).

Based on the clinical evaluation on the late-phase test subset (Fig. 2), the generalist CNN is slightly preferable also for late-phase data, with no or only minor corrections

Tab. 1. Summary of the quantitative segmentation performance (mean and standard deviation) for the generalist CNN (G) vs. the specialized late-phase CNN (S).

Test Cases	CNN	Dice Score	CDice 5 mm	MSD	HD
All	G	0.955 ± 0.029	0.907 ± 0.061	1.76 ± 1.13	29.2 ± 13.1
	S	0.909 ± 0.155	0.837 ± 0.161	5.23 ± 16.3	43.5 ± 31.2
Late phase	G	0.955 ± 0.038	0.915 ± 0.072	1.83 ± 1.50	30.3 ± 15.8
	S	0.955 ± 0.027	0.902 ± 0.070	1.91 ± 1.25	33.3 ± 13.6
Other phases	G	0.954 ± 0.014	0.899 ± 0.046	1.69 ± 0.53	28.0 ± 9.6
	S	0.863 ± 0.208	0.773 ± 0.197	8.56 ± 22.5	53.7 ± 39.4

(ratings 4 and 5) required for 16/20 test cases, vs. 14/20 test cases for the specialized late-phase CNN.

Six exemplary test cases (Fig. 3) show the similar performance of both CNNs on late-phase images (top row), and the superiority of the generalist CNN on other contrast phases (bottom row). The main challenges, which are currently not solved by either CNN, are the correct exclusion of larger vessels (aorta, portal vein, hepatic artery), and in some cases the correct inclusion of tumors located at the liver boundary.

In summary, we can conclude that training across DCE-MRI contrast phases not only increases the robustness of the CNN concerning heterogeneous image data, but also achieves the same performance as a specialized late-phase CNN on the corresponding late-phase test subset in our study.

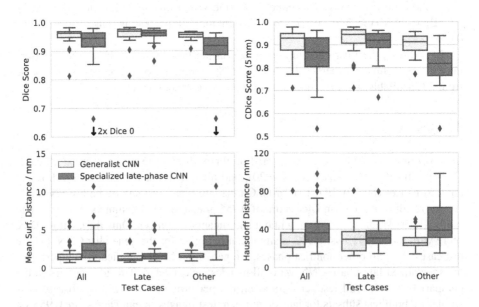

Fig. 1. Quantitative evaluation of liver segmentation. For better visibility of the differences between both CNNs, two outliers with Dice score 0 are cut off as indicated.

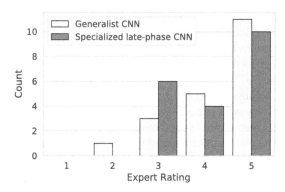

Fig. 2. Clinical expert rating of the contours by both CNNs on the late-phase test subset (N=20), judging the correction effort on a scale from 1 (unsuitable for correction) to 5 (no corrections).

4 Discussion

Our results indicate that a generalist CNN trained across DCE-MRI contrast phases can robustly segment the liver in heterogeneous image data. In particular, no loss in performance was seen on the late hepatobiliary phase compared to a specialized late-phase CNN. Based on the Dice score, our results on heterogeneous image data (mean

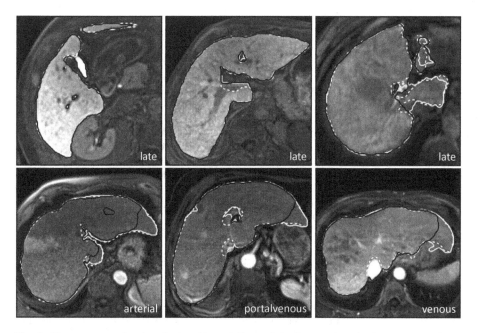

Fig. 3. Six test cases showing the late hepatobiliary phase (top row) and other contrast phases (bottom row), with the phase indicated in each image. The contours correspond to reference segmentation (white dashed), generalist CNN (yellow solid), and specialized late-phase CNN (black solid).

0.955 ± 0.029) are similar to recent results from literature, which were based on the late hepatobiliary phase (0.951 ± 0.018 [3], 96 ± 1.9% [4]).

A remaining challenge is that hypo- or hyperintense structures at the liver boundary, such as larger vessels or tumors, may be incorrectly segmented. To some extent, this could be due to the fact that the relative intensity of these structures to the liver parenchyma changes with the contrast phase. A solution could be to increase the training set either by collecting and annotating more data or by registering and correcting the available manual liver segmentations to other contrast phases of the same study. Furthermore, it could be beneficial to encode information about the contrast phase into the training, e.g. as additional network input. The current global evaluation measures do not explicitly consider such details.

For future work, it would be desirable to evaluate the "generalist vs. specialist" approach on a larger scale by using more annotated data per contrast phase and by training specialized CNNs for other important phases of HCC diagnosis, such as the arterial phase.

Acknowledgement. This work was funded by the BMBF project STRIKE (grant number 13GW0369C). We thank Christiane Engel from Fraunhofer MEVIS for providing ground truth segmentations.

References

1. Bilic P et al. The liver tumor segmentation benchmark (LiTS). arXiv e-prints. 2019. arXiv:1901.04056.
2. Roberts LR, Sirlin CB, Zaiem F, Almasri J, Prokop LJ, Heimbach JK et al. Imaging for the diagnosis of hepatocellular carcinoma: a systematic review and meta-analysis. Hepatology. 2018;67(1):401–21.
3. Chlebus G, Schenk A. Automatic liver and tumor segmentation in late-phase MRI using fully convolutional neural networks. Procs CURAC. 2018:195–200.
4. Winther H, Hundt C, Ringe KI, Wacker FK, Schmidt B, Jürgens J et al. A 3D deep neural network for liver volumetry in 3T contrast-enhanced MRI. RoFo. 2021;193(3):305–14.
5. Strehlow J, Spahr N, Rühaak J, Laue H, Abolmaali N, Preusser T et al. Landmark-based evaluation of a deformable motion correction for DCE-MRI of the liver. Int J Comput Assist Radiol Surg. 2018;13(4):597–606.
6. Ronneberger O, Fischer P, Brox T. U-Net: convolutional networks for biomedical image segmentation. Lect Notes Comput Sci. 2015;9351:234–41.
7. Chlebus G, Schenk A, Hahn HK, Ginneken B van, Meine H. Robust segmentation models using an uncertainty slice sampling based annotation workflow. arXiv e-prints. 2021. arXiv:2109.14879.
8. Chollet F et al. Keras. https://keras.io. 2015.
9. Moltz JH, Hänsch A, Lassen-Schmidt B, Haas B, Genghi A, Schreier J et al. Learning a loss function for segmentation: a feasibility study. Procs ISBI. 2020:957–60.

Abstract: Light-weight Semantic Segmentation and Labelling of Vertebrae in 3D-CT Scans

Hellena Hempe, Mattias P. Heinrich

Institute of Medical Informatics, University of Lübeck
`hellena.hempe@uni-luebeck.de`

In order to facilitate early diagnosis and prevention of osteoporosis and degenerative diseases of the spine, automated opportunistic screening in routine 3D-CT scans can be implemented to assist radiologists in clinical practice. The resource limited clinical setting demands for solutions that emphasise accuracy and robustness while oftentimes being limited by computational resources. The VerSe19 and '20 challenges aim at addressing the task of spine CT analysis but most proposed methods require multiple-stages and are computationally complex. In contrast to prior work for vertebrae segmentation and labelling, we design a light-weight deep learning alternative: a 3D DeepLab [1]. Our proposed patch-based segmentation method comprises a modified MobileNetV2 backbone, Atrous Spatial Pyramid Pooling and a small segmentation head with a single skip connection. To fit our model to this specific task and improve efficiency and accuracy, we have further optimised the network architecture by applying the compound scaling idea of the EfficientNet. Our model was trained and evaluated on the public VerSe19 dataset sampled to isotropic 1.5 mm spacing and is compared to results of the nnUNet as baseline method. Our method yields a multi-label Dice score of $73\pm17\,\%$ and a binary Dice score of $86\pm5\,\%$. In comparison, the nnUNet scored a multi-label Dice score of $81\pm14\,\%$ and a binary Dice score of $90\pm4\,\%$. The Centre-Mass-Distances of each vertebra over each scan are 2.7 ± 2.2 Voxel and 1.9 ± 2.0 Voxel, respectively. However, the inference time of our method is an order of magnitude faster due to the reduced amount of trainable parameters, namely 1.2 M parameters for our method and 32.2 M parameters for the nnUNet. The segmentation outcome of our method can be further employed for down-stream tasks such as detection of fractured vertebrae and degenerative diseases in the context of opportunistic spine assessment. We believe that our memory and time efficient segmentation algorithm is a promising alternative to already existing algorithms and helps facilitate the application of opportunistic screening for osteoporosis and other degenerative deformities of the spine. Code available at: `github.com/multimodallearning/vertebrae-segmentation-classification`.

References

1. Hempe H, Yilmaz EB, Meyer C, Heinrich MP. Opportunistic CT screening for degenerative deformities and osteoporotic fractures with 3D DeepLab. Medical Imaging 2022: Image Processing. SPIE, 2022.

© Der/die Autor(en), exklusiv lizenziert durch
Springer Fachmedien Wiesbaden GmbH, ein Teil von Springer Nature 2022
K. Maier-Hein et al. (Hrsg.), *Bildverarbeitung für die Medizin 2022*,
Informatik aktuell, https://doi.org/10.1007/978-3-658-36932-3_4

Few-shot Unsupervised Domain Adaptation for Multi-modal Cardiac Image Segmentation

Mingxuan Gu, Sulaiman Vesal, Ronak Kosti, Andreas Maier

Pattern Recognition Lab, Friedrich-Alexander-Universität Erlangen-Nürnberg (FAU), Erlangen, Germany
mingxuan.gu@fau.de

Abstract. Unsupervised domain adaptation (UDA) methods intend to reduce the gap between source and target domains by using unlabeled target domain and labeled source domain data, however, in the medical domain, target domain data may not always be easily available, and acquiring new samples is generally time-consuming. This restricts the development of UDA methods for new domains. In this paper, we explore the potential of UDA in a more challenging while realistic scenario where only one unlabeled target patient sample is available. We call it Few-shot Unsupervised Domain adaptation (FUDA). We first generate target-style images from source images and explore diverse target styles from a single target patient with Random Adaptive Instance Normalization (RAIN). Then, a segmentation network is trained in a supervised manner with the generated target images. Our experiments demonstrate that FUDA improves the segmentation performance by 0.33 of Dice score on the target domain compared with the baseline, and it also gives 0.28 of Dice score improvement in a more rigorous one-shot setting. Our code is available at https://github.com/MingxuanGu/Few-shot-UDA.

1 Introduction

As manual contouring of medical images is tedious and time-consuming, automatic medical image segmentation is more desirable [1]. While deep learning methods often suffer from performance degradation when a domain gap is observed between training (source) and testing (target) data. UDA methods tackle this problem by reducing the domain gap with a variety of techniques, for example, discrepancy reduction [2], adversarial learning [3], image translation [4], etc. These methods are conditioned on the availability of a large amount of target data which, however, is quite scarce.

In this work, we consider a more realistic and practical scenario where we still have sufficient labeled source data, while we only have one unlabeled target data for training. To this end, a style transfer method called Random Adaptive Instance Normalization (RAIN) [5] is used to generate diverse target-style images from a single target patient data. Then, a segmentation module can be trained in a supervised manner with generated images. Our contributions are: (1) we explore the potential of FUDA for multi-modal

Springer Fachmedien Wiesbaden GmbH, ein Teil von Springer Nature 2022
K. Maier-Hein et al. (Hrsg.), *Bildverarbeitung für die Medizin 2022*,
Informatik aktuell, https://doi.org/10.1007/978-3-658-36932-3_5

cardiac CMR segmentation and it shows better performance compared with its baseline model and other recent UDA methods, (2) we extend our method to one-shot learning and demonstrate the possibility of FUDA with only one slice of target data available.

2   Materials and methods

2.1   Dataset

We assess the proposed FUDA on MS-CMRSeg [6] 2019 challenge dataset, which consists of 45 short-axis bSSFP, T2-weighted and LGE scans from patients diagnosed with cardiomyopathy. The ground-truth contours are generated by two experts and include right ventricle (RV) cavity, left ventricle (LV) cavity, and myocardium (Myo) region. Only affine transformation (rotation, translation, shearing, etc.) is applied and the sequences are normalized using min-max normalization. Then, the sequences are center-cropped to 224×224 pixels to have only region-of-interest (ROIs) areas.

2.2   Problem statement

In UDA for semantic segmentation, a set of labeled data in source domain $\mathcal{D}^s(x^s, y^s)$ is given, where x^s represents one sample, and y^s the corresponding label in $\mathcal{D}^s$. Whereas

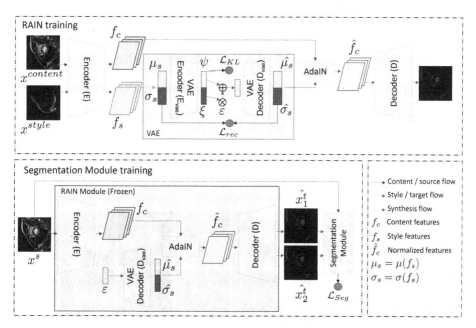

Fig. 1. Overview of the proposed FUDA segmentation framework. RAIN is first pre-trained with x^{content} (bSSFP) and x^{style} (T2). Then during training of the segmentation module, stylized target images will be generated by RAIN with source images and ε generated from target image(s). After that, the segmentation module can be trained using the source and stylized images. The ε is iteratively updated to generate more difficult stylized images.

for target domain ($\mathcal{D}^t$) only unlabeled target images (x^t) are given. The goal is to improve the performance of the segmentation by reducing the distribution gap between the source and target domain. In our case, we consider only one unlabeled target patient data (x^t) being available.

2.3 RAIN Module

RAIN is developed on the basis of Adaptive Instance Normalization (AdaIN) [7]. AdaIN has an encoder-decoder architecture. It generates stylized images which have the appearance of the style image while preserving the structure of the content images by re-normalizing the features of content images with Equation 1

$$\text{AdaIN}(f_c, f_s) = \sigma(f_s)(\frac{f_c - \mu(f_c)}{\sigma(f_c)}) + \mu(f_s) \tag{1}$$

where f_c, f_s are the latent features of the content and style image, $\mu(.)$ and $\sigma(.)$ denote channel-wise mean and standard deviation. To achieve realistic image transfer, a content loss $\mathcal{L}_c$ and a style loss $\mathcal{L}_s$ [7] is employed.

RAIN takes advantage of the style transfer in AdaIN and involves a style variational auto-encoder (VAE) in between the encoder and the decoder. The style-VAE is composed of an encoder E_{vae} and a decoder D_{vae}. E_{vae} encodes $\mu(f_s) \oplus \sigma(f_s)$ to $N(\psi, \xi)$, where $\oplus$ denotes concatenation, and D_{vae} aims to reconstruct the original style with $\mu(\widetilde{f_s}) \oplus \sigma(f_s) = D_{\text{vae}}(\varepsilon)$, where $\varepsilon \sim N(\psi, \xi)$. Kullback-Leibler (KL) divergence loss is applied to enforce $N(\psi, \xi)$ to be normal distributed. Furthermore, L2 loss is applied between $\mu(f_s) \oplus \sigma(f_s)$ and $\mu(\widetilde{f_s}) \oplus \sigma(f_s)$ to force identity reconstruction $\mathcal{L}_{\text{Rec}}$.

Thus, the overall loss function to train RAIN can be formulated as $\mathcal{L}_{\text{RAIN}} = \mathcal{L}_c + \lambda_s \mathcal{L}_s + \lambda_{\text{KL}} \mathcal{L}_{\text{KL}} + \lambda_{\text{Rec}} \mathcal{L}_{\text{Rec}}$ where λ_s, λ_{KL} and λ_{Rec} denote the weights for the losses.

2.4 Few-shot UDA for cardiac MRI segmentation

The proposed FUDA framework is constructed based on ASM [5] implementation and is shown in Figure 1. To train the segmentation module and explore styles from a single

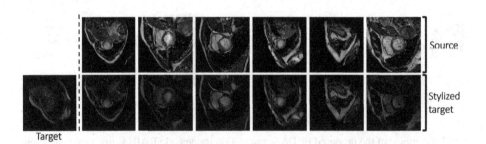

Fig. 2. Qualitative results of RAIN on bSSFP → LGE. The first column shows a LGE axial slice as the style image. The first row shows the bSSFP images as the content images, the second row shows the corresponding stylized LGE images.

target image, we first generate the latent distribution $\mathcal{N}(\psi, \xi)$ from the input image x^t. Then we sample an ε_0 from $\mathcal{N}(\psi, \xi)$. After that, we can generate stylized images $\hat{x}^t$ from any source image x^s. Then the style transfer can be formulated as

$$\hat{x}^t = D(\text{AdaIN}(E(x^s), D_{\text{vae}}(\varepsilon))) \tag{2}$$

Furthermore, the segmentation module can be trained in a supervised manner with x^s and the corresponding $\hat{x}^t$.

We train the segmentation module with a combination of cross-entropy loss (CE) and jaccard distance loss (JD) as $\mathcal{L}_{\text{seg}} = \mathcal{L}_{\text{CE}} + \mathcal{L}_{\text{JD}}$. To enforce the segmentation module to produce domain invariant features between x^s and the corresponding $\hat{x}^t$, $\mathcal{L}_{\text{con}} = ||z^s - z^t||_2$ is applied as a consistency loss, where $z^{s/t}$ are the latent features of the source and the corresponding generated target image from the bottleneck layer of the segmentation module. Then the overall loss function for the segmentation module is

$$\mathcal{L}_S = \mathcal{L}_{\text{seg}} + \lambda \mathcal{L}_{\text{con}} \tag{3}$$

where λ is the weight of $\mathcal{L}_{\text{con}}$. Finally, to generate more diverse and increasingly difficult target images , ε is updated in the direction that makes the segmentation module perform worse on segmentation with

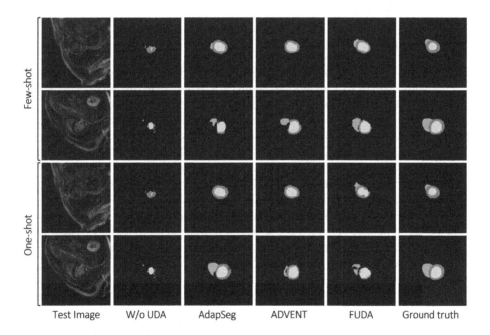

Fig. 3. A visual comparison of segmentation output results produced by different methods for test LGE images under one and few-shot learning settings. The first two rows show the results for few-shot models and the last two rows are for one-shot respectively. **LV** is shown in yellow, **Myo** in brown and **RV** in light-blue colors.

Tab. 1. Dice coefficient (DC) and Hausdorff distance (HD) measures for the proposed FUDA together with baseline (W/o UDA) method, inter-observer study and the performance of the two successful UDA methods AdaptSeg [8] and ADVENT [3]. Baseline is trained with bSSFP images and tested directly on LGE images. For few-shot learning, we take the whole LGE squence of patient 10 as the training target data. For one-shot learning, we only use slice 13 of patient 10 as the training target data. Best results are *emphasized*.

Method	Data	DC (↑)				HD [mm] (↓)			
		Myo	LV	RV	AVG	Myo	LV	RV	AVG
W/o UDA	N/A	0.24	0.40	0.27	0.30	31.7	31.0	45.0	35.9
AdaptSeg	Few	0.39	0.63	0.58	0.53	39.1	28.7	25.6	31.1
ADVENT	Few	0.39	0.59	0.52	0.50	38.4	35.3	37.9	37.2
Proposed	Few	*0.46*	*0.77*	*0.65*	*0.63*	*24.5*	*13.7*	*22.4*	*20.2*
AdaptSeg	One	*0.45*	0.65	0.52	0.54	*32.3*	34.3	36.4	34.3
ADVENT	One	0.37	0.61	0.51	0.50	42.7	26.9	35.0	34.9
Proposed	One	0.39	*0.73*	*0.63*	*0.58*	36.2	*19.0*	25.6	*26.9*
Observer	N/A	0.76	0.88	0.81	0.82	12.0	14.3	21.5	15.9

$$\varepsilon_{i+1} = \varepsilon_i + \alpha \nabla_{\varepsilon_i} \mathcal{L}_{\text{seg}}(\hat{x^t}, y^s) \tag{4}$$

where i is the iteration number, y^s represents the corresponding source label for $\hat{x^t}$ and α denotes the learning rate.

2.5 Training

The training process has two stages. First, we use bSSFP-MRI as content images and T2-weighted-MRI as style images to pretrain the RAIN module. Since it does not involve any target images (LGE), this process makes it convenient to train RAIN anytime before training the segmentation module. In the second stage, the RAIN model is frozen, and we employ Dilated-Residual UNet (DR-UNet) [9] as the segmentation module. We first pretrain the DR-UNet with bSSFP images and the generated LGE-style images in a supervised manner for 40-50k iterations. Then the model is trained together with ε being iteratively updated for another 40-50k iterations. We used stochastic gradient descent (SGD) with a momentum of 0.9 and a weight decay of $5e - 4$ as the optimizer. We empirically set the hyper-parameters of $\lambda_s = 5, \lambda_{\text{KL}} = 1, \lambda_{\text{Rec}} = 5$ and $\lambda = 2e - 3$. The proposed method is trained and tested on one Geforce 1080Ti GPU. The training of RAIN and segmentation module takes 2 hours and 21 hours respectively. Overall inference takes 23 seconds in average for each patient.

3 Results

Figure 2 shows the qualitative results of the pretrained RAIN. We can observe that RAIN successfully captures the features of target images. Tabular 1 summarizes the quantitative results of different methods. Baseline method achieved the lowest average volumetric Dice (0.30) and an HD (35.9 mm). With a few-shot UDA setting, our proposed method achieved the best overall Dice (0.63) and the best lowest HD (20.2 mm). Subsequently, we demonstrate the results for one-shot UDA, and our proposed method achieved the highest Dice (0.58) and the lowest HD (26.9 mm). Figure 3 illustrates qualitative examples of different segmentation approaches. Compared with other methods, the proposed method is able to produce more complete and precise segmentation maps.

4 Discussion

In this work, we presented a few-shot UDA (FUDA) for multi-modal CMR image segmentation while restricting the experiments in a more challenging yet realistic scenario where only one target sample is available. By comparing the proposed method with other approaches under the same settings, we show that FUDA highly reduced the domain gap with only a few target slices. We also demonstrated that the proposed few-shot method produces promising results with the more rigorous one-shot setting. We find for conventional UDA methods like AdaptSeg and ADVENT, performance on one-shot and few-shot settings only has a slight difference. This can be attributed to the fact that the slices of one patient only have a small distribution shift, hence the knowledge learned by the model from target slices of one patient is limited. While for FUDA, the model has the ability to explore unseen styles of the target images, hence more data provided results in more diverse target styles. Consequently, better segmentation performance could be achieved. Furthermore, we believe there is still room to improve the quality of the segmentation prediction. As a result, in the future, we will explore feasible techniques like contrastive learning and attention to improve the performance of the proposed FUDA.

References

1. Kurzendorfer T, Forman C, Schmidt M, Tillmanns C, Maier A, Brost A. Fully automatic segmentation of left ventricular anatomy in 3-D LGE-MRI. Comput Med Imaging Graph. 2017;59:13–27.
2. Gretton A, Borgwardt K, Rasch M, Schölkopf B, Smola AJ. A kernel method for the two-sample-problem. Advances in neural information processing systems. 2007:513–20.
3. Vu T, Jain H, Bucher M, Cord M, Pérez P. ADVENT: adversarial entropy minimization for domain adaptation in semantic segmentation. CVPR. 2019:2512–21.
4. Zhu J, Park T, Isola P, Efros AA. Unpaired image-to-image translation using cycle-consistent adversarial networks. ICCV. 2017:2242–51.
5. Luo Y, Liu P, Guan T, Yu J, Yang Y. Adversarial style mining for one-shot unsupervised domain adaptation. Advances in Neural Information Processing Systems. Vol. 33. Curran Associates, Inc., 2020:20612–23.
6. Zhuang X. Multivariate mixture model for myocardial segmentation combining multi-source images. IEEE Trans Pattern Anal Mach Intell. 2019:1–1.
7. Huang X, Belongie S. Arbitrary style transfer in real-time with adaptive instance normalization. ICCV. 2017:1510–9.
8. Tsai Y, Hung W, Schulter S, Sohn K, Yang M, Chandraker M. Learning to adapt structured output space for semantic segmentation. CVPR. 2018:7472–81.
9. Vesal S, Ravikumar N, Maier A. Automated multi-sequence cardiac MRI segmentation using supervised domain adaptation. STACOM. 2020:300–8.

Unsupervised Anomaly Detection in the Wild

David Zimmerer[1], Daniel Paech[2], Carsten Lüth[3], Jens Petersen[1], Gregor Köhler[1], Klaus Maier-Hein[1]

[1]Division of Medical Image Computing, German Cancer Research Center (DKFZ)
[2]Division of Radiology, German Cancer Research Center (DKFZ)
[3]Interactive Machine Learning, German Cancer Research Center (DKFZ)
d.zimmerer@dkfz.de

Abstract. Unsupervised anomaly detection is often attributed great promise, especially for rare conditions and fast adaptation to novel conditions or imaging techniques without the need for explicitly labeled data. However, most previous works study different methods in a constrained research setting with a limited number of common types of pathologies. Here, we want to explore a more realistic setting and target the incidental findings in a large-scale population study with 10000 participants using a recent anomaly detection approach. Despite the difficulties in selecting a proper training set in such scenarios, we were able to produce promising quantitative results and detected 31 anomalies which were not reported previously. Evaluation by a radiologist revealed remaining open challenges when it comes to the detection of less conspicuous anomalies.

1 Introduction

Unsupervised anomaly detection, also known as out-of-distribution detection, strives to identify samples that deviate from the distribution of samples defined to be normal. In medical imaging settings, this often aims at pathological cases and includes the precise *localization* of anomalies in the image. The unsupervised setting promises to be largely independent of labeled data and as such not needing a time- and cost-intensive labeling effort. Especially in the medical imaging domain, the labeling has to be performed by specialists, who often don't have sufficient time or data to create a large number of high-quality labels. Furthermore, even experts can be vulnerable to so-called inattentional-blindness. Experiments have shown that the majority of trained radiologists might miss anomalies that they were not expecting [1]. Consequently, with the claim to be independent of such labels, unsupervised anomaly detection approaches have been proposed and have shown promising results on multiple different imaging sequences and pathologies with a primary focus on brains and brain tumors and lesions [2–5]. However, most of the previous performance evaluations were performed in setups where training data could be ensured to be purely healthy and where test sets were homogeneously consisting of one type of pathology. While this can be helpful to further develop new methods, it also comes with some limitations in terms of validity and generalization to real-world settings:

© Der/die Autor(en), exklusiv lizenziert durch
Springer Fachmedien Wiesbaden GmbH, ein Teil von Springer Nature 2022
K. Maier-Hein et al. (Hrsg.), *Bildverarbeitung für die Medizin 2022*,
Informatik aktuell, https://doi.org/10.1007/978-3-658-36932-3_6

1. The claim to be "unsupervised" does not take account of the fact that normal scans, i.e. scans without pathology, are required for training and that these need to be carefully selected. In a truly unsupervised setting, a normal scan refers to a person without known medical conditions, as for example provided in a population-based representative sample. In general, the definition of normal and abnormal is often not "black-and-white" and depends on the assessment protocol of the dataset, which, for example, might not guarantee that none of the existing anomalies will be missed during curation.

2. Current approaches are often tested on the same and very limited set of anomalies, in particular brain tumors and lesions. While this is probably due to the frequent occurrence of such conditions and the availability of corresponding annotated datasets, this can raise two questions for unsupervised anomaly detection: first, whether there is a need for unsupervised techniques for those explicit pathologies and second, whether there is a bias in the developed techniques towards these anomalies. This holds especially true in cases where generalization to other anomalies is not shown, even though large and high-quality datasets exist. The capabilities of an approach in detecting any, including rare or unknown, conditions or bio-markers reflects a medically highly relevant task.

3. Often the used datasets contain a fixed but not realistic ratio of normal and abnormal samples. The most extreme case is still very prominent in literature, in which a dataset either only contains normal data or only data with a certain kind of pathology. Moreover, in some studies, these datasets are stemming from different sources, which can further cause issues as they inherently encompass domain shifts, which can cause a bias in the results. Despite the previously mentioned constraints, a controlled research setting can be very helpful for method development and as a reference baseline. However, here we want to answer the question of how current anomaly detection algorithms would perform in a more realistic setting, in particular, the detection of anomalies in a large scale population study (LSPS). In contrast to previous works, the 10000 participants of the LSPS are sampled representatively and contain a variety of different anomalies. All images were previously reviewed by radiologists, allowing to make additional statements about the labeling performance and definition of normality by radiologists.

2 Methods

2.1 Anomaly detection

For anomaly detection, we focused on a VAE-based method, the ceVAE [5], which have shown good performance in recent studies [2, 5, 6]. A ceVAE augments VAEs with self-supervised learning, in particular context encoding. A VAE optimizes a lower bound (known as evidence lower bound, ELBO) on the log-likelihood of a data sample: $\mathcal{L}_{\text{VAE}} = D_{\text{KL}}(q(z|x)\|p(z)) - \mathbb{E}_{z \sim q(z|x)}[\log p(x|z)] \leq \log p(x)$. In practise, $q(z|x)$ is chosen as a Normal distribution which is paramterized via an CNN encoder $f(x) = \mu_z, \sigma_z$, $p(z)$ is chosen as an isotropic Gaussian with zero mean and variance 1, the expectation is resolved using MC sampling with a sample size 1 and $p(x|z)$ is chosen to be Gaussian as well with a fixed variance and a mean given by a CNN decoder g :

$p(x|z) = \mathcal{N}(x|g(z), c)$. As a result the VAE-loss $\mathcal{L}_{VAE}$ can be computed analytically and is optimized over the training set. For the ceVAE in addition to the VAE-loss $\mathcal{L}_{VAE}$ a reconstruction loss between the reconstructions of perturbed input samples $\tilde{x}$ and the unperturbed samples x is added: $L_{ce} = L_{rec}(x, g(f(\tilde{x})))$. This was shown to produce a slightly more discriminative latent space/features [5]. As anomaly score we use the gradients of D_{KL} with respect to the input image x as proposed by [5] since it, in contrast to a reconstruction loss, is more independent of the pixel-value magnitudes. Similar to [2], we further post-processed the predictions with a Gaussian filter of size 3 and cropped the predictions to the brain region only. For the model architecture, we used a symmetric en- and decoder consisting of 3D Convolutions. We chose an input size of 112^3 and a features size of 1024.

2.2 Metrics

As metrics, we used the commonly used and recommended average precision (AP) [2, 7, 8]. We also use AUROC and the Dice by choosing a binarization threshold, which we term *detection-threshold*, that achieves the best Dice on the validation set.

2.3 Datasets

The major part of this work was performed on an LSPS dataset. The study data consists of 10000 T1-weighted (T1) and FLAIR brain scans and reported reference Incidental Findings (refIFs). The T1 and FLAIR scans were co-registered using FSL and the brain was extracted using BET and then were z-score normalized. The refIFs were given as a single point, for which we manually added a radius. All findings that were not in the brain region were excluded. This resulted in 84 refIF. We further chose 3 gradings: *C1*: Very conspicuous, should definitely be found, *C2*: Partially conspicuous, could be found, *C3*: unobtrusive, without context and/or expert knowledge hard to detect. To create a near real-world setting, we randomly chose 5000 test images from the resulting images, which, together with the refIFs, compose the test set. From the remaining images, we chose 4800 images for training and 200 for validation. As it was shown in [8] that already simple toy anomalies give a good indication of performance, similarly to [8] we created a validation set with 100 samples with very simple "toy-sphere"anomalies to facilitate the problem of model and threshold selection. The study was approved by the IRB committee and all participants gave informed consent.

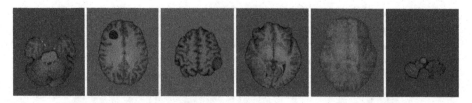

Fig. 1. Anomaly Detection results. Image 1&2 show not detected reported IFs, 3&4 detected reported IFs, 5&6 detected and not reported anomalies.

2.4 Model and parameter selection

To validate the methods during development and compare them with the reported results, in analogy to [5], we trained them on the HCP dataset [9] and validated them on the BraTS17 [10] dataset and an in-house dataset. We resampled and z-score normalized the datasets to a common data distribution. On the Brats17 dataset the 3D ceVAE model, with an AUROC of 0.934 and an AP of 0.24, achieves comparable performance to our slice-wise transversal 2D model as well as the reported scores in [5]. We also compared the 3D ceVAE model to a 2D ceVAE model on an in-house dataset, where the 3D model outperformed the 2D model by a large margin. As a result, we chose to use the 3D model for the real-world scenario evaluation.

3 Experiments and results

We first look at the prediction from the trained model using conventional metrics and then compare them with metrics based on ratings by a radiologist.

3.1 Basic metrics

First, we calculated the dataset AUROC and AP on the refIF scans only. Here, the AUROC is 0.838 and the AP is 0.312, which appear to be similar to the results on the BraTS17 dataset (please note that the results are not completely comparable since for the LSPS we approximated the refIF segmentation by a sphere). While this at a first glance may seem promising, especially since the AP, which is correlated to Dice, is even higher, some peculiarities of the metrics come into play which may lead to overly optimistic conclusions. Since AUROC, AP and Dice are not defined if there is only one class, those metrics are undefined for a normal scan. As a consequence, the scores are often reported on a dataset level (i.e. throwing all pixels into one bucket) rather than an aggregated per-scan level (i.e. calculating the score for all pixels in one scan and taking the mean over all scans). Thus, for the refIF scans only, there is already a stark contrast between the dataset Dice of 0.382 and the per-scan Dice of 0.061 and the dataset AP of 0.312 and the aggregated per-scan AP of 0.108, as is more detailed in the AP histogram (Fig. 2): for most scans, the algorithm fails while for a few it seems to work. However, the cases for which it works are cases with the largest amount of labeled pixels, i.e. scans with large and easy to detect anomalies. This leads to the large and easy-to-detect anomalies dominating the dataset AP score and overshadowing the performance of arguably more medically interesting, harder to detect, and smaller anomalies. Therefore, to get a more direct performance metric of anomaly detection (which arguably is more important than a pixel-level delineation), a radiologist manually reviewed the predictions made by the algorithm.

3.2 Expert evaluation

Here, the predictions which exceeded the "detection-threshold" were, together with the corresponding scans, presented to an expert radiologist ($\sim$ 10 years of experience in neuroimaging). Overall, the algorithm detected 83 suspicious regions in the whole dataset (training + validation + test set). The expert was asked to classify them into one of the five classes: "False Positive", "Brain Extraction Failure", "Imaging Artifact", "Not Medically Relevant Anomaly", "Incidental Finding", for which we considered the first two cases to be an algorithm failure and the latter three a correct anomaly detection. We compared the detections with the refIFs, and overall 19 of 84 refIFs were found, but almost all (16/19) were $C1$. However, still a large amount (21/37 ,> 50%) of $C1$ findings were not detected. We also investigated if some findings were detected, which were not reported in the refIFs. The algorithm was able to detect 31 findings that were not reported previously. Of those, 22/31 were in the test set, 2/31 in the validation set, and 7/31 in the training set, indicating some robustness to outliers but also an expected bias towards detecting a higher percentage of anomalies in the test set, which can be attributed to overfitting (Fig. 1).

4   Discussion

The presented results question the direct applicability of anomaly detection methods in medical practice. However, the algorithm could still detect 31 abnormal samples, which were not reported. It is unclear whether these cases were actually overlooked or whether there were some discrepancies in the reporting, data management, or labeling protocol (e.g. the conditions were noted previously/elsewhere). Given these (at least) 31 abnormal not reported data samples in the LSPS datasets and even one abnormal data sample in the well-curated HCP dataset it's important for the algorithms to be able to handle such cases during training. Furthermore, for use "in the wild", robustness to some anatomical variations which occur with aging might be needed or a more context-specific model. Overall, the results showed that only very prominent anomalies were detected. In addition, even these conditions were not detected reliably enough. The more frequently overlooked and potentially more benefiting anomalies were hardly detected by the used algorithm. Consequently, this makes it hard to recommend the tested models for day-to-day clinical use. However, the detection of imaging artifacts and large anomalies might make it a viable prefiltering step for fully automated diagnosis pipelines, i.e., detecting OoD data on which a consecutive algorithm might fail or behave unexpectedly

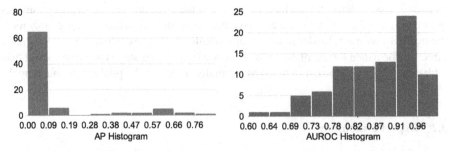

Fig. 2. Left: histogram of per-scan AP scores. Right: histogram of per-scan AUROC scores.

or as a backup check in such a LSPS setting. Overall, we believe that for translation, we need to rethink the alignment of the medical objective and the used metrics, and the assumptions made, and if they are realistic.

5 Conclusion

Here, we evaluated the performance of an unsupervised anomaly detection method, 3D ceVAE, in a realistic large-scale population study setting. Despite the promising scorings by classically used metrics such as AP, DICE, and AUROC, an evaluation by a radiologist showed that the approach is far from expert performance in a day-to-day setting and that it might only be useful as a second opinion for the expert when pinpointing findings that might have been overseen by the expert. Overall, this outlines open points for further research: anomaly detection metrics, robustness to training data anomalies, and detection of less conspicuous anomalies.

Acknowledgement. The present contribution is supported by the Helmholtz Association under the joint research school "HIDSS4Health – Helmholtz Information and Data Science School for Health" and the Helmholtz Imaging Platform (HIP).

References

1. Drew T, Vo MLH, Wolfe JM. The invisible gorilla strikes again: sustained inattentional blindness in expert observers. Psychol Sci. 2013;24(9):1848–53.
2. Baur C, Denner S, Wiestler B, Navab N, Albarqouni S. Autoencoders for unsupervised anomaly segmentation in brain MR images: a comparative study. Med Image Anal. 2021;69:101952.
3. Uzunova H, Schultz S, Handels H, Ehrhardt J. Unsupervised pathology detection in medical images using conditional variational autoencoders. Int J Comput Assist Radiol Surg. 2019;14(3):451–61.
4. Schlegl T, Seeböck P, Waldstein SM, Schmidt-Erfurth U, Langs G. Unsupervised anomaly detection with generative adversarial networks to guide marker discovery. IPMI. (Lect Notes Comput Sci). 2017:146–57.
5. Zimmerer D, Petersen J, Isensee F, Maier-Hein K. Context-encoding variational autoencoder for unsupervised anomaly detection. International Conference on Medical Imaging with Deep Learning – Extended Abstract Track. London, United Kingdom, 2019.
6. Bengs M, Behrendt F, Krüger J, Opfer R, Schlaefer A. 3-Dimensional deep learning with spatial erasing for unsupervised anomaly segmentation in brain MRI. arXiv:2109.06540 [cs, eess]. 2021.
7. Ahmed F, Courville A. Detecting semantic anomalies. arXiv:1908.04388 [cs]. 2019.
8. Zimmerer D, Petersen J, Köhler G, Jäger P, Full P, Roß T et al. Medical out-of-distribution analysis challenge. 2020. Publisher: Zenodo.
9. Van Essen DC, Ugurbil K, Auerbach E, Barch D, Behrens TEJ, Bucholz R et al. The human connectome project: a data acquisition perspective. NeuroImage. 2012;62(4):2222–31.
10. Menze BH, Jakab A, Bauer S, Kalpathy-Cramer J, Farahani K, Kirby J et al. The multi-modal brain tumor image segmentation benchmark (BRATS). IEEE Trans Med Imaging. 2015;34(10):1993–2024.

Epistemic and Aleatoric Uncertainty Estimation for PED Segmentation in Home OCT Images

Timo Kepp[1], Julia Andresen[1], Helge Sudkamp[2], Claus von der Burchard[3], Johann Roider[3], Gereon Hüttmann[4,5], Jan Ehrhardt[1,6], Heinz Handels[1,6]

[1]Institute of Medical Informatics, University of Lübeck, Lübeck, Germany
[2]Visotec GmbH, Lübeck, Germany
[3]Department of Ophthalmology, University of Kiel, Kiel, Germany
[4]Institute of Biomedical Optics, University of Lübeck, Lübeck, Germany
[5]Airway Research Center North (ARCN), Großhansdorf, Germany
[6]German Research Center for Artificial Intelligence, Lübeck, Germany
timo.kepp@uni-luebeck.de

Abstract. New innovative low-cost optical coherence tomography (OCT) devices enable flexible monitoring of age-related macular degeneration (AMD) at home. In combination with current machine learning algorithms like convolutional neural networks (CNNs), assessment of AMD-related biomarkers such as pigment epithelial detachment (PED) can be supported by automatic segmentation. However, limited availability of medical image data as well as noisy ground truth does not guarantee a high generalizability of CNN models. Estimating a segmentation-related uncertainty can be used to evaluate the confidence of the prediction. In this work, two types of uncertainties are analyzed for the segmentation of PED in home OCT image data. Epistemic and aleatoric uncertainties are determined by dropout and augmentation at test time, respectively. Evaluations are performed using pixel-wise as well as structure-wise uncertainty metrics. Results show that test-time augmentation produces both more accurate segmentations and more reliable uncertainties.

1 Introduction

Age-related macular degeneration (AMD) is the leading cause of vision loss and blindness among adults over 60 in the Western world. In the wet form of AMD, nutritional undersupply of photoreceptor cells leads to uncontrolled growth of abnormal fragile blood vessels, causing tissue displacement and fluid leakage into the retina. Optical coherence tomography (OCT) can be used to detect retinal disease activity long before subjective visual impairment occurs. Using modern OCT systems, characteristic retinal changes of AMD can be visualized in high resolution and used as biomarkers. However, the examination intervals of current treatment regimens are often too long and inflexible to ensure early detection of pathological changes. Therefore, novel low-cost OCT systems [1] offer the possibility of self-examination, allowing independent control at home. In combination with current machine learning methods diagnostics of AMD can be supported and optimized.

The vast majority of current segmentation methods for AMD biomarker detection and quantification are based on convolutional neural networks (CNNs) [2]. Despite the great success of CNN-based approaches, it remains challenging to make reliable predictions due to the broad variability of pathological structures and limited image quality or imaging artifacts. Consequently, the determination of segmentation uncertainties is critical in order to indicate possibly mispredicted regions. In general, one distinguishes between epistemic and aleatoric uncertainty. Where epistemic uncertainty describes the lack of knowledge of a model resulting from insufficient training data, aleatoric uncertainty describes the inherent uncertainty due to probabilistic variability such as noise in the training data. Based on [3], in this work a CNN architecture relying on the U-Net is used to segment pigment epithelium detachment (PED), an important AMD biomarker, in 2D cross-sectional images (B-scans) of home OCT scans. Similar to [4], corresponding epistemic and aleatoric uncertainties are estimated. In addition to the segmentation performance, the quality of the estimated epistemic and aleatoric uncertainties is evaluated and compared using pixel-wise as well as structure-wise uncertainty measures.

2 Materials and methods

2.1 Segmentation of PED and uncertainty estimation

Epistemic uncertainty can be estimated via Bayesian deep learning [5], where dropouts are used within CNNs as an approximation of Gaussian processes. To do this, test-time dropout (TTD) is utilized to produce Monte Carlo (MC) samples by N stochastic forward steps of the same input image. The drawn samples can then be averaged to obtain a final segmentation and measures like standard deviation, variance or entropy between the samples to provide a pixel-wise estimate of epistemic uncertainty.

To determine aleatoric uncertainty, test-time augmentation (TTA) is used [6]. Instead of using activated dropouts, the CNN receives N different augmented versions of the same test image as input to generate corresponding MC samples. Horizontal flips, similarity transforms and gamma correction are used for augmentation. Note that in case of geometric transformations, the respective inverse transformation must be applied to the MC samples before computation of final segmentation and uncertainty.

For segmentation of PEDs, the Densely-Connected U-Net (DCU-Net) is deployed, a U-Net-based fully convolutional network that uses additional skip-connections for feature reuse. A detailed description of the architecture can be found in [7]. For its Bayesian version (BDCU-Net) additional dropout layers are integrated after each densely-connected block to allow the estimation of epistemic uncertainties.

2.2 Metrics for quantification and evaluation uncertainties

For pixel-wise assessment of the segmentation uncertainty, the global entropy is determined among the softmax probabilities p of the N generated samples, which is given by

$$U(\boldsymbol{x}) = \sum_C -\frac{1}{N} \sum_{i=1}^{N} p_i(\boldsymbol{x}) \log(p_i(\boldsymbol{x})) \tag{1}$$

where C denotes the number of classes. In addition, the entropy maps are normalized to the range [0, 1]. Low values of the entropy map represent a high confidence with respect to the predicted segmentation estimate and vice versa.

For quality evaluation of pixel-wise uncertainties, the filtering method proposed in [8] is used. Here, uncertain image pixels are filtered using several uncertainty thresholds $T \in [0, 1]$ and are not considered in both prediction and ground truth for further evaluation. Changes in Dice as well as the filtering of correctly classified pixels (filtered true positives or negatives, FTPs/FTNs) will be traced. In the best case, filtering should show increasing dice and slowly increasing FTPs and FTNs as T decreases. The resulting curves are used to determine a final score for uncertainty assessment, which can be calculated from the individual area under the curves (AUCs): $U_{Score} = \frac{1}{3}(AUC_{Dice} + (1 - AUC_{FTP}) + (1 - AUC_{FTN}))$.

Furthermore, two metrics presented in [9] are used to assess the uncertainty of a particular structure (here PED) rather than each pixel and are computed between the N MC samples. The first measure determines the Dice overlap between all pairs of segmentation samples $\tilde{y}_i$ and $\tilde{y}_j$

$$\text{pwDice} = E\left[\left\{\text{Dice}\left(\tilde{y}_i, \tilde{y}_j\right)\right\}_{i<j}\right] \tag{2}$$

As a second measure, the coefficient of variation is used to examine the volume variation between MC samples:

$$CV = \frac{\sigma}{\mu} \tag{3}$$

Here μ and σ denote mean and standard deviation of the sample volumes.

3   Experiments and results

Experiments were performed on single 2D B-scans derived from OCT images of 39 patients with AMD. In comparison to [3], images are acquired by a modified prototype home OCT system during a follow-up study [10]. Since, the partner eye was also imaged in some cases, the image dataset includes OCT scans of 68 eyes in total, of which 59 % of the B-scans contain PED. All scans have a volume size of 250×968×608 pixels ($1.44{\times}2.92{\times}1.8$ mm^3). PED has been annotated in 30 equidistant B-scans per OCT volume by a medical expert. Image data is preprocessed using adaptive histogram equalization and moving average filter to increase the signal-to-noise ratio. Furthermore, images are resampled for training.

Evaluation is performed via four-fold cross-validation. Per fold, the BDCU-Net is trained for 300 epochs using generalized Dice loss. A dropout rate of 0.3 is used and the number of MC samples is set to 20 for both TTD and TTA.

An exemplary qualitative segmentation result including pixel-wise entropy as uncertainty estimate is shown Figure 1. One can observe that most of the epistemic uncertainties are located close to the edges of the PED segmentation. The same applies to aleatoric uncertainty, in which challenging areas such as motion artifacts are displayed in addition to edge regions. Moreover, magnitudes of aleatoric uncertainty are comparatively smaller.

Two qualitative examples of uncertainty filtering for $T = \{1.00, 0.75, 0.50, 0.25\}$ are shown in Figure 2. With decreasing uncertainty threshold, an accumulation of filtered and therefore uncertain pixels can be observed, which as expected spread out from the edge regions. For $T = 0.25$ almost all FPs and FNs disappear due to filtering of the segmentations computed by TTA. However, at the same time the proportion of filtered TPs increases significantly and appears slightly higher in contrast to the segmentation examples of the TTD method.

These observations are confirmed by quantitative evaluation of the filtering procedure, which is shown in Figure 3, visualizing changes in Dice, FTP, and FTN. Without filtering ($T = 1.00$), a Dice of 0.621 for TTA and 0.607 for TTD is achieved, steadily increasing when lowering the threshold. Due to the higher entropy values of epistemic uncertainties, more TPs of TTD segmentations are filtered quite early ($T > 0.5$). Then, for $T < 0.50$ comparatively more TPs in the TTA segmentations are marked as uncertain. The amount of FTNs increases very slowly and is almost the same for TTA and TTD. Overall, a mean total score U_{score} of 0.814 is obtained for the aleatoric uncertainties and is slightly higher compared to the score for the epistemic uncertainty ($U_{score} = 0.808$).

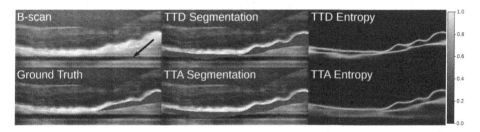

Fig. 1. Visualization of PED segmentation including uncertainty estimation. A motion artifact is indicated by the black arrow.

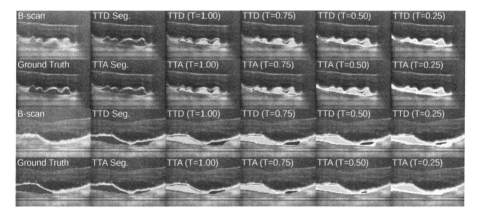

Fig. 2. Illustration of the effect of various uncertainty thresholds on two exemplary PED segmentations (the first and last two rows, respectively). Color coding is as follows: segmentation in purple, TP in green, FP in blue, FN in red and uncertain pixels in yellow.

Despite this small difference, statistical significance can be verified by a Wilcoxon rank sum test ($p=0.019$).

A final experiment is conducted to investigate the correlation between high Dice values and low uncertainties and vice versa. The size of the individual PEDs is also taken into account in the experiment. For this purpose, the structure-wise uncertainty metrics related to Dice values calculated between mean segmentation and ground truth are shown as scatter plots in Figure 4, wherein each data point represents a B-scan containing PED. Compared to TTD, scatter plots of TTA show stronger linear correlations with higher r values for pwDice as well as CV. Based on the color coding, one can see that mainly mid-sized PEDs are segmented with higher accuracy and reliability, as indicated by the accumulation of data points (light blue to orange) in the lower right area. In contrast, data points of smaller PEDs (dark to light blue) are predominantly located in the upper regions of the point clouds as well as widely fanned out at the left side, indicating

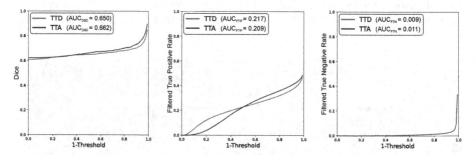

Fig. 3. Effect of altering the uncertainty threshold on Dice, FTP, and FTN. AUCs are given in the respective legend.

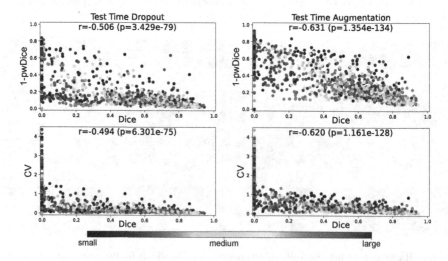

Fig. 4. Scatter plots of the structure-wise uncertainty metrics pwDice and CV versus Dice determined on B-scans containing PEDs with corresponding correlation coefficient. Data points are color coded based on the respective PED size.

less reliable segmentation estimates. Despite the low agreement between segmentation of (very) large PEDs (orange to dark red) and ground truth, the confidence of their prediction is relatively high, which might be related to their the low representation in the dataset.

4 Discussion

This work investigates epistemic and aleatoric uncertainties for PED segmentation in home OCT image data. Evaluations reveal that using TTA produces both more accurate segmentations as well as qualitatively better uncertainties than the TTD method. However, uncertainty estimates of very small or large PEDs do not always reflect the confidence level of the segmentation model, which will be tackled by calibration techniques in future work.

Overall, the evaluations of pixel-wise and structure-wise uncertainties represent important tools for understanding machine learning models and also provide important feedback for patient safety in relation to AMD home diagnostics.

References

1. Sudkamp H, Koch P, Spahr H et al. In-vivo retinal imaging with off-axis full-field time-domain optical coherence tomography. Opt Lett. 2016;41(21):4987–90.
2. Bogunović H, Venhuizen F, Klimscha S et al. RETOUCH-The retinal OCT fluid detection and segmentation benchmark and challenge. IEEE Trans Med Imaging. 2019;38:1858–74.
3. Kepp T, Sudkamp H, von der Burchard C et al. Segmentation of retinal low-cost optical coherence tomography images using deep learning. Medical Imaging 2020: Computer-Aided Diagnosis. Vol. 11314. SPIE, 2020:113141O.
4. Joy TT, Sedai S, Garnavi R. Analyzing epistemic and aleatoric uncertainty for drusen segmentation in optical coherence tomography images. AIII Workshop on Trustworthy AI for Healthcare. 2021.
5. Kendall A, Gal Y. What uncertainties do we need in bayesian deep learning for computer vision? Advances in Neural Information Processing Systems. Vol. 30. 2017:5580–90.
6. Wang G, Li W, Aertsen M et al. Aleatoric uncertainty estimation with test-time augmentation for medical image segmentation with convolutional neural networks. Neurocomputing. 2019;338:34–45.
7. Kepp T, Droigk C, Casper M et al. Segmentation of mouse skin layers in optical coherence tomography image data using deep convolutional neural networks. Biomed Opt Express. 2019;10(7):3484–96.
8. Mehta R, Filos A, Gal Y, Arbel T. Uncertainty evaluation metric for brain tumour segmentation. Medical Imaging with Deep Learning (MIDL). 2020.
9. Roy AG, Conjeti S, Navab N, Wachinger C. Bayesian QuickNAT: model uncertainty in deep whole-brain segmentation for structure-wise quality control. NeuroImage. 2019;195:11–22.
10. von der Burchard C, Moltmann M, Tode J et al. Self-examination low-cost full-field OCT (SELFF-OCT) for patients with various macular diseases. Graefes Arch Clin Exp Ophthalmol. 2021;259(6):1503–11.

Quality Monitoring of Federated Covid-19 Lesion Segmentation

Camila González[1], Christian L. Harder[1], Amin Ranem[1], Ricarda Fischbach[2], Isabel J. Kaltenborn[2], Armin Dadras[2], Andreas M. Bucher[2], Anirban Mukhopadhyay[1]

[1]Medical and Environmental Computing, Technische Universität Darmstadt
[2]Institut für Diagnostische und Interventionelle Radiologie, Universitätsklinikum Frankfurt
camila.gonzalez@gris.tu-darmstadt.de

Abstract. Federated Learning is the most promising way to train robust Deep Learning models for the segmentation of Covid-19-related findings in chest CTs. By learning in a decentralized fashion, heterogeneous data can be leveraged from a variety of sources and acquisition protocols whilst ensuring patient privacy. It is, however, crucial to continuously monitor the performance of the model. Yet when it comes to the segmentation of diffuse lung lesions, a quick visual inspection is not enough to assess the quality, and thorough monitoring of all network outputs by expert radiologists is not feasible. In this work, we present an array of lightweight metrics that can be calculated locally in each hospital and then aggregated for central monitoring of a federated system. Our linear model detects over 70% of low-quality segmentations on an out-of-distribution dataset and thus reliably signals a decline in model performance.

1 Introduction

The Covid-19 pandemic has strained medical resources across the world while demonstrating the value of time-saving workflow enhancements. Deep Learning solutions for the quantification of clinically relevant infection parameters, which segment Covid-19-characteristic lesions in CTs, have shown promising results.

Yet sufficient maturity for clinical use is frequently not reached by present approaches [1]. This is mainly due to neural networks failing silently coupled with a lack of appropriate quality controls. Scanner models and acquisition protocols vary between and within hospitals, changing image distribution. This causes Deep Learning models to produce low-quality outputs with high confidence [2].

Covid-19-related ground glass opacities and consolidations can occur in various forms, from covering multiple small regions to diffuse affection of the entire lung. Identifying low-quality segmentation masks is very time consuming and requires extensive experience, but thorough monitoring of all network outputs by expert readers is not logistically feasible.

Automated quality assurance for segmentation masks is not yet a developed field. Existing approaches include the training of a CNN on the logits of the segmentation

Springer Fachmedien Wiesbaden GmbH, ein Teil von Springer Nature 2022
K. Maier-Hein et al. (Hrsg.), *Bildverarbeitung für die Medizin 2022*,
Informatik aktuell, https://doi.org/10.1007/978-3-658-36932-3_8

prediction [3] or the concept of a Reverse Classification Algorithm [4] to predict segmentation quality. These are either computationally expensive or depend on rigid target shapes, which is not given in the case of Covid-19 lesions. Failed segmentations can however be identified by observing certain properties in the segmentation masks.

We propose an array of lightweight yet reliable quality metrics for segmentation masks that do not require ground truth annotations. These can be calculated locally without the need for expert reader review and then aggregated for each hospital for central monitoring of federated systems, as illustrated in Figure 1.

2 Materials and methods

We implemented our code with Python 3.8 and PyTorch 1.6 and performed a retrospective study using several open-source datasets, as well as in-house data. The code can be found at github.com/MECLabTUDA/QA_Seg.

2.1 Data

To obtain a dataset of predicted segmentations, we extracted predictions from an nnU-Net [5] trained on the COVID-19 Lung Lesion Segmentation Challenge (*Challenge*) dataset [6]. We also predicted segmentations on *MosMed* [7], as well as in-house data with further 50 cases. Images were interpolated to dimension (50,512,512). Further details can be found in Table 1. We partitioned the predictions into in-distribution (ID) for the Challenge and in-house datasets (with which we trained our classifiers) and out-of-distribution (OOD) for MosMed. The ID datasets were randomly divided into *ID train* and *ID test*. We considered the Dice between ground truth and predicted masks as a measure of segmentation quality, as it is the most-used metric for segmentation overlap. As shown in Table 1, the ID data is heavily skewed towards good-quality segmentations. We define a *failed* segmentation as having a Dice lower than 0.6 (following Valindria et al. [4]) and report their prevalence in Table 1.

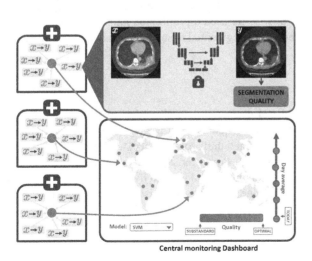

Central monitoring Dashboard

Fig. 1. Quality features are extracted and an SVM model is used to perform inference locally at several hospitals. These quality scores are aggregated for each site and visualized at a central dashboard. In the entire process, only the privacy-preserving aggregated scores leave the institutions.

Tab. 1. Data distribution, including ratio of infection within the segmented lung volume [8], nnU-Net performance and number of failed segmentation masks.

Property	Challenge	In-house	MosMed
Nr. cases (train, test)	199 (160, 39)	50 (40, 10)	50 (0, 50)
Mean resolution	(68.87,512.0,512.0)	(266.64,819.20,825.68)	(40.98,512.00,512.00)
Infection ratio	0.061 ± 0.093	0.275 ± 0.274	0.016 ± 0.015
nnU-Net Dice (train)	0.75 ± 0.14	0.59 ± 0.2	N.A.
nnU-Net Dice (test)	0.71 ± 0.18	0.68 ± 0.1	0.47 ± 0.19
Failed masks (train)	24	12	N.A.
Failed masks (test)	8	1	37

2.2 Proposed features

Inspired by van Rikxoort et al. [9], we looked to predict the quality of segmentation masks - in the form of Dice coefficient - using only four features (Fig. 2), defined as follows:

- *Connected Components*: While lung lesions may occupy several components, failed segmentations are often more disconnected. We counted the number of connected components using *Scikit-Image*, defining a component as one with a maximal distance of 3 by the City Block Metric to other voxels.
- *Intensity Mode*: Observing the intensity values in the CT, we can identify tissue that is very unlikely to be infected. Inspired by Kalka et al. [10], we fitted a Gaussian distribution over the largest component and returned its mean.
- *Segmentation Smoothness*: Even though Covid-19 lesions are diffuse in nature, in a correct segmentation mask we expect two consecutive slices to have a high overlap and thus a high two-dimensional Dice. We computed the smoothness for every component by taking the average Dice scores for all consecutive slices that were not identical. We then averaged the smoothness over all components.
- *Lesions within Lungs*: A correct segmentation mask should be completely contained within the lung. To factor this in, we used a pre-trained lung segmentation model [8] and recorded the percentage of segmented tissue that is inside of the lung.

2.3 Models and training

With these features, we trained and evaluated several models to predict the segmentation quality. We directly regressed the quality with a Ridge Regression (RR) and a Support Vector Regression (SVR) (trained until convergence) as well as a Multi-Layer-Perceptron (MLP) with (50,100,100,50) layers for 200 epochs minimizing the Mean Squared Error. We also discretized the quality values into five bins and performed classification with Support Vector Machine (SVM) and Logistic Regression (LR) models, using balanced class weights. Unless otherwise stated, we used the default *Scikit-learn* library implementations.

2.4   Evaluation

As we were primarily interested in detecting failed segmentations, we report the sensitivity of all 5 models on this task. We also report the specificities for identifying the correct quality interval (averaged over 5 bins) on all ID and OOD datasets. In addition, we report the Mean Absolute Error as a metric than quantifies the ability of all models to directly predict the segmentation quality.

3   Results

In terms of sensitivity (detection of faulty segmentations) the classifiers (LR and SVM) outperformed the regression models by a large margin (Tab. 2). This can be attributed to the class weights of the LR and SVM models balancing the disparately appearing classes in the training data, which improved their performance on differently distributed data. Though we were unable to detect the single failed segmentation out of 10 on the in-house dataset, we highlight the performance of the LR model, which detects over 60% of failed segmentations on both of the bigger Challenge and MosMed datasets. All models showed a high specificity of over 0.8 on all datasets. The regression models achieved a lower mean absolute error but seemed to overfit the good-quality segmentations on the training dataset, which might explain their worse sensitivity.

We further evaluated the LR model using 10000 bootstrapping runs, sampling 192 data points from the training set and evaluating the model's sensitivity trained on these samples on the ID and OOD datasets for every run. We achieved 95% confidence intervals for the sensitivity covering a range from 0.22 to 1.0. Furthermore, using a p-valued test with a significance level of 0.05, we can reject every null hypothesis stating that the sensitivity of the LR model is below 0.28.

In order to evaluate the individual contribution of each feature, we performed an ablation study where we left out each of the features for LR models. The Intensity Mode feature proved to be the least useful. Leaving it out allows us to correctly identify 5 more

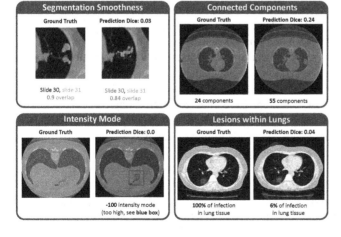

Fig. 2. Exemplary subjects and slides for the four features used to assess segmentation quality.

Tab. 2. Sensitivity of finding failed segmentations (Dice < 0.6), specificity of identifying the correct quality interval (avg. over 5 bins) and Mean Absolute Error (mean+/- std) results for each model for ID and OOD datasets.

		Classifiers		Regressors		
		LR	SVM	RR	SVR	MLP
Sensitivity	Challenge	0.63 (5/8)	0.38 (3/8)	0.38 (3/8)	0.13 (1/8)	0.25 (2/8)
	In-house	0.0 (0/1)	0.0 (0/1)	0.0 (0/1)	0.0 (0/1)	0.0 (0/1)
	MosMed	0.76 (28/37)	0.68 (25/37)	0.14 (5/37)	0.35 (13/37)	0.35 (13/37)
Specificity	Challenge	0.84	0.85	0.88	0.87	0.87
	In-house	0.8	0.83	0.95	0.9	0.9
	MosMed	0.8	0.83	0.82	0.84	0.85
MAE	Challenge	0.29 ± 0.22	0.26 ± 0.22	0.1 ± 0.1	0.11 ± 0.11	0.18 ± 0.13
	In-house	0.24 ± 0.12	0.26 ± 0.14	0.08 ± 0.09	0.1 ± 0.07	0.09 ± 0.07
	MosMed	0.33 ± 0.19	0.29 ± 0.23	0.22 ± 0.16	0.21 ± 0.18	0.23 ± 0.18

high-quality segmentations as such, though 9 faulty segmentations less are detected. All in all, using all four features achieves the best sensitivity-to-specificity trade-off.

We attribute most of the falsely classified segmentations to the low representation of bad segmentations in the training data and to these displaying plausible shapes. For example, segmentation masks covering only a few spots of healthy lung tissue, containing intensity values of possibly infected areas, while maintaining a smooth shape, were not detected.

4 Discussion

We introduced a simple method to monitor performance of an nnU-Net trained to detect lung infections onset by Covid-19. We designed four features and found that a LR model using these reliably detects faulty segmentation masks. All the features are lightweight and do not require ground truth annotations, and so they can be used to monitor the deployment of a distributed, federated learning system.

Our findings have some limitations. First, we tested our methods retrospectively on a statically trained nnU-Net. This allowed us to accurately evaluate our methods, as we had access to ground truth test annotations, but a prospective study on a federated system with a few participating institutions would better emulate real deployment.

Secondly, the CT data was acquired on ICU patients, thus introducing considerable bias in patient demographics which are likely not representative of the general Covid-19 population. This also suggests that a measure other than Dice may be better suited for the general population, as the expressiveness of Dice is heavily dependent on lesion size.

Finally, each dataset was annotated by a different group of experts, so the definitions of the findings may vary across datasets. This is often the case when evaluating with OOD data but should be taken into account when considering the differences in performance.

In conclusion, training models in a federated fashion allows to leverage heterogeneous data sources without compromising patient privacy. However, it is necessary to constantly monitor the quality of the model outputs. In this work, we introduced an array of lightweight quality metrics that can be calculated locally and aggregated for central monitoring. These are particularly well-suited to the use case of lung lesion segmentation in chest CTs, as lesions vary greatly in terms of form and location and verifying their correctness is time-intensive even for trained radiologists. Future work should expand the metric catalogue and assess the effectiveness of the proposed methods in a model deployed across multiple hospitals. Our results present a first step towards an effective quality control of federated lung lesion segmentation.

References

1. Roberts M, Driggs D, Thorpe M, Gilbey J, Yeung M, Ursprung S et al. Common pitfalls and recommendations for using machine learning to detect and prognosticate for covid-19 using chest radiographs and ct scans. Nat Mach Intell. 2021;3(3):199–217.
2. Gonzalez C, Gotkowski K, Bucher A, Fischbach R, Kaltenborn I, Mukhopadhyay A. Detecting when pre-trained nnU-Net models fail silently for covid-19 lung lesion segmentation. Med Image Comput Comput Assist Interv. Springer. 2021:304–14.
3. Chen X, Men K, Chen B, Tang Y, Zhang T, Wang S et al. CNN-based quality assurance for automatic segmentation of breast cancer in radiotherapy. Front Oncol. 2020;10:524.
4. Valindria VV, Lavdas I, Bai W, Kamnitsas K, Aboagye EO, Rockall AG et al. Reverse classification accuracy: predicting segmentation performance in the absence of ground truth. IEEE Trans Med Imaging. 2017;36(8):1597–606.
5. Isensee F, Jaeger PF, Kohl SA, Petersen J, Maier-Hein KH. nnU-Net: a self-configuring method for deep learning-based biomedical image segmentation. Nat Methods. 2021;18(2):203–11.
6. Roth H, Xu Z, Diez CT, Jacob RS, Zember J, Molto J et al. Rapid artificial intelligence solutions in a pandemic - the covid-19-20 lung CT lesion segmentation challenge. Res Sq. 2020.
7. Morozov S, Andreychenko A, Pavlov N, Vladzymyrskyy A, Ledikhova N, Gombolevskiy V et al. Mosmeddata: chest ct scans with covid-19 related findings dataset. arXiv preprint arXiv:2005.06465. 2020.
8. Hofmanninger J, Prayer F, Pan J, Röhrich S, Prosch H, Langs G. Automatic lung segmentation in routine imaging is primarily a data diversity problem, not a methodology problem. Eur Radiol Exp. 2020;4(1):1–13.
9. Rikxoort EM van, Hoop B de, Viergever MA, Prokop M, Ginneken B van. Automatic lung segmentation from thoracic computed tomography scans using a hybrid approach with error detection. Med Phys. 2009;36(7):2934–47.
10. Kalka N, Bartlow N, Cukic B. An automated method for predicting iris segmentation failures. 2009 IEEE 3rd International Conference on Biometrics: Theory, Applications, and Systems. IEEE. 2009:1–8.

Detection of Large Vessel Occlusions Using Deep Learning by Deforming Vessel Tree Segmentations

Florian Thamm[1,2], Oliver Taubmann[2], Markus Jürgens[2], Hendrik Ditt[2], Andreas Maier[1]

[1]Friedrich-Alexander University Erlangen-Nuremberg, Erlangen, Germany
[2]Siemens Healthcare GmbH, Forchheim, Germany
florian.thamm@fau.de

Abstract. Computed Tomography Angiography is a key modality providing insights into the cerebrovascular vessel tree that are crucial for the diagnosis and treatment of ischemic strokes, in particular in cases of large vessel occlusions (LVO). Thus, the clinical workflow greatly benefits from an automated detection of patients suffering from LVOs. This work uses convolutional neural networks for case-level classification trained with elastic deformation of the vessel tree segmentation masks to artificially augment training data. Using only masks as the input to our model uniquely allows us to apply such deformations much more aggressively than one could with conventional image volumes while retaining sample realism. The neural network classifies the presence of an LVO and the affected hemisphere. In a 5-fold cross validated ablation study, we demonstrate that the use of the suggested augmentation enables us to train robust models even from few data sets. Training the EfficientNetB1 architecture on 100 data sets, the proposed augmentation scheme was able to raise the ROC AUC to 0.85 from a baseline value of 0.56 using no augmentation. The best performance was achieved using a 3D-DenseNet yielding an AUC of 0.87. The augmentation had positive impact in classification of the affected hemisphere as well, where the 3D-DenseNet reached an AUC of 0.93 on both sides.

1 Introduction

Computed Tomography Angiography (CTA) is a commonly used modality in many clinical scenarios including the diagnosis of ischemic strokes. An ischemic stroke is caused by an occluded blood vessel resulting in a lack of oxygen in the affected brain parenchyma. An occlusion in the internal carotid artery (ICA), proximal middle cerebral artery (MCA) or basilar artery is often referred to as large vessel occlusion (LVO). These LVOs are visible in CTA scans as a discontinuation of contrast agent in the vascular tree, which is a complex system of arteries and veins and varies from patient to patient. Consequently the diagnosis takes time and requires expertise. Clinics and patients would therefore benefit from an automated classification of LVOs on CTA scans.

Prior research in that field is described in literature. Amukotuwa et al. detected LVOs in CTA scans with a pipeline consisting of 14 steps and tested their commercially

© Der/die Autor(en), exklusiv lizenziert durch
Springer Fachmedien Wiesbaden GmbH, ein Teil von Springer Nature 2022
K. Maier-Hein et al. (Hrsg.), *Bildverarbeitung für die Medizin 2022*,
Informatik aktuell, https://doi.org/10.1007/978-3-658-36932-3_9

available algorithm on two different data cohorts, reporting a performance of 0.86 ROC AUC in the first trial with 477 patients [1] and 0.94 in the second trial [2] with 926 patients. Stib et al. [3] computed maximum-intensity projections of segmentations of the vessel tree based on multi-phase CTA scans (three CTA scans covering the arterial, peak venous and late venous phases), and trained a 2D-DenseNet [4] on 424 patients to classify the presence of an LVO. They report ROC AUC values between 0.74 and 0.85 depending on the phase. Luijten et al.'s work [5] investigated the performance of another commercially available LVO detection algorithm based on a Convolutional Neural Network (CNN) and determined a ROC AUC of 0.75 on 646 test patients.

In all studies, very large data cohorts were available. This appears mandatory to train (and test) AI-based detection algorithms, since in case-wise classification the number of training samples equals the number of available patients. In this work we present a data-efficient method that achieves performance comparable to what is seen in related work while relying on only 100 data sets for training.

2 Materials and methods

2.1 Data

Altogether, 168 thin-sliced (0.5 to 1 mm) head CTA data sets were available. Of these, 106 patients were LVO positive due to an occlusion either in the middle cerebral artery or the internal carotid. Regarding the affected hemisphere, 54 (52) LVOs were located on the left (right) side. The data was acquired from a single site with a Somatom Definition AS+ (Siemens Healthineers, Forchheim, Germany).

2.2 Methodology

The method we propose is based on the idea of aggressively augmenting the vessel tree segmentations in order to artificially extend the amount of trainable data. The classification pipeline itself (Fig. 1), consists of three subsequent steps. In the first step, the cerebrovascular tree is segmented using segmentation approach published by Thamm et al. [6]. Additionally, the algorithm prunes the vessel tree to the relevant arteries by masking out all vascular structures which are a walking distance (geodesic distance w.r.t. vessel center lines) of more than 150 mm away from the Circle of Willis. Thereby veins, which are not relevant in the diagnosis of LVOs, like the Sinus Sagittalis are mostly excluded from further processing. In the second step, the original CTA scan is non-rigidly registered to the probabilistic brain atlas by Kemmling et al. [7]. The registration is based on Chefd'hotel et al.'s method [8] but may be done using other, publicly available registration methods as well. The resulting deformation field is used to transform the segmentation mask into the atlas coordinate system. An accurate registration between an atlas and the head scan is not crucial in our work as variations in the vessel tree are present in all patients anyway. Once the volumes are in the atlas coordinate space, they are equally sized with $182 \times 205 \times 205$ voxels with isotropic spacing of 1 mm in all dimensions. The primary purpose of the registration is to consistently orient and somewhat anatomically "normalize" the segmentation for the next step, in which a convolutional neural network classifies the presence of an LVO. The network receives the binary segmentation masks volume-wise and predicts a softmax activated vector of length 3, representing the three classes: No LVO, left LVO and right LVO. In our work, we tested a 3D-version of DenseNet [9] ($\approx$ 4.6m parameters) and EfficientNetB1 [10] ($\approx$ 6.5m parameters) where the channel dimension has been repurposed as the z-Axis. Cross entropy serves as the loss optimized with Adam on which is minimized using the Adam optimizer [11]. Our implementation is based on PyTorch 1.6 [12] and Python 3.8.5.

2.3 Augmentation

From patient to patient, the cerebrovascular anatomy follows coarsely the same structure. However, anatomical variations (e.g., absence ICA, accessory MCA) combined with the individual course of the vessels lead to a wide variety of configurations in intracranial vascular systems such that no vessel tree is quite like another. Considering this, augmentations can be used in order to artificially generate more vessel trees and from a network's perspective visually new patients. Therefore, we propose to elastically and randomly deform the segmentation masks for training. While the use of elastic deformation for augmentation per se is not a novel technique [13], in our setup we are uniquely able to apply it much more aggressively than otherwise possible, enabling us to dramatically increase its benefit compared to typical use cases. This is possible due to the fact that only vessel segmentations are used as input for our CNN-based classifier model. Whereas strong deformations on a conventional image volume will quickly introduce resampling artifacts that render the image unrealistic, masks remain visually

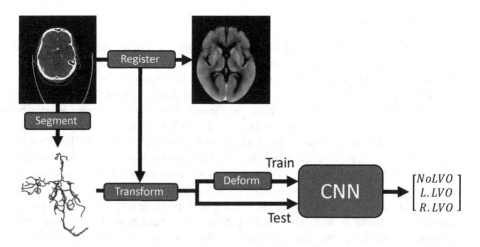

Fig. 1. Proposed pipeline. In the first step, the CTA volume is registered to a probabilistic brain atlas. The cerebrovascular vessel tree is then segmented and transformed into the atlas coordinate system by applying the resulting deformation vector field. For augmentation purposes, the vessel tree segmentation masks are elastically deformed for training only. A network predicts the three mutually exclusive classes: No LVO, left or right LVO.

comparable to the original samples even when heavily deformed. As the segmentation is performed on full volumes, an online augmentation, i.e. deforming while the network is trained, is computationally too expensive and would increase the training time to an impractical level. Instead, we suggest to elastically deform the segmentation masks prior to the training for a fixed number of random fields for each original volume. As masks, unlike regular image volumes, are highly compressible, this does not notably increase data storage requirements as would typically be associated with such an approach.

In this work we aim to demonstrate the impact of this data augmentation on the performance for the classification of LVOs. Using the RandomElasticDeformation of TorchIO [14] which interpolates displacements with cubic B-splines, we randomly deformed each segmentation mask 10 times with 4 and 10 times with 5 random anchors, all 20 augmentations with a maximal displacement of 90 voxels (Examples in Figure 2). Additionally, we mirror the original data sets sagitally and again apply the above procedure to create 20 variants, which flips the right/left labels but has no effect if no LVO is present. We thus create 40 samples out of one volume, resulting in a total of 6720 vessel tree samples generated from 168 patients.

3 Results

We investigated the impact on the elastic augmentations in an ablation study considering two architectures, where we systematically disable features (deformation and mirroring). For a fully 3D variant we evaluated the 3D-DenseNet architecture [9] and alternatively a 2D variant where the channel axis of the input is used for the axial (z) dimension

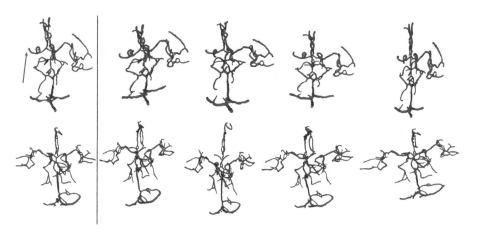

Fig. 2. Two examples with four augmentations of the original tree on the left, all viewed axially caudal with the same camera parameters. The upper row shows a case with an occlusion in the left middle cerebral artery, indicated by the arrow. The lower row shows an LVO-negative vessel tree. Instead of binary masks, surface meshes of the deformed masks were rendered for a sharper and clearer visualization. For each row, the augmentation on the far right shows an extreme example of a possible deformation.

Tab. 1. ROC AUCs with 95% confidence intervals (by determined by bootstrapping) in brackets for the 3D-DenseNet and EfficientNetB1 architecture. The abbreviation "D" stands for "deformation" and "M" for "mirroring". To computeFor the computation of "AUC Left", the right and no-LVO class were combined to one class enabling a binary classification. "AUC Right" was calculated analogously.

Setup	AUC LVO	AUC Left	AUC Right
3D-DenseNet + D + M	0.87 [0.81, 0.92]	0.93 [0.87, 0.97]	0.93 [0.88, 0.97]
3D-DenseNet + D	0.84 [0.77, 0.90]	0.89 [0.84, 0.94]	0.94 [0.90, 0.97]
3D-DenseNet	0.77 [0.69, 0.84]	0.85 [0.78, 0.91]	0.85 [0.78, 0.92]
EfficientNetB1 + D + M	0.85 [0.79, 0.90]	0.86 [0.79, 0.91]	0.90 [0.84, 0.96]
EfficientNetB1 + D	0.83 [0.77, 0.89]	0.85 [0.79, 0.91]	0.91 [0.85, 0.96]
EfficientNetB1	0.56 [0.47, 0.65]	0.59 [0.49, 0.68]	0.68 [0.58, 0.78]

using the EfficientNetB1 architecture [10]. We evaluated both architectures in a 5-fold cross validation setup with a 3-1-1 split ratio for training, validation and testing, where on average, 100 original data sets were used for training per cycle. The baseline (no augmentation) was trained for 200 epochs, a variant using the original and the deformed, but not mirrored data sets was trained for 100 epochs, and finally, as the proposed setting, models were trained for 50 epochs using the original, the deformed and mirrored data. Epoch numbers differ as there are more samples available when augmentation is used. All models overfitted by the end of their allotted epochs.were overfitting by the end of their allotted epochs, i.e. would not have benefited from further training. The validation loss was used to pick the best performing network out of all epochs. The test data was not augmented to provide a fair comparison between all setups. Both architectures significantly benefit from the deformation-based augmentation (Tab. 1); in particular, EfficientNet failed to grasp the problem at all without it. Overall, the 3D-DenseNet trained with deformed and mirrored data sets outperformed the other setups by a significant margin, especially in detecting LVOs and left LVOs. Depending on the chosen threshold, this variant achieved a sensitivity of 80% (or 90%) and a specificity of 82% (or 60% respectively) for the detection of LVOs.

4   Discussion

We presented a method for automated classification of LVOs based on CTA data which makes heavy use of deformation fields for augmentation. With an AUC of 0.87 for LVO detection, we achieved a performance comparable to that of other DL-based approaches while using as few as 100 patient data sets for training. While not novel in itself, elastic deformation for the purpose of augmentation could be applied much more aggressively in our setup compared to regular use cases as our model relies exclusively on segmented vessel tree masks as input; for these, even strong deformations—that would cause severe resampling artifacts when applied to regular image volumes—still lead to anatomically meaningful representations that are virtually indistinguishable from real samples. In an ablation study we showed that the performed augmentation was crucial for the ability of state-of-the-art models to properly learn the task at hand from a small number of data sets. This leads us to the conclusion that a learning-based detection of LVOs stands and falls with the number of training data sets. The cerebrovascular system is highly patient-specific, which is why the use of sophisticated augmentation techniques offers great potential. We postulate that also larger data pools could benefit from more extensive data augmentation if applied meaningfully.

References

1. Amukotuwa SA, Straka M, Smith H, Chandra RV, Dehkharghani S, Fischbein NJ et al. Automated detection of intracranial large vessel occlusions on computed tomography angiography: a single center experience. Stroke. 2019;50(10):2790–8.
2. Amukotuwa SA, Straka M, Dehkharghani S, Bammer R. Fast automatic detection of large vessel occlusions on CT angiography. Stroke. 2019;50(12):3431–8.
3. Stib MT, Vasquez J, Dong MP, Kim YH, Subzwari SS, Triedman HJ et al. Detecting large vessel occlusion at multiphase CT angiography by using a deep convolutional neural network. Radiology. 2020;297(3):640–9.
4. Huang G, Liu Z, Van Der Maaten L, Weinberger KQ. Densely connected convolutional networks. Proceedings of the IEEE conference on computer vision and pattern recognition. 2017:4700–8.
5. Luijten SP, Wolff L, Duvekot MH, Doormaal PJ van, Moudrous W, Kerkhoff H et al. Diagnostic performance of an algorithm for automated large vessel occlusion detection on CT angiography. J Neurointerv Surg. 2021.
6. Thamm F, Jürgens M, Ditt H, Maier A. VirtualDSA++-automated segmentation, vessel labeling, occlusion detection, and graph search on CT angiography data. VCBM. 2020:151–5.
7. Kemmling A, Wersching H, Berger K, Knecht S, Groden C, Nölte I. Decomposing the hounsfield unit. Clin Neuroradiol. 2012;22(1):79–91.
8. Chefd'Hotel C, Hermosillo G, Faugeras O. Flows of diffeomorphisms for multimodal image registration. Proceedings IEEE International Symposium on Biomedical Imaging. IEEE. 2002:753–6.
9. Hara K, Kataoka H, Satoh Y. Can spatiotemporal 3D CNNs retrace the history of 2D CNNs and ImageNet? Proceedings of the IEEE Conference on Computer Vision and Pattern Recognition (CVPR). 2018:6546–55.
10. Tan M, Le Q. Efficientnet: rethinking model scaling for convolutional neural networks. International Conference on Machine Learning. PMLR. 2019:6105–14.
11. Kingma DP, Ba J. Adam: a method for stochastic optimization. arXiv preprint arXiv:1412.6980. 2014.
12. Paszke A, Gross S, Massa F, Lerer A, Bradbury J, Chanan G et al. Pytorch: an imperative style, high-performance deep learning library. arXiv preprint arXiv:1912.01703. 2019.
13. Nalepa J, Marcinkiewicz M, Kawulok M. Data augmentation for brain-tumor segmentation: a review. Front Comput Neurosci. 2019;13:83.
14. Pérez-García F, Sparks R, Ourselin S. TorchIO: a Python library for efficient loading, preprocessing, augmentation and patch-based sampling of medical images in deep learning. Comput Methods Programs Biomed. 2021:106236.

Abstract: nnDetection

A Self-configuring Method for Medical Object Detection

Michael Baumgartner[1], Paul F. Jäger[2], Fabian Isensee[3], Klaus H. Maier-Hein[1,4]

[1]Division of Medical Image Computing, German Cancer Research Center, Heidelberg, Germany
[2]Interactive Machine Learning Group, German Cancer Research Center
[3]HIP Applied Computer Vision Lab, German Cancer Research Center
[4]Pattern Analysis and Learning Group, Heidelberg University Hospital
m.baumgartner@dkfz.de

Simultaneous localisation and categorization of objects in medical images, also referred to as medical object detection, is of high clinical relevance because diagnostic decisions often depend on rating of objects rather than e.g. pixels. For this task, the cumbersome and iterative process of method configuration constitutes a major research bottleneck. Recently, nnU-Net has tackled this challenge for the task of image segmentation with great success. Following nnU-Net's agenda, in this work we systematize and automate the configuration process for medical object detection. The resulting self-configuring method, nnDetection, adapts itself without any manual intervention to arbitrary medical detection problems while achieving results en par with or superior to the state-of-the-art. We demonstrate the effectiveness of nnDetection on two public benchmarks, ADAM and LUNA16, and propose 11 further medical object detection tasks on public data sets for comprehensive method evaluation. Notably, this work has previously been published at MICCAI 2021 [1]. Code is at https://github.com/MIC-DKFZ/nnDetection.

References

1. Baumgartner M, Jäger PF, Isensee F, Maier-Hein KH. nnDetection: A Self-Configuring Method for Medical Object Detection. Proc MICCAI. 2021:530–9.

Springer Fachmedien Wiesbaden GmbH, ein Teil von Springer Nature 2022
K. Maier-Hein et al. (Hrsg.), *Bildverarbeitung für die Medizin 2022*,
Informatik aktuell, https://doi.org/10.1007/978-3-658-36932-3_10

Machine Learning-based Detection of Spherical Markers in CT Volumes

Disha D. Rao[1], Nicole Maass[2], Frank Dennerlein[2], Andreas Maier[1], Yixing Huang[1]

[1]Pattern Recognition Lab, FAU Erlangen-Nürnberg, Germany
[2]Siemens Healthcare GmbH, Erlangen, Germany
disha.d.rao@fau.de

Abstract. X-ray CT geometry alignment procedures commonly use phantoms with spherical markers to estimate the geometry parameters. Obtaining precise 3D positions of the markers is crucial for an accurate alignment. A typical approach utilizes a 3D version of fast radial symmetry transform for marker detection. This method works only for a given set of radii and tends to be influenced by reconstruction artifacts. With a desire for a more robust solution, a deep learning-based approach is investigated. A 3D version of the region proposal network (RPN) is implemented to determine the position and the diameter of markers in real CT measurements of alignment phantoms. The RPN incorporates a U-Net-based backbone network to capture the multi-scale information present in the volume. Experiments to determine the robustness of the network to distortion-free, limited-angle distortions, and misalignment distortions are presented. In all the three cases, all markers can be localized within the radius precision. The results show that RPN is a promising method to determine the marker positions in distorted CT volumes.

1 Introduction

Phantom-based geometry alignment of cone-beam computed tomography systems often relies on spherical markers to determine geometry parameters. The workflow requires precise knowledge of 3D marker positions and marker sizes for marker correspondence. In a recent work on geometry calibration [1], fast radial symmetry transform (FRST) has been employed to determine the marker positions in projection images. It is possible to utilize the 3D version of FRST for 3D marker detection. This algorithm requires the input of a set of radii and uses local symmetry to highlight the centroid points of the markers. The precision of this method is reduced if the reference scan contains CT reconstruction artifacts that could arise from the loss of symmetry of the markers caused by their bearing structure. In addition to these physical distortions, mathematical artifacts can arise from both misaligned exact CT trajectories and approximate CT trajectories, which naturally reduces the reliability of FRST- based 3D marker detection. This calls for a more robust solution to determine the 3D marker positions.

A natural inclination would be towards machine learning techniques. Owing to the advancement in processing hardware, deep neural networks have shown a tremendous

Springer Fachmedien Wiesbaden GmbH, ein Teil von Springer Nature 2022
K. Maier-Hein et al. (Hrsg.), *Bildverarbeitung für die Medizin 2022*,
Informatik aktuell, https://doi.org/10.1007/978-3-658-36932-3_11

impact in the field of computer vision [2]. Previous works on marker detection using deep learning either take the approach of segmentation, require prior knowledge or are designed for 2D space [3–5]. With segmentation approaches, there is always a question of accuracy with the segmented regions if the objective is to localize the center coordinates from them [3]. Although analysis in 2D is more memory efficient, our work aims to explore the 3D spatial information to compute the centroid coordinates. Region Proposal Networks (RPNs) have been widely used in the detection of lung nodules directly in 3D space [6, 7]. As the markers in phantoms and the majority of nodules outline a spherical shape, our work takes its inspiration from the task of lung nodule detection.

2   Materials and methods

2.1   3D region proposal network

The structure of RPN is illustrated in Figure 1. It is a fully convolutional network consisting of a U-Net-based backbone network interleaved with 3D residual units and a region proposal module. The RPN framework used in this work follows the works of [6]. U-Net enables the network to include multi-scale information effectively, as it is essential to capture different sizes of markers [6]. The backbone network in this work does not include the additional location crop that is attributed to the location information of lung nodules as observed in [6]. The region proposal module slides over the output feature map of the backbone network generating a predefined number of bounding boxes (termed as "anchor boxes"). These boxes are defined based on the distribution of marker diameters. If the bounding box encompasses the marker perfectly, the center coordinates of the box can be representative of the centroid of the marker and its side length can be representative of the diameter of the marker. The objective of RPN is to check whether the anchor boxes contain markers and refine their coordinates to better fit the markers. Each anchor box contributes to 5 parts in the loss function, binary cross-entropy loss to determine the objectness score indicating whether a marker is present or not and smoothed L_1 regression loss for its center coordinates (x, y, z) and side length.

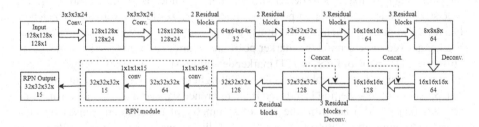

Fig. 1. RPN framework containing a U-Net-based encoder-decoder structure and an RPN module. The number inside boxes are feature map sizes in the format (rows × columns × slices × channels). The numbers above connections indicate (filters × rows × columns × slices). Each residual block in the encoder consists of a standard residual unit [8] and is followed by a max pooling layer. Deconvolution and max pooling operations are performed using a kernel size $2 \times 2 \times 2$ and stride of 2.

2.2 Dataset and experiments

The dataset comprises real CT measurements of 5 different phantoms provided by Siemens Healthcare GmbH, Erlangen. Spherical markers of high attenuation material are embedded in a collinear arrangement using holders as observed in [1]. The difference in the phantoms is attributed to different kinds of holder structure, size, and the number of markers. Some measurements originate from the same phantom but are scanned using different voltage settings. Care was taken not to distribute measurements from the same phantom between the training and the test set. With this, 3 phantoms are used for training and 2 for testing. Three kinds of experiments are performed. The RPN is evaluated on volumes without any distortions, where the markers are dominantly seen with a spherical shape in the reconstructions. The training set was augmented by inducing random Gaussian noise (offline), flipping, and swapping of one of the coordinate axis (online). Additionally, the RPN is evaluated in 72° limited angle tomography followed by geometrical distortion cases. Distortions are artificially introduced during the reconstruction of volumes from the measured projection images. For the limited angle experiment, the training set is augmented using multiple reconstructions of phantoms using different start projection angles. In order to introduce geometrical distortion, the rotation axis is slightly misconfigured. The training set is augmented using two different values of this parameter. These are especially challenging distortions as the markers no longer appeared spherical. The ground-truth 3D locations of the markers are acquired using the FRST algorithm using high-quality volumes where all distortions are minimized with conventional methods.

2.3 Training and testing

The model is trained using the stochastic gradient descent optimization with a momentum of 0.9. The total number of epochs is set to 100 but an early stopping criterion monitors the training. The initial learning rate is set to 0.0001 which decays after every 30 epochs by a decay factor of 0.05. Due to GPU limitations, subvolumes are employed for training and testing. Two kinds of subvolumes are used. 75% of the subvolumes are randomly cropped such that they contain at least one marker and the remaining 25% of the subvolumes do not contain any marker. The latter ensured the coverage of the space of non-marker regions in the phantoms. Additionally, the distribution of marker sizes is unbalanced due to the arrangement observed in [1]. Large markers are less than small ones. To balance this, large markers are sampled more than small markers during subvolume creation. Anchor boxes of sizes $5 \times 5 \times 5$, $10 \times 10 \times 10$, $20 \times 20 \times 20$ and $25 \times 25 \times 25$ are considered in the experiments. For training, RPN assigns a binary class label to each anchor. It gets a positive label if the Intersection over Union (IOU) with a ground truth box is greater than 0.5 or has the highest IOU for a ground truth box. It gets a negative label if the IOU is less than 0.02 and the rest do not contribute to the training process. As there are more negative anchors than positive ones, an online version of hard negative mining [6] is incorporated to create a balance. During testing, non-maximum suppression (NMS) is implemented to rule out overlapping predictions.

Tab. 1. Results of centroid and diameter predictions from distortion-free experiment.

Test Phantom	Total Markers	Marker Radius (mm)	Precision (0.5mm)	Precision (Radius)	Recall (Radius)	MPE (mm)	MPD (mm)
A	4	3.25	75%	100%	100%	0.37±0.14	5.68±0.03
B	20	Small: 1	90%	100%	100%	0.35 ±0.71	2.28±0.05
		Large: 1.5					3.4±0.03

Tab. 2. Results of centroid and diameter predictions from limited angle experiment.

Test Phantom	Total Markers	Marker Radius (mm)	Precision (0.5mm)	Precision (Radius)	Recall (Radius)	MPE (mm)	MPD (mm)
A	4	3.25	50%	100%	100%	0.64±0.43	5.85±0.12
B	20	Small: 1	95%	100%	100%	0.27±0.12	2.03±0.07
		Large: 1.5					2.42±0.07

2.4 Evaluation

Precision and recall are computed to evaluate the ability of RPN in determining the positions of marker centroids. Precision computes the percentage of accurate predictions out of the total predictions. Recall computes the number of accurate predictions over the number of markers in the phantom. A prediction is considered to be accurate if a marker is detected within a distance $R \in \{0.5\,mm, \text{marker radius (mm)}\}$ from its centroid. A mean position error (MPE) computes the mean of Euclidean distances between the ground-truth and the predicted centroid coordinates of all the markers. Mean predicted diameter (MPD) computes the mean of all the predicted marker diameters.

3 Results

Tables 1-3 display the quantitative evaluation results in distortion-free, 72° limited angle, and geometrical distortion cases, respectively, and Figure 2 shows six exemplary detection results. In all the experiments, no false positive markers are detected, nor any markers are entirely missing. In the distortion-free case, 100% precision and recall are observed for centroid prediction within radius distance with MPE around 0.37 mm for both test phantoms. Figures 2a, 2b show the predicted anchor boxes have good overlaps with the markers, which demonstrates the efficacy of RPN in marker localization. However, the MPD still have relatively large error, indicates its limitation for accurate diameter estimation.

In 72° limited angle and geometrical distortion cases, RPN achieves comparable marker detection results, with all the markers detected within the radius distance, while some of them are beyond the 0.5 mm precision range. Figures 2c-2e are three examples where the side lengths of predicted anchor boxes are consistent with the actual marker diameters. Figure 2f is an example where RPN fails to predict the correct marker diameter.

Tab. 3. Results of centroid and diameter predictions from geometrical distortion experiment. g_1 and g_2 represent two different misconfigurations of the rotation axis geometry parameter with the degree of distortion in the order $g_1 < g_2$.

Test Phantom	Total Markers	Marker Radius (mm)	Precision (0.5mm)	Precision (Radius)	Recall (Radius)	MPE (mm)	MPD (mm)
A(g1)	4	3.25	50%	100%	100%	0.63±0.33	4.35±0.06
B(g1)	20	Small: 1	95%	100%	100%	0.26±0.14	2.09±0.06
		Large: 1.5					2.14±0.03
A(g2)	4	3.25	50%	100%	100%	0.64±0.29	4.38±0.06
B(g2)	20	Small: 1	75%	100%	100%	0.34±0.09	2.79±0.42
		Large: 1.5					2.16±0.04

4 Discussion

This work addresses the task of marker detection in alignment phantoms as an object detection task. Although RPN has large inaccuracy in estimating marker diameters, we are able to classify whether a marker is large or small according to its predicted diameter in distortion-free case. This information is beneficial for marker type classification, and

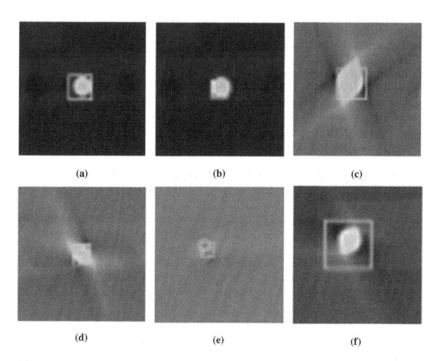

(a)   (b)   (c)

(d)   (e)   (f)

Fig. 2. Visualization of central slices for bounding box predictions. 2a and 2b Distortion-free cases. 2c and 2d 72° limited angle case. 2e Geometrical distortion case. 2f Unsatisfying large side length prediction from 72° limited angle case.

hence for further marker-to-marker correspondence identification. In the limited angle and geometrical distortion cases, reconstructed markers suffer from streak artifacts. Therefore, it is more difficult for RPN to estimate marker diameters. As a consequence, the two marker types are not fully distinguishable.

In general, the results of Test Phantom A, e.g. MPE, are inferior to those of Phantom B. One potential reason is that the amount of training data in the above preliminary experiments is not sufficient, limiting the generalizability of the trained RPN model. More importantly, Phantom A has a different holder structure from the holders in the training set, leading Phantom A to be out-of-distribution of the training dataset.

Despite the above limitations, the preliminary experiments in this work have shown that RPN has the potential to detect markers in CT volumes even when the markers are distorted in shape. In the future, more training data covering a wide range of markers in size, material, holder structure and so on needs to be generated to improve the neural network performance.

Disclaimer. The concepts and information presented in this paper are based on research and are not commercially available.

References

1. Aichert A, Bier B, Rist L, Maier A. Projective invariants for geometric calibration in flat-panel computed tomography. Proc CT-Meeting. 2018:69–72.
2. Chai J, Zeng H, Li A, Ngai EW. Deep learning in computer vision: a critical review of emerging techniques and application scenarios. Mach Learn Appl. 2021.
3. Nguyen V, De Beenhouwer J, Bazrafkan S, Hoang A, Van Wassenbergh S, Sijbers J. BeadNet: a network for automated spherical marker detection in radiographs for geometry calibration. Proc CT-Meeting. 2020:3–7.
4. Qian J, Cheng M, Tao Y, Lin J, Lin H. CephaNet: an improved faster R-CNN for cephalometric landmark detection. 2019 IEEE 16th International Symposium on Biomedical Imaging (ISBI 2019). 2019:868–71.
5. Scherr T, Streule K, Bartschat A, Böhland M, Stegmaier J, Reischl M et al. BeadNet: deep learning-based bead detection and counting in low-resolution microscopy images. Bioinformatics. 2020;36.
6. Liao F, Liang M, Li Z, Hu X, Song S. Evaluate the malignancy of pulmonary nodules using the 3-D deep leaky noisy-OR network. IEEE Trans Neural Netw Learn Syst. 2019;30(11):3484–95.
7. Zhu W, Liu C, Fan W, Xie X. Deeplung: deep 3d dual path nets for automated pulmonary nodule detection and classification. Proc. WACV. 2018:673–81.
8. He K, Zhang X, Ren S, Sun J. Deep residual learning for image recognition. Proc CVPR. 2016:770–8.

A Keypoint Detection and Description Network Based on the Vessel Structure for Multi-modal Retinal Image Registration

Aline Sindel[1], Bettina Hohberger[2], Sebastian Fassihi Dehcordi[2], Christian Mardin[2], Robert Lämmer[2], Andreas Maier[1], Vincent Christlein[1]

[1]Pattern Recognition Lab, FAU Erlangen-Nürnberg
[2]Department of Ophthalmology, Universitätsklinikum Erlangen
aline.sindel@fau.de

Abstract. Ophthalmological imaging utilizes different imaging systems, such as color fundus, infrared, fluorescein angiography, optical coherence tomography (OCT) or OCT angiography. Multiple images with different modalities or acquisition times are often analyzed for the diagnosis of retinal diseases. Automatically aligning the vessel structures in the images by means of multi-modal registration can support the ophthalmologists in their work. Our method uses a convolutional neural network to extract features of the vessel structure in multi-modal retinal images. We jointly train a keypoint detection and description network on small patches using a classification and a cross-modal descriptor loss function and apply the network to the full image size in the test phase. Our method demonstrates the best registration performance on our and a public multi-modal dataset in comparison to competing methods.

1 Introduction

In ophthalmological imaging, different imaging systems, such as color fundus (CF), infrared (IR), fluorescein angiography (FA), or the more recent optical coherence tomography (OCT) and OCT angiography (OCTA), are used. For the diagnosis, often multiple images that might come from different systems or capturing times are used, particularly for long-term monitoring of the progression of retinal diseases, such as diabetic retinopathy, glaucoma, or age-related macular degeneration. Multi-modal registration techniques that accurately align the vessel structures in the different images can support ophthalmologists by allowing a direct pixel-based comparison of the images.

Multi-modal retinal registration methods estimate an affine transform, a homography, or a non-rigid displacement field. Here, we focus on feature-based methods for homography estimation. These methods generally consist of keypoint detection, descriptor learning, and descriptor matching. Conventional methods address the multi-modal keypoint detection and description, for instance by introducing a partial intensity invariant feature descriptor (PIIFD) [1] combined with the Harris corner detector. Deep learning methods replace all or some steps by neural networks. In DeepSPA [2], a convolutional neural network (CNN) is used to classify patches extracted at vascular junctions based on a step pattern representation. GLAMPoints [3] uses a U-Net as keypoint detector with

Springer Fachmedien Wiesbaden GmbH, ein Teil von Springer Nature 2022
K. Maier-Hein et al. (Hrsg.), *Bildverarbeitung für die Medizin 2022*,
Informatik aktuell, https://doi.org/10.1007/978-3-658-36932-3_12

root SIFT descriptors for retinal images. It is trained to maximize the keypoint matching in a self-supervised manner by homographic warping. Wang et al. [4] proposed a weakly supervised learning-based pipeline composed of a multi-modal retinal vessel segmentation network, SuperPoint [5], and an outlier network based on homography estimation.

In this paper, we propose a deep learning method for multi-modal retinal image registration based on jointly learning a keypoint detection and description network that extracts features of the vessel structure. We base our approach on CraquelureNet [6] and transfer the task of learning a cross-modal keypoint detector and descriptor based on crack structures in paintings to the medical domain. For this task, we created a multi-modal dataset with manual keypoint pair and class annotations.

2   Materials and methods

2.1   Network for multi-modal keypoint detection and description

We adopt the CraquelureNet [6] as network architecture for our task of multi-modal retinal image registration, named RetinaCraquelureNet, as shown in Figure 1. The fully-convolutional CraquelureNet consists of a ResNet [7] backbone and two heads.

2.1.1   Detector and descriptor loss functions.
The keypoint detection and description heads are jointly trained with small image patches of size $32 \times 32 \times 3$ using the multi-task loss [6]: $\mathcal{L}_{\text{Total}} = \lambda_{\text{Det}} \mathcal{L}_{\text{BCE}} + \lambda_{\text{Desc}} \mathcal{L}_{\text{QuadB}}$, where $\lambda_{\text{Det}}, \lambda_{\text{Desc}}$ are the weights for the detector and descriptor loss.

The keypoint detection head is trained using the binary cross-entropy loss $\mathcal{L}_{\text{BCE}}$ with the two classes "vessel" and "background", where "vessel" refers to patches centered at a striking position in the vessel structure, such as a bifurcation, intersection, or a sharp bend. Analogously to [6], we randomly sample the same number of patches from each class and each modality per batch.

The description head is trained using the bidirectional quadruplet loss [6], which applies an online in-batch hard negative mining strategy to randomly sample positive

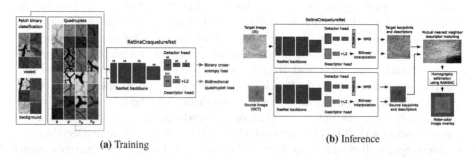

(a) Training   (b) Inference

Fig. 1. Our multi-modal retinal image registration method using a CNN to extract deep features of the vessel structures.

pairs (anchor a and positive counterpart p) for one batch and to select the closest non-matching descriptors in both directions within this batch [6]

$$\mathcal{L}_{\mathrm{QuadB}}(a, p, n_a, n_p) = \max[0, m + d(a, p) - d(a, n_a)] \\ + \max[0, m + d(p, a) - d(p, n_p)] \tag{1}$$

where m is the margin, $d(x, y)$ the Euclidean distance, n_a the closest negative to a, and n_p is the closest negative to p.

2.1.2 Keypoint detection, descriptor matching, and homography estimation. For inference, we feed the complete image to the network at once. The detector output is bicubically upscaled by a factor of 4 and a dense keypoint confidence heatmap is computed by the difference of the two class predictions of the upscaled output. Then, non-maximum suppression with a threshold of 4 pixel is applied and the N_{max} keypoints with the highest confidence values are extracted and the corresponding descriptors are linearly interpolated [6]. Distinctive point correspondences are determined in both images by brute force mutual nearest neighbor descriptor matching and random sample consensus (RANSAC) [8] (reprojection error of 5 pixel) is applied for homography estimation.

2.2 Multi-modal retinal datasets

Our IR-OCT-OCTA dataset, provided by the Department of Ophthalmology, FAU Erlangen-Nürnberg, consists of multi-modal images of the macula of 46 controls measured by Spectralis OCT II, Heidelberg Engineering. For each control, the multi-modal images (IR images, OCT volumes, and OCTA volumes) of the same eye were scanned up to three times a day. For this work, we use the IR image (768×768) and the en-face OCT/OCTA projections of the SVP layer (Par off) of the macula (both 512×512). The image splits for each modality are: train: 89, val: 15, and test: 30. Eyes of the same control are inside one set.

Further, we use a public dataset [9] of color fundus (CF, $576 \times 720 \times 3$) and fluorescein angiography (FA, 576×720) images, which are composed of 29 image pairs of controls

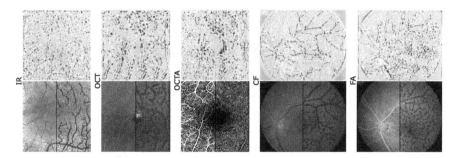

Fig. 2. Keypoint confidence heatmaps (red to blue) and extracted keypoints of our multi-modal registration method RetinaCraquelureNet for both datasets.

and 30 pairs of patients with diabetic retinopathy. The image pair splits are: train: 35, val: 10, and test: 14, where healthy and non-healthy eyes are equally distributed.

We manually annotated N_{kp} matching keypoints at striking vessel positions in each image for each test person, where $N_{kp} >= 21$ for IR-OCT-OCTA and $N_{kp} = 40$ for CF-FA. For the keypoint detection task, we use all keypoints for the vessel class (train: 6273|2800, val: 945|800 for IR-OCT-OCTA|CF-FA) and the same number of points for the background class. For the description task, we build the positive pairs from all multi-modal image pairs (train: 6273|1400, val: 945|400 for IR-OCT-OCTA|CF-FA) and additional for the IR-OCT-OCTA dataset from uni-modal image pairs of scans from different recording times (train: 6021, val: 945). For the test set, we annotated 6 control points per image and computed ground truth homographies.

2.3   Experimental details

We train our RetinaCraquelureNet (using pretrained weights by [6]) for the combination of our IR-OCT-OCTA dataset and the public CF-FA dataset, where we oversample the smaller dataset. We use Adam solver with a learning rate of $\eta = 1 \cdot 10^{-4}$ for 20 epochs with early stopping, a batch size of 576 for detector and 288 for descriptor, $m = 1$, $\lambda_{Det} = 1$, $\lambda_{Desc} = 1$ (analogously to [6]), and online data augmentation (color jittering, horizontal/vertical flipping and for the keypoint pairs additional joint rotation, scaling, and cropping).

We compare our method with SuperPoint [5] and GLAMPoints [3]. We fine-tuned both methods with our combined dataset by extending the training code of [10] for SuperPoint and [3] for GLAMPoints by additionally incorporating multi-modal pairs for the homography warping and picked the best models based on the validation split.

For the experiments, we invert the images of OCT, OCTA, and FA to depict all vessels in dark. For RetinaCraquelureNet, we feed the images in RGB, for GLAMPoints as green channel, and for SuperPoint in grayscale. For all methods, we use the same test settings (descriptor matching, RANSAC, $N_{max} = 4000$).

As metrics we use the success rate of the registration based on the mean Euclidean error $SR_{ME} = \frac{1}{N} \sum_{i=1}^{N} ((\frac{1}{N_j} \sum_{j=1}^{N_j} D_{ij}) <= \epsilon)$ and maximum Euclidean error $SR_{MAE} =$

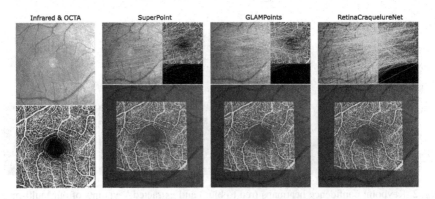

Fig. 3. Qualitative results for one IR-OCTA example.

Tab. 1. Quantitative evaluation for the public CF-FA dataset.

Metrics [%]	SR_{ME} ($\epsilon = 3$)	SR_{MAE} ($\epsilon = 5$)	Rep ($\epsilon = 5$)	MIR ($\epsilon = 5$)
SuperPoint (fine-tuned)	100.0	92.9	53.7	56.5
GLAMPoints (fine-tuned)	78.6	78.6	35.3	27.6
RetinaCraquelureNet	100.0	100.0	78.4	69.2

$\frac{1}{N} \sum_{i=1}^{N} ((\max_{j \in N_j} D_{ij}) <= \epsilon)$ of the $N_j = 6$ control points and the pixel error threshold ϵ. Therefore, we compute the Euclidean error $D_{ij} = \|T(p_{ij}, H_{\text{pred}_i}) - q_{ij}\|_2$ with p_{ij} being the j-th source point and q_{ij} the j-th target point, H_{pred_i} the predicted homography, and $T(p_{ij}, H_{\text{pred}_i})$ the projected j-th source point of image i. Further, we compute the detector repeatability (Rep) as defined in [5] and the matching inlier ratio (MIR) as the fraction of number of RANSAC inliers and number of detected matches per image.

3 Results

Some qualitative results of our RetinaCraquelureNet are shown in Figure 2 that depicts for one example of each modality the confidence keypoint heatmaps and the extracted keypoints that are concentrated on interesting points in the vessel structures. In Figure 3 the registration performance of RetinaCraquelureNet, GLAMPoints, and SuperPoint is visually compared for one IR-OCTA example. RetinaCraquelureNet detects the highest number of correct matches which are densely spread over the images resulting in the most accurate image overlay. GLAMPoints detects densely distributed keypoints which are also located in the background but with fewer correct matches. SuperPoint finds the lowest number of keypoints and correct matches. The image overlays of the competing methods show some misalignments at the left borders.

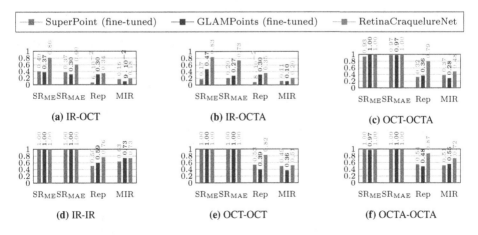

Fig. 4. Quantitative evaluation for our IR-OCT-OCTA dataset using SR_{ME} ($\epsilon = 5$), SR_{MAE} ($\epsilon = 10$), Rep ($\epsilon = 5$), and MIR ($\epsilon = 5$). In (c-f) we use follow-up image pairs.

The quantitative evaluation for the IR-OCT-OCTA dataset is summarized in Figure 4. RetinaCraquelureNet clearly outperforms GLAMPoints and SuperPoint for the multi-modal image pairs in all metrics. Regarding the registration of the follow-up images, all methods reach a success rate of about 100 % with ME <= 5 and MAE <= 10, however our method obtains considerably higher scores in Rep and MIR. Results for the CF-FA dataset in Table 1 also show the advantage of our method, which successfully registers all images with ME <= 3 and MAE <= 5 and gains best scores in Rep and MIR.

4   Discussion

We trained a CNN that extracts features of the vessel structure to jointly learn a cross-modal keypoint detector and descriptor for multi-modal retinal registration. In the experiments, we showed that our method achieves the best registration results for both multi-modal datasets. For the more challenging IR-OCT and IR-OCTA registration, which has a smaller overlap region, we still achieve good success rates while the competing methods show a strong decline. By training our method jointly on two datasets, the network learns to detect distinctive features in five different modalities. Further, we demonstrated that the same trained model can be used to register multi-modal images and follow-up scans. Thus, our method can be very beneficial to support the long time analysis of retinal disease progression. As future work, we will investigate deep learning methods inspired by known operators for our registration pipeline.

References

1. Chen J, Tian J, Lee N, Zheng J, Smith RT, Laine AF. A partial intensity invariant feature descriptor for multimodal retinal image registration. IEEE Trans Biomed Eng. 2010;57(7):1707–18.
2. Lee J, Liu P, Cheng J, Fu H. A deep step pattern representation for multimodal retinal image registration. Proc IEEE ICCV. 2019:5076–85.
3. Truong P, Apostolopoulos S, Mosinska A, Stucky S, Ciller C, Zanet SD. GLAMpoints: greedily learned accurate match points. Proc IEEE ICCV. 2019:10732–41.
4. Wang Y, Zhang J, Cavichini M, Bartsch DUG, Freeman WR, Nguyen TQ et al. Robust content-adaptive global registration for multimodal retinal images using weakly supervised deep-learning framework. IEEE Trans Image Process. 2021;30:3167–78.
5. DeTone D, Malisiewicz T, Rabinovich A. SuperPoint: self-supervised interest point detection and description. Proc IEEE CVPR. 2018.
6. Sindel A, Maier A, Christlein V. CraquelureNet: matching the crack structure in historical paintings for multi-modal image registration. Proc IEEE ICIP. 2021:994–8.
7. He K, Zhang X, Ren S, Sun J. Deep residual learning for image recognition. Proc IEEE CVPR. 2016:770–8.
8. Fischler MA, Bolles RC. Random sample consensus: a paradigm for model fitting with applications to image analysis and automated cartography. Commun ACM. 1981;24(6):381–95.
9. Hajeb Mohammad Alipour S, Rabbani H, Akhlaghi MR. Diabetic retinopathy grading by digital curvelet transform. Comput Math Methods Med. 2012;2021:761901.
10. Jau YY, Zhu R, Su H, Chandraker M. Deep keypoint-based camera pose estimation with geometric constraints. Proc IEEE IROS. 2020:4950–7.

Training Deep Learning Models for 2D Spine X-rays Using Synthetic Images and Annotations Created from 3D CT Volumes

Richin Sukesh[1], Andreas Fieselmann[2], Srikrishna Jaganathan[1], Karthik Shetty[1], Rainer Kärgel[2], Florian Kordon[1,3], Steffen Kappler[2], Andreas Maier[1,3]

[1]Pattern Recognition Lab, FAU Erlangen-Nürnberg, Erlangen
[2]Siemens Healthcare GmbH, Forchheim
[3]Erlangen Graduate School in Advanced Optical Technologies, FAU Erlangen-Nürnberg, Erlangen
richin.sukesh@fau.de

Abstract. When training deep learning models in the medical domain, one is always burdened with the task of obtaining reliable medical data annotated by experts. However, the availability of annotated data is often limited. To overcome such limitations, this paper addresses the idea of using synthetic spine X-ray data to train a deep learning model to aid in the detection of vertebrae. For this purpose, a pipeline for automatic generation of synthetic datasets comprising synthetic X-ray images and their corresponding annotations is developed and evaluated. The results of these experiments show improvements in detection rates of the model when synthetic X-ray data is added to the training dataset.

1 Introduction

Accurate detection and classification of vertebrae in spine X-ray images play a decisive role in the diagnosis of pathological conditions, surgical planning, and post-operative assessment. Studies have shown that using deep learning based object detection models for such purposes has resulted in a positive clinical impact for diagnostic tasks. However, applications employing deep learning based models require a large number of training samples, which must be structured and annotated with respect to the anatomical regions of interest. Acquiring annotations to detect anatomical structures or disease patterns is an expensive and time-consuming process, and more often than not, these limitations are difficult to overcome. When the quantity of available data is insufficient, the CNN models may tend to overfit, ultimately leading to the model not being able to generalize well on unseen data. In this paper, we propose an approach to overcome these constraints by generating synthetic spine X-ray images and corresponding annotations from 3D CT volumes to extend the original dataset. In a similar work by Bier et al. [1], manually annotated synthetic data was used to aid in the detection of pelvic landmarks. Their results indicate that the model trained on synthetic data was able to generalize well on clinically acquired pelvic data.

2   Materials and methods

2.1   Synthetic X-ray image generation

To generate synthetic X-ray images from CT volumes, the digitally reconstructed radiograph (DRR) generator from the DeepDRR [2] framework was used. The DRR generator implements a ray-tracing algorithm to forward project the 3D CT volume onto a 2D image plane. To classify the attenuation characteristics for different regions of the CT volume, material decomposition into air, soft tissue, and bone are achieved by thresholding the Hounsfield Unit (HU) values. Based on the photon count set by the user, a Poisson noise model is used to estimate the quantum noise in the image. To simulate the pixel crosstalk, which flat-panel detectors suffer from, the quantum noise of neighboring pixels is correlated by convolving the noise signal with a blurring kernel. The electronic readout noise is simulated by an additive Gaussian noise. The 2D projection image from the DRR generator then undergoes nonlinear multi-scale image enhancement (NOMSIE) [3]. This image enhancement aims to adjust the image such that the visual information contained in the image is optimized for human perception, making the image suitable for visual analysis. The post-processing algorithm also allows the user to vary the magnitude of enhancement applied to the image by changing the parameters associated with NOMSIE.

2.2   Annotation generation

To generate a complete synthetic dataset, annotations need to be generated along with the synthetic X-ray images. This process begins by feeding the CT volume data as input to an application that makes use of a learning-based approach [4] for vertebra center localization and labeling in 3D space. Once the vertebra centers have been detected in the CT volume, it is then projected onto the 2D space of the generated synthetic image. To estimate the bounding boxes for each vertebra, a statistical model of the vertebra was developed using an X-ray dataset (500 images) with vertebra corner annotations. The statistical model aimed at finding a correlation between bounding box parameters (height and width) and the Euclidean distance between centers of adjacent vertebrae. Once this correlation was established for all the vertebrae, the data was used to train a linear regression model to predict the height and width of the bounding box given the detected centers and labels for each vertebra.

2.3   Vertebra detection with Faster R-CNN

The faster R-CNN [5] object detection model was selected to evaluate the viability of using the generated synthetic X-ray images for training models in real-world scenarios. The main goal of the model is the detection and classification of the spine vertebrae (T1-L5). The centerline of the spine is also estimated by fitting a cubic spline through the centers of predicted bounding boxes. The Faster R-CNN object detector with a ResNet-50 backbone was used. Pixel values of the input images were normalized to values between 0 and 1. The images were resized to 600×600 pixels, preserving their original aspect ratio. Online data augmentation was implemented by random horizontal flipping, rotation, Gaussian noise, sharpening, brightness, and contrast variations. An additional offline augmentation technique was also employed when generating synthetic data, wherein, multiple variations of an image were generated by varying factors such as X-ray source viewing angles in 3D and photon count. Stochastic gradient descent with momentum is used to optimize the parameters of the Faster R-CNN [5]. The initial learning rate, momentum, and batch size were set at 0.005, 0.9, and 4 respectively and run for 200 epochs with early stopping criteria to avoid overfitting. A learning rate decay was also set where the learning rate changes for every 20 epochs with a decay factor of 0.1. The model was trained multiple times on varying combinations of training data comprising of the real X-ray and synthetic X-ray datasets:

1. 25% of real data
2. 25% of real data + 100% of synthetic data
3. 50% of real data
4. 50% of real data + 100% of synthetic data
5. 75% of real data
6. 75% of real data + 100% of synthetic data
7. 100% of synthetic

Each of the aforementioned scenarios was validated using 5-fold cross-validation where 25% of available real data was used for validation.

2.4 Dataset

To carry out the different experiments, primarily two groups of datasets were required, i.e., a dataset of real X-ray images and a dataset of CT volumes to generate the synthetic X-ray images. They will be henceforth termed as the "real dataset" and "synthetic dataset" respectively in this paper. The real dataset consisted of 609 spinal anterior-posterior (AP) X-ray images from the AASCE MICCAI 2019 challenge [6] and a proprietary dataset of 294 full spine AP X-ray images. The four corners of each vertebra were annotated as landmarks for every image. Both these datasets include X-ray images of scoliotic patients.

The synthetic dataset consists of multiple CT volume sets: 1) 214 publicly available CT volumes were obtained from the VerSe 2020 grand challenge [7]. These CT volumes were paired with vertebra center annotations. 2) CT Lymph node dataset consisting of 176 CT images of mediastinum and abdomen [8]. 3) 117 thoracic CT images focusing on the coronavirus disease (COVID-19) positive patients [9]. 4) 213 spine-focused CT scans from the "Microsoft Spine Web Dataset" paired with vertebra center annotations [10] and lastly, 5) an internally available dataset of 283 whole body and chest CT images. After filtering through all the datasets to remove CT volumes focusing on unwanted anatomical regions, a total of 730 CT volumes were selected to generate synthetic X-ray images.

2.5 Evaluation

The bounding box estimator was evaluated against 128 annotated X-ray images from the real dataset using: 1) Root mean square error (RMSE) with respect to height and width of the boxes and 2) Intersection over Union (IoU) metrics. The success detection rate (SDR) and RMSE with the associated standard deviation (SD) were used to evaluate the performance of the Faster R-CNN model. SDR is defined as the ratio of the number of accurate predictions to the total number of predictions. A prediction is considered accurate only if the distance between the centers of ground truth and prediction bounding boxes is less than d $\in$ {2 mm, 4 mm, 6 mm} precision. The SDR is formulated as

$$SDR = \frac{\#\{j : \| L_d(j) - L_g(j) \| < d\}}{\#\Omega} \times 100\% \tag{1}$$

where L_d and L_g represent the coordinates of the detected and ground truth landmarks respectively. $\#\Omega$ stands for the number of predictions made, and $j \in \Omega$ indicates the jth sample. In the case of the Faster R-CNN model, L_d and L_g are the center points of the prediction and ground truth bounding boxes respectively. The predicted label of the vertebra also has to be correct in order to be considered as a valid prediction. All the trained instances of the model were tested on images from the real X-ray dataset.

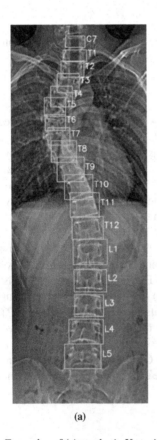

(a)

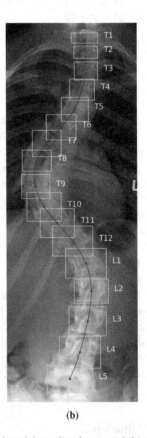

(b)

Fig. 1. Examples of (a) synthetic X-ray image with ground truth bounding boxes and (b) vertebra detection on a real X-ray image.

3 Results

The linear regressor used in ground truth bounding box estimation for the synthetic data was validated against 628 annotated X-ray images from the real dataset. The RMSE with respect to the height and width of the bounding boxes were found to be 2.50 ± 0.35 mm and 4.01 ± 1.20 mm respectively. 94.45% of the estimated bounding boxes had an IoU value greater than 0.9. An example of the generated synthetic X-ray image along with its bounding box annotation is shown in Figure 1a.

Figure 1b shows an example of the results generated by the Faster R-CNN model on a real X-ray image. Figure 2 shows the summarized results of performing 5-fold cross validation on the Faster R-CNN model. In the case of training the model solely on synthetic data, the detection rate is found to be considerably low especially for SDR with low precision values. In the case of the other scenarios, it can be observed that augmenting the original dataset with synthetic data resulted in improvement with respect to the SDR values.

4 Discussion

The experiments and evaluations conducted in this paper address the topic of how adding synthetic data could impact training a deep learning model. To this end, a pipeline was set up that was able to automatically generate synthetic X-ray images from 3D CT data and their accompanying annotations in 2D space. The pipeline also employs numerous augmentation techniques, thus, increasing the size of the created synthetic dataset. Various experimental scenarios were considered to validate the performance of the model when the generated synthetic data was added to the training set of the model. The

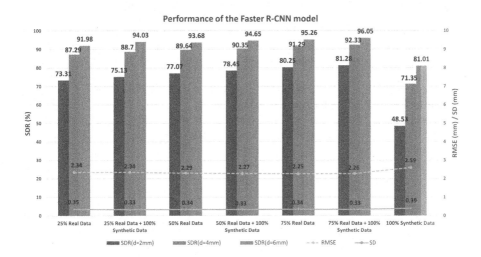

Fig. 2. Mean results of 5-fold cross validation when using synthetic data in the training set. The model was validated using SDR at multiple precision values $d \in \{2mm, 4mm, 6mm\}$ and RMSE.

results show promising evidence that adding synthetic X-ray images to extend the dataset can help in improving detection accuracy. It is also observed that the model trained only on synthetic data was unable to generalize well on to images showing high degrees of scoliosis. The reason for the performance degradation in this case can be attributed to two factors: 1) There was an inherent error in the ground truth produced when automatically generating the ground truth annotations which might make it difficult for the model to adapt during training and 2) there was an under-representation of scoliotic cases in the synthetic dataset. Generating more synthetic images with scoliotic cases that better represents the training set and evaluation on a larger test dataset would be useful to further solidify these findings.

Disclaimer. The concepts and information presented in this paper are based on research and are not commercially available.

References

1. Bier B, Unberath M, Zaech J, et al. X-ray-transform invariant anatomical landmark detection for pelvic trauma surgery. Proc MICCAI. Springer, 2018:55–63.
2. Unberath M, Zaech J, Lee SC, et al. DeepDRR: a catalyst for machine learning in fluoroscopy-guided procedures. Proc MICCAI. Springer, 2018:98–106.
3. Stahl M, Aach T, Dippel S. Digital radiography enhancement by nonlinear multiscale processing. Med Phys. 2000;27(1):56–65.
4. Zhan Y, Jian B, Maneesh D, et al. Cross-modality vertebrae localization and labeling using learning-based approaches. Spinal Imaging and Image Analysis. Springer, 2015:301–22.
5. Shaoqing R, Kaiming H, Ross G, et al. Faster R-CNN: towards real-time object detection with region proposal networks. Proc NeurIPS. Vol. 28. Curran Associates, Inc., 2015:91–9.
6. Wu H, Bailey C, Rasoulinejad P, et al. Automatic landmark estimation for adolescent idiopathic scoliosis assessment using BoostNet. Proc MICCAI. Springer, 2017:127–35.
7. Kirschke J, Jan S, Löffler M, et al. VerSe 2020. CoRR. 2021;abs/2001.09193.
8. Roth H, Lu L, Seff A, et al. A new 2.5D representation for lymph node detection using random sets of deep convolutional neural network observations. Proc MICCAI. Springer, 2014:520–7.
9. Tsai E, Simpson S, Lungren MP, et al. Data from the MIDRC - RICORD - 1a - chest CT Covid. The Cancer Imaging Archive. 2020.
10. Glocker B, Zikic D, Konukoglu E, et al. Vertebrae localization in pathological spine CT via dense classification from sparse annotations. Proc MICCAI. Springer, 2013:262–70.

Robust Intensity-based Initialization for 2D-3D Pelvis Registration (RobIn)

Stephanie Häger[1], Annkristin Lange[1], Stefan Heldmann[1], Jan Modersitzki[1,2], Andreas Petersik[3], Manuel Schröder[3], Heiko Gottschling[3], Thomas Lieth[4], Erich Zähringer[4], Jan H. Moltz[1]

[1]Fraunhofer Institute for Digital Medicine MEVIS, Lübeck / Bremen
[2]Institute of Mathematics and Image Computing, Universität zu Lübeck
[3]Stryker Trauma GmbH, Schönkirchen
[4]Stryker Leibinger GmbH & Co. KG, Freiburg
stephanie.haeger@mevis.fraunhofer.de

Abstract. In image-guided orthopedic procedures, 2D-3D registration is an essential tool to align intra-operative 2D X-ray images with pre-operative 3D CT data. Since this is a non-convex problem, appropriate initialization is important. Here, we introduce RobIn, a robust and solely intensity-based initialization method for intervention support for pelvic fractures. Key to RobIn's robustness is the focus on the bony pelvis region in the 2D X-ray images, which is determined by automatic segmentation. First validation studies on simulated X-rays demonstrate that RobIn successfully retrieves ground truth in about 99.7% of the cases.

1 Introduction

Image registration is crucial for many clinical applications and excellent solutions can be found in the literature, e.g. [1, 2]. However, since the problem is non-convex and ill-posed, proper initialization is crucial but still an open question. This applies in particular to the so-called 2D-3D registration, where data of different dimensions are to be aligned. Examples include radiation therapy, cardiac and endovascular interventions, or orthopedic procedures.

In this paper, we propose the new robust initialization method (RobIn) for assisting screw placement in pelvic fractures. In this application, an intra-operative 2D X-ray image from a C-arm device and a pre-operative 3D CT are to be registered. RobIn provides estimates for rigid parameters. We assume that the translational parameters can be sufficiently estimated by a heuristic for X-rays capturing the entire pelvis and focus on the three rotation angles. In contrast to other initialization schemes that depend on additional information such as landmarks [3, 4], fiducial markers [5] or RGBD-Cameras [6], RobIn is based solely on image intensities. As we are focusing on a robust initialization scheme for a conventional 2D-3D registration, a comparison with direct deep-learning-based 2D-3D registration approaches is not within the scope of this paper.

A key component for RobIn's robustness is the focus on a region of interest (ROI) in the X-ray image. This ROI is determined by an automatic segmentation of the bony pelvis, defined by the hip bones and the sacrum. Particularly, our segmentation also excludes occlusions by surgical instruments. Therefore, RobIn provides an outstanding starting point for a subsequent fine registration, e.g. the one described in [7].

© Der/die Autor(en), exklusiv lizenziert durch
Springer Fachmedien Wiesbaden GmbH, ein Teil von Springer Nature 2022
K. Maier-Hein et al. (Hrsg.), *Bildverarbeitung für die Medizin 2022*,
Informatik aktuell, https://doi.org/10.1007/978-3-658-36932-3_14

Tab. 1. Data sources used for training of the automatic segmentation of 3D CT data and 2D X-ray data as well as for generation of ground truth data for our studies; D3 and D4 from the Stryker Orthopaedic Modeling and Analytics (SOMA) database [11].

Dataset	Source	Contained data
D1	CTPEL [12]	90 segmented CT pelvis scans of unfractured pelvises
D2	JHU [13]	40 segmented CT pelvis scans of unfractured pelvises
D3	SOMA [11]	99 segmented CT pelvis scans of unfractured pelvises
D4	SOMA [11]	60 CT pelvis scans of fractured pelvises

Currently, we only have access to pre-operative CTs with expert segmentations but we are lacking the corresponding X-rays. Therefore, we also present a concept to simulate corresponding intra-operative X-rays. The simulated data provide ground truth spatial correspondence of 2D and 3D data as well as the possibility to transfer the 3D expert segmentation into 2D (Fig. 2).

The paper reports first validation studies which demonstrate that RobIn successfully retrieves the ground truth in 99.7% of the cases (details in Section 3).

2   Materials and methods

Focusing on the bony pelvis ROI is crucial for our robust registration scheme. For the 3D CT segmentation, we train a nnU-Net [8] on data sets D1–D3 including expert segmentations (Tab. 1).

As we do not have access to X-ray data with expert segmentations, we train a nnU-Net [8] for 2D X-ray segmentation on simulated X-ray (sXR) images with projected expert segmentations. To simulate X-rays that cover the variability in both fractures and occlusion from surgical instruments, we suggest the following steps (Fig. 2).

In the first step, we derive digitally reconstructed radiographs (DRRs) [9] with expert segmentation from the 3D CT data of D3. To transform these DRRs into more realistic simulated X-rays, we add various artifacts such as scissors to the 3D CT before computing the DRR and subtract the artifact projection from the corresponding 2D segmentation. Furthermore, we crop the DRR images to the typical disk shape of a C-arm image, and apply a cycle GAN to mimic X-ray appearance; see [10] for details.

Conceptually, RobIn depends on six pose parameters (three for translation, three for rotation) as well as two parameters for the distances source to detector and pelvis to detector (Fig. 1).

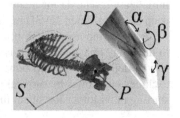

Fig. 1. DRRs are parameterized by a square detector (D) in a plane that is orthogonal to the ray from the source (S) through the bounding box center of the pelvis segmentation (P), with specified distances S to D and P to D, respectively. The ray is parameterized by the Eulerian angles $\eta = (\alpha, \beta, \gamma)$ with respect to the coordinate system of the CT data centered at P.

However, we assume that the two distances can be readout from the X-ray device. In addition, we assume that for X-ray images capturing the entire pelvis, the translation is sufficiently approximated by P, i.e. the bounding box center of our 3D segmentation (more details in Section 4). In future work, we will generalize the estimation of the translation parameters such that we can also handle cases of close-up X-rays that only capture parts of the pelvis. For the remaining three rotation parameters, we perform an exhaustive search based on sampled intervals. In detail, RobIn determines a minimizer of an image distance between the parameterized DRR and the X-ray image on the ROI. Normalized gradient fields (NGF) [14] is used to measure the multi-modal image distances.

3   Results

The starting point for our validation studies is fractured pelvis data from D4 (60 CT scans) from which we obtain DRRs that are augmented by adding instruments, by cropping and adding instruments, and by applying a cycle GAN to create sXRs. For each of these four classes, we consider inlet (top view) as well as outlet (bottom view) images, which results in a total of $60 \cdot 4 \cdot 2 = 480$ images. The ground truth parameters are set as follows. The distance source to detector is set to 1200 mm and the distance pelvis to detector to 360 mm, the pelvis center (i.e. translation parameter) is obtained from the automatic 3D segmentation and the ground truth parameters for rotation are set according to the

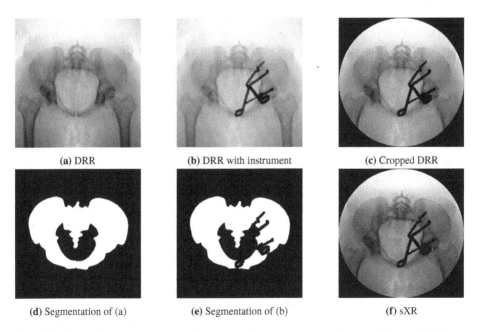

      (a) DRR   (b) DRR with instrument   (c) Cropped DRR

(d) Segmentation of (a)   (e) Segmentation of (b)   (f) sXR

Fig. 2. Different X-ray simulations and corresponding segmentations for an arbitrary DRR from data set D3. Simulations are used to create training data for the 2D segmentation from D3 and RobIn validation data from D4.

Tab. 2. Results for the full range, close range, and offset studies in Section 3 and four different DRR classes: plain DRR, DRR with added instrument (DRR-I), cropped DRR with added instrument (DRR-C), and simulated X-ray (sXR); each class comprises 120 images. Results are reported for RobIn and a variant of RobIn that does not focus the distance measure to the pelvis ROI (no-ROI). The performance is given by $n(\varepsilon)$, where n is the number of successful ground truth retrievals (zero error for the full and close range experiments, below sampling spacing for the offset experiment) and ε is the maximal rotation error.

DRR class	Full range study		Close range study		Offset study	
	RobIn	no-ROI	RobIn	no-ROI	RobIn	no-ROI
plain DRR	120 (0°)	120 (0°)	119 (1°)	119 (1°)	120 (1.5°)	120 (1.5°)
DRR-I	120 (0°)	120 (0°)	119 (1°)	119 (1°)	120 (1.5°)	115 (13.5°)
DRR-C	120 (0°)	119 (3°)	119 (1°)	119 (1°)	120 (1.5°)	81 (13.5°)
sXR	120 (0°)	118 (15°)	120 (0°)	119 (1°)	120 (1.5°)	85 (13.5°)

literature [15]: $\eta = (-125°, 0°, 180°)$ for inlet images and $\eta = (-55°, 0°, 180°)$ for outlet images, respectively.

We study the performance of RobIn for three different scenarios: a full range exploration, a close range exploration, and an offset exploration. Results are summarized in Table 2. In each study, each of the three rotation parameters in η is explored on equidistantly spaced sampling points in a specific interval. To demonstrate the importance of the 2D pelvis segmentation, we also compare the results of RobIn to a version of the same method that computes image distances on the entire images instead of focusing on the bony pelvis ROI.

The full range study demonstrates that RobIn is able to recover ground truth for the simulated data. Based on [15], we explore angles in a range of $\pm 15°$. More precisely, we use a sampling width of 3° for the interval $[\theta^* - 15°, \theta^* + 15°]$, where θ^* denotes the corresponding ground truth value. The total run-time for one case is about 130 seconds on a current laptop computer and includes $11^3 = 1\,331$ computations of DRRs and their NGF distance to the X-ray. The automatic pelvis segmentation only takes 1–2 seconds. Focusing on the ROI, RobIn recovered ground truth in all 480 cases. On the other hand, if we do not focus on the ROI, ground truth could not be determined for one cropped DRR and two sXR cases.

For the close range perspective, we use a sampling width of 1° for the interval $[\theta^* - 1°, \theta^* + 1°]$ to see if ground truth can also be recovered with an accuracy of 1°. RobIn on the ROI recovers ground truth in 477 cases (Tab. 2), the other three cases belong to the same CT scan. Figure 3 shows the NGF values of all sampled angle combinations for one of the failing cases. If we do not focus on the ROI, ground truth could not be determined for four cases belonging to this CT.

Lastly, we perform an offset study. Here, we use a sampling width of 3° for the interval $[\theta^* - 13.5°, \theta^* + 13.5°]$, such that the grid does not contain the ground truth value θ^*. For all 480 cases, RobIn performed successfully, i.e. determined a value $\hat{\theta}$ which is below grid spacing: $|\hat{\theta} - \theta^*| < 3°$. However, when the distance is computed on the entire image, the scheme failed for 5 DRRs with added instrument, for 39 cropped DRRs, and for 35 simulated X-ray image. An exemplary result is shown in Figure 4.

4 Discussion

The novel fully automated and robust initialization method RobIn for 2D-3D registration of 2D X-ray and 3D CT data is presented. RobIn is solely based on image intensities and does not require any external devices, fiducials, or landmarks. The key to the success of RobIn is the focus on a bony pelvis ROI, which is obtained by automatic 2D and 3D segmentations. Assuming that the entire pelvis is captured in the X-ray, these segmentations enable us to sufficiently estimate translation parameters and to identify an educated guess for the rotation angles that is further refined by an exhaustive search. We present different experiments to demonstrate the performance of RobIn. In an ideal setting, where the ground truth is contained in the sampling grid, RobIn retrieves ground truth in about 99.7% of the cases. In a more realistic setting, when the sampling grid does not contain the ground truth, the error is below the sampling width in all cases. Our studies also highlight another major advantage of the ROI-based approach: Intensity gradients from outside the ROI do not affect the image comparison. This applies to both types of artefacts, occlusions by surgical instruments as well as cropping (Fig. 4).

A major difficulty both for training the 2D segmentation and for our validation is the current lack of paired real data (acquisition is in preparation). In the paper, we bypassed this difficulty by simulating X-ray images. In future work, we aim to generalize the

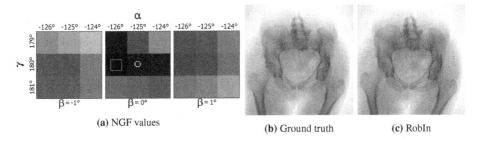

(a) NGF values   (b) Ground truth   (c) RobIn

Fig. 3. Results for cropped DRR inlet image in close range study for which RobIn does not recover ground truth: (a) NGF values of all angle combinations; values are better for darker shades. RobIn result marked by red square, ground truth marked by green circle. (b) DRR computed with ground truth, (c) DRR computed with angle combination recovered by RobIn.

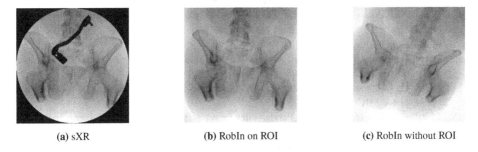

(a) sXR   (b) RobIn on ROI   (c) RobIn without ROI

Fig. 4. Exemplary results for the offset study, highlighting the importance of the ROI: (a) input sXR, (b) RobIn results on ROI (accurate to sampling width), and (c) without ROI (failure).

estimation of the translation parameters such that we can also handle cases of close-up X-rays that only capture parts of the pelvis.

With RobIn we achieved a first milestone on the way towards improved image guidance for orthopedic interventions.

Acknowledgement. This work was funded by the German Federal Ministry for Economic Affairs and Energy (project KI-SIGS, funding code: 01MK20012Q).

References

1. Sotiras A, Davatzikos C, Paragios N. Deformable medical image registration: a survey. IEEE Trans Med Imaging. 2013;32(7):1153–90.
2. Markelj P, Tomaževič D, Likar B, et al. A review of 3D/2D registration methods for image-guided interventions. Med Image Anal. 2012;16(3):642–61.
3. Gao C, Grupp RB, Unberath M, et al. Fiducial-free 2D/3D registration of the proximal femur for robot-assisted femoroplasty. Proc SPIE Medical Imaging. 2020;11315:113151C.
4. Miao S, Lucas J, Liao R. Automatic pose initialization for accurate 2D/3D registration applied to abdominal aortic aneurysm endovascular repair. Proc SPIE Medical Imaging. 2012;8316:83160Q.
5. Russakoff DB, Rohlfing T, Mori K, et al. Fast generation of digitally reconstructed radiographs using attenuation fields with application to 2D-3D image registration. IEEE Trans Med Imaging. 2005;24(11):1441–54.
6. Fotouhi J, Fuerst B, Johnson A, et al. Pose-aware C-arm for automatic re-initialization of interventional 2D/3D image registration. Int J Comput Assist Radiol Surg. 2017;12(7):1221–30.
7. Lange A, Heldmann S. Intensity-based 2D-3D registration using normalized gradient fields. Proc BVM. 2020:163–8.
8. Isensee F, Jaeger PF, Kohl S, et al. nnU-Net: a self-configuring method for deep learning-based biomedical image segmentation. Nat Methods. 2021;18:203–11.
9. Russakoff DB, Rohlfing T, Jr JRA, et al. Intensity-based 2D-3D spine image registration incorporating a single fiducial marker. Acad Radiol. 2005;12(1):37–50.
10. Himstedt M, Häger S, Heldmann S, et al. DRR to C-arm X-ray image translation with application to trauma surgery. Proc CARS. 2021:S22.
11. Schmidt W, LiArno S, Khlopas A, et al. Stryker orthopaedic modeling and analytics (SOMA): a review. Surg Technol Int. 2018;32:315–24.
12. Wang C, Connolly B, Oliveira Lopes PF de, et al. Pelvis segmentation using multi-pass U-Net and iterative shape estimation. Proc Computational Methods and Clinical Applications in Musculoskeletal Imaging. 2018:49–57.
13. Han R, Uneri A, Silva TD, et al. Atlas-based automatic planning and 3D–2D fluoroscopic guidance in pelvic trauma surgery. Phys Med Biol. 2019;64(9):095022.
14. Haber E, Modersitzki J. Intensity gradient based registration and fusion of multi-modal images. Proc MICCAI. 2006:726–33.
15. Murphy A. Reference articles: Pelvis (inlet view) + Pelvis (outlet view). (accessed on 18 Oct 2021). 2016. URL: https://radiopaedia.org/articles/45242, https://radiopaedia.org/articles/45218.

Learning an Airway Atlas from Lung CT Using Semantic Inter-patient Deformable Registration

Fenja Falta, Lasse Hansen, Marian Himstedt, Mattias P. Heinrich

Institute of Medical Informatics, University of Lübeck
fenja.falta@student.uni-luebeck.de

Abstract. Pulmonary image analysis for diagnostic and interventions often relies on a canonical geometric representation of lung anatomy across a patient cohort. Bronchoscopy can benefit from simulating an appearance atlas of airway cross-sections, intra-patient deformable image registration could be initialised using a shared lung atlas. The diagnosis of pneumonia, COPD and other respiratory diseases can benefit from a well defined anatomical reference space. Previous work to create lung atlases either relied on tedious and often ambiguous manual landmark correspondences and/or image features to perform deformable inter-patient registration. In this work, we overcome these limitations by guiding the registration with semantic airway features that can be obtained straightforwardly with an nnUNet and dilated training labels. We demonstrate that accurate and robust registration results across patients can be achieved in few seconds leading to high agreement of small airways of later generations. Incorporating the semantic cost function improves segmentation overlap and landmark accuracy.

1 Introduction

Creating lung atlases from inter-subject registration of CT scans has already been studied nearly two decades ago [1]. Yet this work relied on manual one-to-one correspondences that are difficult to obtain and might be ambiguous with respect to the topology of the airway tree. Newer work [2] established an elaborated inter-subject registration pipeline that aims to tackle the challenges of large deformations across anatomical variation based on keypoint alignment and demonstrated discrimination capabilities for COPD (chronic obstructive pulmonary disease) and calcifications.

Establishing airway atlases can be beneficial for large-scale analysis of anatomical topologies like tree structures, that have been shown to be statistically applicable in medical diagnosis [3], and may be applied to further use cases like bronchoscopy guidance.

Deformable inter-patient registration is widely used in medical image analysis to define dense correspondences across different subjects. Recent work on fast 3D medical registration [4] has demonstrated the benefits of directly incorporating deep learning based segmentation features into conventional (discrete) optimisation algorithms. For

© Der/die Autor(en), exklusiv lizenziert durch
Springer Fachmedien Wiesbaden GmbH, ein Teil von Springer Nature 2022
K. Maier-Hein et al. (Hrsg.), *Bildverarbeitung für die Medizin 2022*,
Informatik aktuell, https://doi.org/10.1007/978-3-658-36932-3_15

inter-patient abdominal CT alignment the best supervised deep-learning registration approach [5] was matched in [4] by decoupling semantic feature extraction and optimisation.

In this work we propose a modular technique that is easy to reproduce and yields promising results for creating an airway atlas based on fast large-deformation estimation and learned binary airway features. Our contribution is three-fold: First, we adapt the loss for the well-established nnUNet framework [6] using dilated airway labels to improve accuracy for smaller structures. Second, we combine these airway features with handcrafted image features and incorporate them into a GPU-accelerated registration framework and evaluate the accuracy on unseen images using both multi-label structural overlap and landmark errors. Third, we demonstrate that airway keypoints are also beneficial within a purely geometric registration approach.

2 Materials and methods

Our method aims to incorporate semantic information for inter-patient lung registration to yield an improved atlas. We obtain semantic information using a segmentation network and employ two different frameworks for inter-patient registration. Figure 1 depicts a schematic representation of our method.

2.1 Dataset and segmentation

All experiments are performed using a public dataset containing 40 thoracic CT scans from the LIDC-IDRI Dataset [7] as well as 20 scans from the EXACT'09 Challenge Dataset [8]. Annotations for these cases have been provided by [9]. A total of 31 (primary, secondary and tertiary) individual bronchi as well as the trachea are distinguished.

We train a full-resolution 3D U-Net architecture in the nnUNet framework [6] to segment the airway divided into singular bronchi (32 unique labels). To improve the performance on smaller bronchi, we dilate segmentations by 1 mm. Prior to training, images have been resampled to isotropic resolution and cropped around the lung area. In regards to data augmentation, mirroring has been disabled to provide the network with further contextual information to distinguish left and right bronchi. The numerical evaluation of the segmentation accuracy is given in Section 3.

2.2 Inter-patient registration

The quality of building an anatomical CT atlas mainly depends on accurate inter-patient registration. Previous methods for lung atlases have been restricted to either using manual correspondences or solely relying on intensity-based similarity metrics. We incorporate the semantic information of the automatic airway segmentation in two different ways. 1) We sample 64 keypoints from each predicted label class via farthest point sampling, resulting in a total of 2048 keypoints inside the predicted airway. 2) We use one-hot encodings of the predicted labels on unseen test images as structural airway features.

We combine structural airway information with two frameworks for deformable image registration that are able to decouple feature learning and fast optimisation.

The first registration approach we employ is sparse loopy belief propagation (sLBP) [10], which is a geometric method using sampled keypoints instead of a dense voxel grid to calculate displacement fields. It incorporates a large displacement correspondence search that uses the input features (defined for each node) to calculate the cost term for keypoint displacements. The graph-based inference algorithm, loopy belief propagation, is used to obtain smooth displacements by enforcing pairwise constraints. The global solution for all keypoints is jointly found using a message passing scheme and discrete optimisation. Keypoint displacements are then extrapolated to obtain a dense displacement field. By using the proposed sampling strategy, the algorithm focusses directly on the geometrically relevant regions of the airway tree. Besides airway keypoints, we may additionally use Förstner keypoints inside of a lung mask as proposed in [10]. Moreover, we can make use of MIND-SSC features [11] (that work well in inhale-exhale lung registration) and semantic airway features (based on nnUNet predictions) to determine the similarity-based cost function for each keypoint displacement.

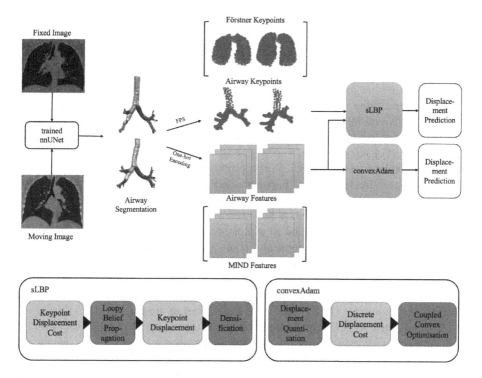

Fig. 1. Out methods consists of extraction of semantic airway information and subsequent image registration. We predict nnUNet airway segmentations of fixed and moving images, which are then used to generate airway keypoints and airway features. In addition to airway keypoints and features we use Förstner keypoints as well as MIND features directly derived from the grey value images. These keypoints and features are applied in registration using a geometric (sLBP) and a dense registration approach (convexAdam). These methods differ regarding how possible displacements are determined as well as optimisation of image similarity and displacement smoothness.

Tab. 1. Dice score coefficients (and standard deviations across cases) for multilabel nnUNet segmentation, averaged over bronchi of the same depth.

	Trachea	Primary	Secondary	Tertiary	Average	Binary
Dice (%)	94.6 (0.03)	92.9 (0.04)	83.1 (0.13)	73.0 (0.21)	78.0 (0.04)	94.2 (0.02)

The second registration approach uses a regular grid and hence cannot directly benefit from the airway tree geometry for the transformation model. It combines convex optimisation of discrete displacements [12] with Adam optimisation and performed second best in the 2021 Learn2Reg challenge[1]. Possible displacements for each voxel are limited within a quantised set of displacements, for which a cost term is defined using input features for each voxel. The resulting cost minimisation problem is globally solved using coupled convex optimisation. A subsequent refinement step is realized by gradient descent using the well-known Adam optimiser. We calculate the cost function for possible displacements using MIND-SSC features as well as our proposed semantic airway features.

3   Results

All cases (individual patients) have been randomly split into 40 training and 20 test cases. Segmentation results on the unseen test cases are presented in Table 1. Segmenting the airway divided into multiple bronchi labels and subsequent binarisation provides comparable results to directly learning a binary segmentation network (Dice: 94.6%).

To evaluate our contribution, we compared the registration quality in several different setups. We explore the benefits of using the proposed airway derived keypoints compared to more generic interest points (Förstner), and we evaluate the impact of including the semantic nnUNet features in comparison to the more general handcrafted features (MIND). Each registration method has been evaluated on a total of 60 pairs of test images (inter-patient). In addition to evaluating the overlap of airway structures, we algorithmically located 34 anatomical landmarks for each scan based on the ground truth airway annotations, each corresponding to the position of a bi- or trifurcation in the airway tree. Note, that we are not using these landmarks to drive the registration (as done in [1]), because it would bias our analysis. We only use these landmarks to calculate target registration error (TRE) in the airway area. Results are presented in Table 2.

For geometric registration, the incorporation of airway keypoints has a very positive influence on registration accuracy in the corresponding area. Using semantic features as cost function improves performance even further. Combining MIND-SSC with semantic airway features yields the best results for all employed methods. While dense registration performs best with regard to overall overlap of the semantic segmentations, sLBP yields better results for the target registration error of specific anatomical bifurcation landmarks. Dense registration of the airway can also be improved with only binary airway features in addition to MIND features (TRE: 7.62px, Dice: 51.4%), though using multilabel features yields better results. Each registration runs in around 1 second at test time on an

---

[1]https://github.com/multimodallearning/convexAdam/

Tab. 2. Average performance of the proposed methods for 60 inter-patient registrations. Dice score is calculated using dilated ground truth airway segmentations and averaged over all 32 labels. Target registration error (TRE) is averaged over 34 landmarks at bifuractions of airways. 1 px corresponds to 1 mm in the fixed image.

	TRE (px) ↓			Dice (%) ↑		
	MIND	Label	MIND+Label	MIND	Label	MIND+Label
Initial	17.25			5.7		
Sampling	MIND	Label	MIND+Label	MIND	Label	MIND+Label
Förstner keypoints	11.13	20.00	9.77	13.3	23.1	27.3
Airway keypoints	8.20	6.47	6.25	40.8	45.5	50.4
Airway+Förstner keypoints	13.30	23.05	7.02	15.2	2.9	51.0
Dense grid (convexAdam)	9.15	13.27	6.92	37.7	56.1	62.6

Nvidia RTX GPU. A visual result of convexAdam registration with MIND and airway features is presented in Figure 2.

4 Discussion

We performed inter-patient lung registration incorporating learned semantic airway information. By decoupling feature learning from fast optimisation of the registration cost function, we obtain state-of-the-art performance without complicated multi-level or cascaded registration architectures. Our results show that high-quality automatic airway segmentation (up to tertiary bronchi) with a simple adaptation (dilation of ground truth segmentations) works well using the 3D nnUNet.

Registration results demonstrate the importance of combining learned semantic information with intensity-based image features for robust and accurate registration. Clear improvement for semantic sampling of keypoints in graph-based registration (+3.5px better TRE, +23% points better Dice) as well as large improvement for using airway features in dense registration (+2.2px better TRE, +25% points better Dice) compared to current state-of-the-art in CT lung registration has been made. We have

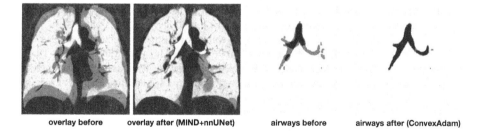

overlay before   overlay after (MIND+nnUNet)   airways before   airways after (ConvexAdam)

Fig. 2. Visual result of proposed semantic inter-patient registration of lung CT (coronal slice of 3D). The overlay shows fixed in blue and warped/moving scan in orange colours (good alignment appears greyish). The alignment of airways before and after registration confirms the good registration quality of our numerical results.

also shown that large improvements are possible when using semantic features derived from binary labels. This can substantially ease the manual annotation task and make it less dependent on the distribution of certain topological variants of airway trees in the training population.

Geometric registration performance surpassing dense image registration in regards to landmark error suggests further employing point cloud-based registration approaches for regular image registration tasks and confirms the relevance of keypoint information for generating anatomical atlases.

Inter-patient registration incorporating learned airway features depicts a first step in generating an airway atlas. In order to create a shared lung atlas, further work, especially regarding statistical analysis and modelling, is required.

References

1. Li B, Christensen GE, Hoffman EA, McLennan G, Reinhardt JM. Establishing a normative atlas of the human lung: intersubject warping and registration of volumetric CT images. Acad Radiol. 2003;10(3):255–65.
2. Xu K, Gao R, Khan MS, Bao S, Tang Y, Deppen SA et al. Development and characterization of a chest CT atlas. Proc SPIE Int Soc Opt Eng. Vol. 2021. NIH Public Access. 2021.
3. Feragen A, Owen M, Petersen J, Wille MM, Thomsen LH, Dirksen A et al. Tree-space statistics and approximations for large-scale analysis of anatomical trees. Inf Process Med Imaging. Springer. 2013:74–85.
4. Hansen L, Heinrich MP. Revisiting iterative highly efficient optimisation schemes in medical image registration. Med Image Comput Comput Assist Interv. Springer. 2021:203–12.
5. Mok TC, Chung AC. Large deformation diffeomorphic image registration with Laplacian pyramid networks. Med Image Comput Comput Assist Interv. Springer. 2020:211–21.
6. Isensee F, Jaeger PF, Kohl SA, Petersen J, Maier-Hein KH. nnU-Net: a self-configuring method for deep learning-based biomedical image segmentation. Nat Methods. 2021;18(2):203–11.
7. Armato III SG, McLennan G, Bidaut L, McNitt-Gray MF, Meyer CR, Reeves AP et al. The lung image database consortium (LIDC) and image database resource initiative (IDRI): a completed reference database of lung nodules on CT scans. Med Phys. 2011;38(2):915–31.
8. Lo P, Van Ginneken B, Reinhardt JM, Yavarna T, De Jong PA, Irving B et al. Extraction of airways from CT (EXACT'09). IEEE Trans Med Imaging. 2012;31(11):2093–107.
9. Tan Z, Feng J, Zhou J. SGNet: structure-aware graph-based network for airway semantic segmentation. Med Image Comput Comput Assist Interv. Springer. 2021:153–63.
10. Hansen L, Heinrich MP. Deep learning based geometric registration for medical images: how accurate can we get without visual features? Inf Process Med Imaging. Springer. 2021:18–30.
11. Heinrich MP, Jenkinson M, Papież BW, Brady M, Schnabel JA. Towards realtime multimodal fusion for image-guided interventions using self-similarities. Med Image Comput Comput Assist Interv. Springer. 2013:187–94.
12. Heinrich MP, Papież BW, Schnabel JA, Handels H. Non-parametric discrete registration with convex optimisation. Biomed Image Registration Proc. Springer. 2014:51–61.

Abstract: Guided Filter Regularization for Improved Disentanglement of Shape and Appearance in Diffeomorphic Autoencoders

Hristina Uzunova[1], Heinz Handels[1,2], Jan Ehrhardt[2]

[1]German Research Center for Artificial Intelligence, Lübeck
[2]Institut für Medizinische Informatik, Universität zu Lübeck
hristina.uzunova@dfki.de

The disentanglement of shape and appearance is a prominent computer vision task, that has become relevant in the medical imaging domain in recent years. Medical images are often acquired in different hospitals, by different devices and using different parameters, resulting in varying intensity profiles. However, when performing population-based analysis over various datasets, e.g. from different hospitals, it is important to be able to distinguish between changes in the anatomical shapes and device-dependent intensity changes. Diffeomorphic and deforming autoencoders are commonly applied for appearance and shape disentanglement. Both models are based on the deformable template paradigm, however, they show some weaknesses for the representation of medical images. On the one hand, diffeomorphic autoencoders generate a global template for the whole dataset, however, they only consider spatial deformations. On the other hand, deforming autoencoders also regard changes in the appearance, yet, no uniform template is generated for the whole training dataset and the appearance is modeled using only a very few parameters. In the presented work [1], we propose a method that represents images based on a global template, where next to the spatial displacement, the appearance is modeled as the pixel-wise intensity difference to the unified template. To ensure that the generated appearance offsets adhere to the shape defined by the template, a guided filter smoothing of the appearance map is integrated into an end-to-end training process. In the experiments performed on brain MRIs, this regularization approach shows significant improvement of the disentanglement of shape and appearance. Furthermore, the generated templates are crisper and improved registration accuracy can be achieved. Our experiments also underline that the proposed approach can be utilized in the field of automatic population analysis.

References

1. Uzunova H, Handels H, Ehrhardt J. Guided filter regularization for improved disentanglement of shape and appearance in diffeomorphic autoencoders. Proc Mach Learn Res. 2021;143:774–86.

Abstract: Automatic Path Planning for Safe Guide Pin Insertion in PCL Reconstruction Surgery

Florian Kordon[1,2,3], Andreas Maier[1,3,4], Benedict Swartman[5], Maxim Privalov[5], Jan S. El Barbari[5], Holger Kunze[1,2]

[1]Pattern Recognition Lab, Universität Erlangen-Nürnberg (FAU), Erlangen
[2]Siemens Healthcare GmbH, Forchheim
[3]Erlangen Graduate School in Advanced Optical Technologies (SAOT), Universität Erlangen-Nürnberg (FAU), Erlangen
[4]Machine Intelligence, Universität Erlangen-Nürnberg (FAU), Erlangen
[5]Department for Trauma and Orthopaedic Surgery, BG Trauma Center Ludwigshafen, Ludwigshafen
florian.kordon@fau.de

Reconstruction surgery of torn ligaments requires anatomically correct fixation of the graft substitute on the bone surface. Several planning methodologies have been proposed to standardise the surgical workflow by localising drill sites or defining the drill tunnel orientation. A precise drill tunnel is of high clinical relevance to prevent detrimental changes in the reconstructed ligament's biomechanics as well as early wall breakout with the risk of damaging neurovascular structures. Unfortunately, the practical implementation of these guidelines is limited by the often complex and time-consuming nature of the planning steps. In this work, we propose an automatic solution to support the trauma surgeon in guide pin path planning in double-bundle posterior cruciate ligament (PCL) reconstruction surgery on the lateral tibia [1]. A two-stage algorithm is proposed that operates on a single intra-operative 2D X-ray image: First, key anatomic cues are extracted from the image using a multi-task deep learning algorithm. Then, these cues are forwarded to a geometric pipeline in which a logical partitioning of the bone contour is used to orient the drilling path optimally and ensure a safe distance between the drill tunnel and the bone edge. In contrast to a single-stage algorithm that directly calculates the tunnel positioning parameters, this allows the user to adjust the location of the inferred anatomical features interactively and enables low-latency modification of the path proposal. We evaluate the approach on 38 radiographs of the tibia where we observe a median path angulation error of $0.37°$ and a median localisation error of 0.96 mm for the ligament attachment centre. The results suggest further clinical validation and comparison to the accuracy of manual plannings.

References

1. Kordon F, Maier A, Swartman B et al. Automatic path planning for safe guide pin insertion in PCL reconstruction surgery. Proc MICCAI. 2021:560–70.

© Der/die Autor(en), exklusiv lizenziert durch
Springer Fachmedien Wiesbaden GmbH, ein Teil von Springer Nature 2022
K. Maier-Hein et al. (Hrsg.), *Bildverarbeitung für die Medizin 2022*,
Informatik aktuell, https://doi.org/10.1007/978-3-658-36932-3_17

Heads up

A Study of Assistive Visualizations for Localisation Guidance in Virtual Reality

Jan Hombeck[1], Nils Lichtenberg[2], Kai Lawonn[1]

[1]University of Jena
[2]University of Tübingen
jan.hombeck@uni-jena.de

Abstract. In minimally invasive surgery, surgeons always rely on camera-based techniques as, unlike in open surgery, they cannot see directly into the patient's body. Providing the necessary equipment for surgeons to become accustomed to these types of devices can be expensive and time-consuming. A much more cost-effective and versatile approach to train surgeons or prepare already trained surgeons for upcoming operations is to create surgical simulations in Virtual Reality (VR). To establish VR in the field of minimally invasive surgery, we need to consider some VR-specific limitations. Although virtual reality provides better depth perception and localization of objects compared to a conventional desktop application, it still needs to be improved to match real-life. Our approach to reduce these offsets in VR is to use different assistive visualizations. Therefore, we conducted a quantitative user study with 19 volunteers each performing 40 trials of five different visualizations. Our results indicate that two of the five visualizations (*Heatmap with Isolines* and *Arrow Glyphs*) are able to reduce the occurrent error, making training in Virtual Reality more suitable for minimally invasive surgery.

1 Introduction

In the field of abdominal and liver surgery, minimally invasive procedures, especially laparoscopy, have come to play an important role. In this procedure, small incisions are made inside the abdominal cavity with the aid of an optical instrument (endoscope). The image generated by the endoscope is then displayed on an external monitor inside the operation room.

Providing the necessary equipment for surgeons to become accustomed to these types of devices can be expensive and time-consuming. This is where virtual reality (VR) technology steps in and can provide a cost-effective, portable, and easy-to-set-up alternative for training or preparing surgeons without the need for large machines. Although these simulations may not fully replace clinical trials yet, they provide an environment for the surgeon to become a) accustomed to potential upcoming complications, b) to become familiar with the technical setup, and c) improve the surgeon's performance during clinical trials [1]. Despite the benefits of VR, the majority of VR applications

Springer Fachmedien Wiesbaden GmbH, ein Teil von Springer Nature 2022
K. Maier-Hein et al. (Hrsg.), *Bildverarbeitung für die Medizin 2022*,
Informatik aktuell, https://doi.org/10.1007/978-3-658-36932-3_18

suffer from a bias in depth perception [2], distance judgment [3], and accurate local-ization of objects [4], resulting in an inaccurate representation of the environment. For common VR applications such as video games or industrial applications, this small error does not affect the usefulness of the application itself. For medical applications, these errors are unacceptable. Misperceiving the location of a tumor by a few centimeters can affect the chosen treatment and have a direct impact on the outcome of surgery. While the benefits of VR are substantial, we must first address these problems to establish VR in the surgical training domain. The work by Hombeck et al. [5] has shown that assistive visualizations such as Arrow Glyphs can help to reduce depth and distance errors in simple VR applications. We intend to expand this work by evaluating how the assistive visualizations perform within a simplified endoscopic scenario with consideration of different distances between user and virtual object.

2 Materials and methods

The following section describes the three assistive visualization techniques Pseudo-chromadapth, Heatmaps with Isolines and Arrow Glyphs (Fig. 1), as well as the en-doscopy setup used in our study. The visualizations were selected based on their promis-ing results in a similar study [5]:

- *Pseudo-chromadepth.* Pseudo-chromadepth (PCD) was originally designed by Ropinski et al. [6] to improve depth perception of vascular structures for desktop applications. PCD encodes depth information using color within a color spectrum ranging from red to magenta to violet and blue. The outermost point of the vessel volume closest to the viewer is red, while the furthest point is given the color blue. Each vertex between these points is determined by interpolation.

- *Heatmap with Isolines.* Heatmaps are commonly used in 2D applications to encode quantitative data such as the population of a city or gaze hotspots on websites. However, mapping heatmaps to 3D objects has gained some traction in the medical field, e.g. Eulzer et al. [7] utilized heatmaps effectively to visualize the extent to which the mitral valve is closed. In our case, the Heatmap is used to show the distance of a tumor to a given surface. The closer the tumor is to that surface, the redder the surface is rendered. Since coding quantitative data with color alone is often insufficient, five equally spaced isolines are added to the Heatmap. As the isolines are not continuously visible, recurrent isolines are prone to mismatches.

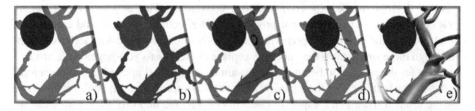

Fig. 1. Vessel with a) Flat Rendering, b) PCD, c) Heatmap, d) Arrow Glyphs, e) Phong.

To improve differentiation between isolines and avoid mismatches, the thickness of every other isoline is thickened.

- *Arrow Glyphs.* The Arrow Glyphs use the space between a specific location, e.g., a tumor, and a specific surface, e.g., the vasculature of the liver. Thereby, all arrows have the same direction; they point from the reference point to the surface (Fig. 1e). The arrows include multiple small spheres spaced 2 cm apart. This allows a relative estimation of distance. To avoid cluttering the view, the spheres are removed and the arrows are reduced in size for smaller distances. In addition to the shape of the arrow, its color is also used as a distance indicator. Here, similar to the Heatmaps, the closer the tumor is to the surface, the redder the arrow. To prevent glyphs from simply appearing or disappearing, smooth blending is achieved through transparency. The sharper the angle or the greater the distance, the more transparent the glyph is displayed.

- *Heads-Up-Visualization.* Expanding the potential use cases of the presented visualizations, we implemented a camera-display setup similar to the once used in endoscopic procedures. For this purpose, a virtual screen was embedded in the background of the VR environment. Initially, the endoscopic camera was attached to the left controller allowing the participant to change the view rendered on the endoscopic display. However, the pilot study indicated that less comparable results are obtained with this setup. The view of the virtual endoscopic screen, here called head-up visualization (HUV), differed too much between participants to draw sound conclusions. Therefore we removed the ability to freely control the endoscopic camera and tied the view to the position of the Head-Mounted Display. The HUV now shows a magnified view of the original image. By pressing a controller button the HUV can be frozen.

2.1 Study setup

This study was conducted within a customized framework for virtual reality rendering based on C++, OpenGL and OpenVR. The VR setup consists of the HTC Vive and its controllers. The vascular data was obtained from a real clinical trial and has been pre-processed for this study. For better visibility and usability, we scaled the vessel model by a factor of ten with regard to its real size, resulting in a mesh size of approximately 1.5 m in virtual space. Unless otherwise stated, we always refer to this scaled scene. Since light effects such as reflections or shadows can impact the perception of visualizations, we combined our visualization with a flat shading. This way our results are purely based on the performance of the visualizations. To draw more detailed conclusions about the effect of reflections or shadows we included one visualization with light effects (Phong shading) and one without (flat shading). In total we compare five visualization techniques (Fig. 1): Flat shading, Phong shading, Pseudo-chromadepth, Heatmaps with Isolines, and Arrow Glyphs. We conducted the study as an in-lab study with fixed participant positions, which increases internal validity and allows to ensure similar distances from participants to the vessel and tumor as well as similar viewing angles. To provide similar difficulties for all trials we performed a pilot study with eight different tumor positions. From those eight positions we choose four with similar error results to increase comparability. Each tumor is presented at two different distance levels, near distance (D_{near}) and far distance (D_{far}). In surgical procedures, the surgeon's operating range is usually defined between a nearly extended arm and a bent arm (the average human arm reach is about 85 cm). D_{near} and D_{far} represent the lower and upper limits for the operating range in surgical procedures. All structures within D_{near} have an average distance of 40 cm, while all structures in D_{far} have an average distance of 70 cm. The study task was divided into two phases:

- *Preparation Phase* (Phase$_{prep}$): Each participant is presented with the vascular mesh combined with one of the five visualizations. In addition, one of four predefined tumor locations, here represented as red spheres, is displayed. The HUV is rendered in the background of the scene and shows a magnified rendering focused on the tumor. During the Phase$_{prep}$, the participant was allowed to move their upper body while still be seated. Once the participant confirms, the view is switched to Phase$_{exe}$.

- *Execution Phase* (Phase$_{exe}$) : The tumor is removed and the participant is instructed to place a second tumor at the previously indicated location. The HUV has captured the last image seen during Phase$_{prep}$ and renders it as a still image, including the position and visualization of the previous tumor. Once the participant has placed the tumor and confirmed the result, the next trial begins immediately.

During the study, we measured the time it took participants to perform Phase$_{prep}$ and Phase$_{exe}$, as well as the distance offset (D_{offset}) by calculating the distance between the original tumor position and the one placed by the participant. Two different factors have been considered for this study: VIS (the five different types of visualization) and DISTANCE (the distance level D_{near} and D_{far}. The experimental design consists of: 5 × VIS, 2 × DISTANCE, 4 × tumor location = 40 × Trials per participant. We recruited participants from different computer science courses at our university, therefore all participants had at least a minor technical background and some experience in the field of medical visualizations. As a result of our recruitment, we found 19 volunteers (14 male, 5 female) with an average age of 25 years.

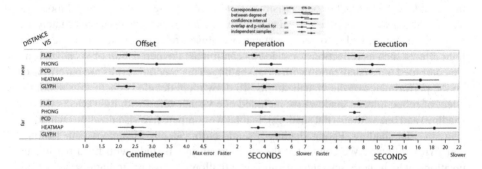

Fig. 2. Measurement of D_{offset} and completion time of Phase$_{prep}$ and Phase$_{exe}$ in a 95% bootstrapped confidence interval sorted by DISTANCE and VIS.

3 Results

To avoid dichotomous thinking regarding study results, we report our findings as confidence intervals and not as p-values as suggested by the APA [8]. Our results (Fig. 2), represent the estimation of a 95 % bootstrapped confidence interval that contains the true mean at 95% of the time and incorporates the effect size.

Within D_{near}, Phong indicates the highest margin of error (MOE), representing a greater uncertainty in the results than any of the other visualizations. While Flat and PCD had similar distance offsets, Glyphs performed minimally better than Flat and PCD. Heatmaps performed best with a slightly smaller error compared to Glyphs and a moderately reduced error compared to Flat and PCD. The results for D_{far} indicate similarly large confidence intervals for most VIS, except for Flat and PCD, where the confidence interval is larger. Heatmap and Glyphs were able to outperform Phong, Flat and PCD. PCD, Flat, and Phong shows similar distance offsets. Both Glyphs and Heatmap moderately reduced the distance offset compared to all other VIS, with Heatmap indicating a slight superiority over Glyphs.

Comparing D_{near} and D_{far}, the results show that the MOE of all visualizations increased with increased distance, with the exception of Phong. While PCD, Heatmap, and Glyphs show slightly increased MOE, Flat shows a large increase and Phong shows a large decrease. Ping et al. [9] found that the distance judgment of Phong shading can vary according to the size of the model. Although the actual size of the vascular model did not change between D_{near} and D_{far}, the number of pixels used to represent the model did. We suspect that the change in "size" corresponds to the change in distance bias. Since flat shading and PCD show similar results, we can conclude that the unique depth encoding of PCD does not have a major impact for our VR application and can be neglected. The color differences within neighboring regions of the mesh is minor and has almost the same effect as flat shading. While almost all visualizations performed slightly superior in D_{near}, Heatmaps and Glyphs consistently performed better than all other visualizations.

While the temporal performance between D_{near} and D_{far} varies only slightly, some major differences between the different visualizations can be observed. The time required for participants to grasp the visualization and sufficiently explore the environment was similar for most VIS, with PCD being the slowest. For the execution time the results indicate some major difference between visualizations, with Glyphs and Heatmap requiring considerably more time. Compared to Flat, Phong and PCD, Heatmap and Glyphs have a more complex structure and more features that need to be matched. While Heatmap uses surface color and isolines, Glyphs offer arrow position, angle, color, and transparency as potential features that must be matched.

4 Discussion

In summary, our work provides evidence on how Flat visualization, Phong shading, Pseudo-chromadepth, Heatmaps with Isolines, and Arrow Glyph affect distance and localization judgments within an endoscopic Virtual Reality application. For our quantitative study, participants were asked to remember a given tumor location and reconstruct the scene using different visualization as well as an endoscopic display. For applications targeting smaller areas of interest, such as precise tumor detection, we can show that PCD has no major impact on distance and localization judgments compared to common renderings. The color difference in adjacent areas is not sufficient to make an informed decision about the exact tumor location. Visualizations with multidimensional distance coding, such as Heatmaps with Isolines and Arrow Glyphs, can improve localization of objects at near and far (still reachable) distances. Both visualizations were able to severely reduce the distance offset compared to all other visualizations, but they also required the most time. With these visualizations, users can trade completion time for better accuracy, which is especially important for medical applications. The distance between the participant and the tumor shows an effect on the performance of the different visualizations. While the effect is quite dominant for the distance and localization judgments, the completion time does not vary as much. In general, our work contributes to establishing Virtual Reality applications in minimally invasive endoscopy for training and preparation purposes by reducing localization errors common to Virtual Reality by using Heatmaps with Isolines or Arrow Glyphs.

Acknowledgement. The work was supported by the German Research Foundation (DFG) project LA 3855/1-1.

References

1. Dawson DL, Meyer J, Lee ES, Pevec WC. Training with simulation improves residents' endovascular procedure skills. J Vasc Surg. 2007;45(1):149–54.
2. Jones A, Swan JE, Singh G, Kolstad E. The effects of VR, AR, and motion parallax on egocentric depth perception. 2008 IEEE VR. 2008;1(212):267–8.
3. Jones A, Swan JE, Singh G, Ellis SR. Peripheral visual information and its effect on distance judgments in virtual and augmented environments. Proc ACM SIGGRAPH. 2011:29–36.
4. Van der Veer AH, Longo MR, Alsmith AJ, Wong HY, Mohler BJ. Self and body part localization in virtual reality: comparing a headset and a large-screen immersive display. Front Robot AI. 2019;6:33.
5. Hombeck JN, Lichtenberg N, Lawonn K. Evaluation of spatial perception in virtual reality within a medical context. BVM. Springer, 2019:283–8.
6. Ropinski T, Steinicke F, Hinrichs K. Visually supporting depth perception in angiography imaging. Symposium on Smart Graphics. Springer. 2006:93–104.
7. Eulzer P, Engelhardt S, Lichtenberg N, De Simone R, Lawonn K. Temporal views of flattened mitral valve geometries. IEEE. 2019;26(1):971–80.
8. American Psychological Association. The publication manual of the american psychological association. 6th. Washington, DC, 2013.
9. Ping J, Thomas BH, Baumeister J, Guo J, Weng D, Liu Y. Effects of shading model and opacity on depth perception in optical see-through augmented reality. J Soc Inf Disp. 2020;28(11):892–904.

Support Point Sets for Improving Contactless Interaction in Geometric Learning for Hand Pose Estimation

Niklas Hermes[1,2], Lasse Hansen[1], Alexander Bigalke[1], Mattias P. Heinrich[1]

[1]Institute of Medical Informatics, Lübeck University
[2]gestigon GmbH, Lübeck
n.hermes@student.uni-luebeck.de

Abstract. Estimation of the hand pose of a surgeon is becoming more and more important in the context of computer assisted surgery. Previous point cloud-based neural network methods for this task usually estimate offset fields to infer the 3D joint positions. Occlusions of important hand parts and inconsistencies in the point clouds, e.g. caused by uneven exposure from the depth sensor, pose a challenge to these methods. We propose to simplify the optimization problem by only estimating a weight for each point of the cloud, such that the inferred joint position is given as the weighted sum over the input points. To better capture the directional information, we define a support point set that expands the convex hull of the hand point set and enter the union of both sets as input to our network. We propose a hierarchical graph CNN, whose graph structure enables optimal information flow between the two point sets. With a mean joint error of 9.43 mm, our approach outperforms most comparable state-of-the-art methods with an average reduction by 19%, while also reducing the computational complexity.

1 Introduction

The determination of the hand pose is becoming increasingly important in computer assisted surgery as well as in other fields of application [1]. The main focus here is on contactless interaction with devices either to ensure sterile working conditions or to enable treatments from a distance. This requires accurate and robust determination of the hand pose in real time, which is still challenging despite the progress made so far.

Until recently, 3D hand pose estimation has been dominated by methods relying on depth images [2–4]. Depth maps enable the processing by powerful CNNs while simultaneously including 3D information [5]. However, they still constitute a projection of 3D data onto a 2D plane, so direct regression of a 3D pose is a highly nonlinear task that is difficult to learn.

On the contrary 3D point clouds preserve the original 3D structure and thus enable a more natural representation for 3D pose estimation. This has been leveraged in multiple works [4, 6], which directly regress the 3D pose from 3D geometric input domains [7]. Specifically for raw 3D point clouds as input, most of the methods predict the 3D pose by estimating offset vectors or fields with respect to the input points. This procedure suffers from two problems: First, estimating offset vectors is still a complex problem that requires complex network architectures. Second, occlusions are still a major problem, since joints with larger distance from the point cloud are more prone to faulty offset predictions. This is a severe limitation, since the focus is on the patient and his treatment, and an optimal camera position is only secondary. Therefore, self-occlusion is a common issue in medical applications.

As illustrated in Figure 1, we address these challenges by making the following three contributions: Firstly, we propose to estimate the position of a joint as the weighted sum of all input points. So instead of an offset vector, we only need to learn a scalar weight for each input point. This is a substantially simpler task that can be solved with a less complex network. However, this procedure only allows estimating joints inside the convex hull of the input cloud, which is quite limited. Therefore, secondly, we propose to complement the input point cloud by a support point set, which is arranged around the input cloud and thus enables a more comprehensive prediction of joint locations. To jointly process the unified set, we develop a hierarchical graph CNN whose graph structure enables information flow between hand points and support points. In particular, geometric information is propagated from the hand points to the surrounding support points, which in turn can improve joint prediction.

2 Materials and methods

We aim to estimate the 3D hand pose which is equivalent to finding the location of all hand joints. The input to our proposed method is a set of points $\mathbf{P} \in \mathbb{R}^{N_p \times 3}$ with $N_p \in \mathbb{N}_+$ being the number of points. We assume that the given point set only contains a hand, where parts of the hand can be missing due to occlusions. The output is a set of joint positions $\mathbf{H} \in \mathbb{R}^{J \times 3}$ with the number of joints $J \in \mathbb{N}_+$.

2.1 Support point sets

A core concept of our method is to estimate the position of the hand joints as the weighted sum over the input point set $\mathbf{P}$. Specifically, we define the position of joint j as

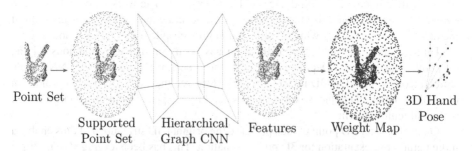

Fig. 1. Overview of the proposed method. We propose to extend the input point cloud by a support point set. The supported point cloud is fed into a hierarchical graph CNN that connects the hand and the support point set and shares their information. The resulting features are transferred into a weight map to infer the final 3D hand pose as weighted sum over all points.

$$\mathbf{H}_j(\mathbf{P}, \mathbf{W}) = \frac{\sum_{i=1}^{N_p} w_{ij} \mathbf{p}_i}{\sum_{i=1}^{N_p} w_{ij}} \tag{1}$$

where the weights $w_{ij} \in [0, 1]$, represented by $\mathbf{W}$, need to be inferred from the input cloud. However, this joint representation has the limitation that it only maps to positions that lie within the convex hull of the given set of points $\mathbf{P}$. When point clouds are generated from a single view depth image, usually some parts of the hand are occluded and not reflected in the point cloud. These occluded hand joints mostly cannot be mapped using representation (1).

In order to solve this problem we create an additional point set to expand the convex hull of the hand. We define a support point set $\mathbf{U}$ by randomly choosing $N_b \in \mathbb{N}_+$ points from the unit sphere $\{x \in \mathbb{R}^3 : \|x\|_2 = 1\}$. To better capture the shape of a hand we scale these support points depending on the standard deviation vector σ of the hand point set and translate them towards the center μ

$$\mathbf{B} = d(\sigma \circ \mathbf{U}) + \mu \tag{2}$$

where $\circ$ denotes the Hadamard product and d a scaling factor that we empirically set to $d = 5$. This support set is unified with the original input cloud, yielding a supported hand point set $\mathbf{P}_{\text{sup}} = \mathbf{P} \cup \mathbf{B}$.

2.2 Network architecture

While most hierarchical network architectures use a PointNet [8, 9] to compute features, we propose a hierarchical Graph CNN [4] to learn weight maps on supported point sets. A graph has the advantage that it can connect the points of the two semantically different point clouds and thus enables an exchange of information. The combination with the hierarchical network structure [9] ensures that we capture local as well as global features of both sets.

Set abstraction layers are usually used to transfer the features of a point set to a coarser resolution [9]. We propose a modified `GraphAbstraction` layer that takes into account both the hand point set and the support point set. Given an input point set of size N_{in} that consists of $N_{\text{in}}/2$ hand points and $N_{\text{in}}/2$ support points around the hand. The new resolution N_{out} is obtained using farthest-point-sampling on the hand points and support points separately. This ensures that the subsampled point set consists of 50% hand points and the other 50% support points.

Point cloud-based graph networks [4] commonly build the graph based on the K-nearest-neighbor method. However, in our case, this would result in hand and support points not being connected due to their distance. Therefore we modify this approach and enforce that each hand point connects to some support points and the other way around. The input point set and the graph connections are then fed into an EdgeConvolution layer followed by a multi layer perceptron (MLP) to obtain the final features of the coarser resolution.

Our network accepts any D-dimensional supported point set as input, where $D \in \mathbb{N}_+$. Within the first `GraphAbstraction` step the input cloud is subsampled to $N_1 = 1024$ feature points of dimension $C_1 = 32$ that are concatenated to the 3D positions. The two following `GraphAbstraction` layers process these features to an $N_2 \times (D + C_2)$ ($N_2 = 256$ and $C_2 = 128$) and subsequently to an $N_3 \times (D + C_3)$ ($N_3 = 64$ and $C_3 = 256$) dimensional feature tensor. We use the same `FeaturePropagation` layers as proposed in [6] to combine the features of two different resolutions. To this end the features of a coarser resolution N_{r+1} are interpolated to a finer resolution N_r using nearest-neighbor-interpolation, concatenated with the features of the `GraphAbstraction` layer GA$_r$ and fed into an MLP to obtain a feature tensor of dimension $N_r \times C_r$. The final features with input resolution are fed into an MLP that outputs one weight map for each hand joint.

We apply deep supervision when training our hierarchical network by adding MLPs to the output of the `FeaturePropagation` layers, each generating a weight map for all joints. This yields the definition of the following loss function for each training sample

$$\mathcal{L}(\mathbf{P}_{\text{sup}}, \mathbf{H}_t, \mathbf{W}) = \sum_{f=0}^{F-1} \sum_{j=1}^{J} \left\| \mathbf{H}_j(\mathbf{P}_{\text{sup}}, \mathbf{W}_f) - \mathbf{H}_{tj} \right\|^2 \tag{3}$$

with $F \in \mathbb{N}_+$ as number of `FeaturePropagation` layers, the generated weight map of a `FeaturePropagation` layer $\mathbf{W}_f$ and the target positions of the hand joints $\mathbf{H}_t$.

3   Results

We evaluate our proposed method on the public dataset NYU [10]. The NYU [10] hand pose dataset contains 8 252 depth maps of a single person for testing and 72 757 depth maps of two users for training. Besides the depth image the dataset contains the 3D position of 36 hand joints. For a better comparison we follow [3, 10] and perform evaluation on a subset of 14 joints.

We transfer the depth image into a 3D point cloud using the camera intrinsic parameters. We then perform a principal component analysis (PCA) to obtain an orthonormal basis where the variance of the points is small along the axes and map the point cloud to that basis. In a last step we normalize the cloud by dividing it by the longest possible distance along one of the axes and shift it to the root by subtracting the mean of the cloud.

Our network is trained and tested on a computer with a GeForce® RTX 2080 Ti 11GB GPU. For the implementations of the deep neural network modules we use the PyTorch framework. On graph creation we connect each point in the cloud with a total of $K = 8$ other points. To enforce connections between hand and support point set, we connect each hand point with one support point and seven other hand points. Each support point is connected to seven hand points and one other support point. We extend the EdgeConvolution layer by replacing the standard max pooling aggregation function by a combination of multiple aggregation functions (PNA) [11]. During the training of our proposed networks we use the Adam optimizer with the initial learning rate 0.001, $\beta_1 = 0.5$, $\beta_2 = 0.999$ and weight decay $5e^{-4}$. Additionally the learning rate is halved every 30 epochs and training is stopped after 120 epochs.

Based on the number of trained parameters, the reduction of network complexity can be deduced. The specified network contains a total of 1 736 413 trainable parameters and thus has a size of 6.95 MB. Compared to the P2P network [6], which has a total size of 17.2 MB, our network is much smaller.

To demonstrate the accuracy of the proposed approach we compared it with seven state-of-the-art methods on the NYU [10] dataset by computing two metrics. First is the mean Euclidean distance between the ground truth and the estimated joint positions. The second metric is the proportion of successfully predicted frames, where the worst joint error is below a certain threshold [3].

As can be seen in Figure 2, with an average error of 9.43 mm our method achieves comparable state-of-the-art accuracy. Compared to the other methods, this means an average reduction of the error by 19%. Only P2P [6] achieves better results than our approach due to suitable postprocessing. Without this postprocessing, P2P [6] achieves an error of 9.5 mm which leads to the assumption that our method also achieves similar results with suitable optimization. Furthermore, training and testing our network without the support points results in an average error of 11.41 mm, which highlights their contribution to the performance.

The high accuracy of our method is also reflected in the percentage of successfully predicted frames. Up to a maximum allowed distance of 20 mm, we outperform all other methods. With a threshold of 10 mm, we correctly predict 27% of the frames, while the next best approach with the same threshold achieves only 23%. Furthermore, we achieve a proportion of 50% correctly predicted frames with a threshold of 13.5 mm. When the threshold is above 20 mm, P2P [6] has a slightly higher percentage of correct predictions than the proposed method. The same is true for CrossInfoNet [2] when the threshold is above 35 mm.

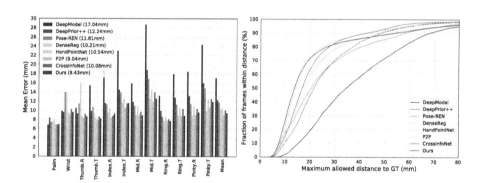

Fig. 2. Evaluation of the proposed method and state-of-the-art methods on the NYU dataset [10]. The figure shows the average error of each joint (left) and the percentage of successfully predicted hand poses (right).

4   Discussion

In this work, we proposed to estimate the 3D hand pose from a point cloud as the union of the input points and a support point set. This enables us to predict the weight maps with an efficient hierarchical graph CNN, which we tailored for optimal information flow between both point sets. That way, we address the problem of occluded joints and reduce the complexity of the optimization problem. Our results demonstrate that the method achieves comparable state-of-the-art accuracy while also reducing the network complexity. By precisely estimating the hand joint positions, the gestures of a person can be detected. This is necessary for contactless interaction with devices, which in turn enables sterile working conditions.

In future work, we will investigate the use of support points in other problem instances. One is the estimation of human body poses on datasets such as the multi-view operating room (MVOR) dataset [12]. Second, we will evaluate the possibility of predicting organ keypoints, such as the position of bifurcations in the lung.

References

1. Hein J, Seibold M, Bogo F, Farshad M, Pollefeys M, Fürnstahl P et al. Towards markerless surgical tool and hand pose estimation. Int J Comput Assist Radiol Surg. 2021;16:799–808.
2. Du K, Lin X, Sun Y, Ma X. Crossinfonet: multi-task information sharing based hand pose estimation. Conf Comput Vis Pattern Recognit Workshops. 2019;2019-June:9888–97.
3. Oberweger M, Wohlhart P, Lepetit V. Hands deep in deep learning for hand pose estimation. CoRR. 2015;abs/1502.06807(July).
4. Wang Y, Sun Y, Liu Z, Sarma SE, Bronstein MM, Solomon JM. Dynamic graph CNN for learning on point clouds. CoRR. 2018;abs/1801.07829.
5. Chatzis T, Stergioulas A, Konstantinidis D, Dimitropoulos K, Daras P. A comprehensive study on deep learning-based 3D hand pose estimation methods. Applied Sciences. 2020;10(19).
6. Ge L, Ren Z, Yuan J. Point-to-point regression pointnet for 3D hand pose estimation. Computer Vision – ECCV 2018. Springer International Publishing, 2018:489–505.
7. Bronstein MM, Bruna J, LeCun Y, Szlam A, Vandergheynst P. Geometric deep learning: going beyond Euclidean data. CoRR. 2016.
8. Qi CR, Su H, Mo K, Guibas LJ. PointNet: deep learning on point sets for 3D classification and segmentation. CoRR. 2016;abs/1612.00593.
9. Qi CR, Yi L, Su H, Guibas LJ. PointNet++: deep hierarchical feature learning on point sets in a metric space. Adv Neural Inf Process Syst. 2017:5100–9.
10. Tompson J, Stein M, Lecun Y, Perlin K. Real-time continuous pose recovery of human hands using convolutional networks. ACM Transactions on Graphics. 2014;33.
11. Corso G, Cavalleri L, Beaini D, Liò P, Velickovic P. Principal neighbourhood aggregation for graph nets. CoRR. 2020;abs/2004.05718.
12. Srivastav V, Issenhuth T, Kadkhodamohammadi A, De Mathelin M, Gangi A, Padoy N. MVOR: a multi-view RGB-D operating room dataset for 2D and 3D human pose estimation. 2018.

Automatic Switching of Organ Programs in Interventional X-ray Machines Using Deep Learning

Arpitha Ravi[1], Florian Kordon[1,2,3], Andreas Maier[1,3]

[1]Pattern Recognition Lab, Universität Erlangen-Nürnberg (FAU), Erlangen
[2]Siemens Healthcare GmbH, Forchheim
[3]Erlangen Graduate School in Advanced Optical Technologies (SAOT), Universität Erlangen-Nürnberg (FAU), Erlangen
arpitha.ravi@fau.de

Abstract. In interventional radiology, the optimal parametrization of the X-ray image and any subsequent software processing strongly depends on the body region being imaged. These anatomy-specific parameters are combined to create customized organ programs and are necessary to obtain an optimal image quality. In today's workflow, these programs have to be switched manually by the surgeon, which can be complex. This paper investigates a deep learning algorithm for automatic switching of organ programs in interventional X-ray machines based on the automatic detection of the imaged anatomy. We compare multiple network architectures for cardiac anatomy classification where the algorithm has to differentiate the left coronary artery, right coronary artery, and left ventricle on radiographs without contrast medium. The best-performing model achieves a micro average F1-score of 0.80. A comparison of the model performance with expert rater annotations shows promising results and recommends further clinical evaluation.

1 Introduction

Optimal parameterization of the acquisition protocol is essential in interventional 2D X-ray imaging to obtain an optimal image quality, and it is dependent on the body region being imaged. For example, the size of the objects deployed is smaller in the brain compared to any other region of the body, and the object velocity is higher in the cardiac region. For a given object size, exposure control must ensure that the resolution is accurate by using small focal spots, short exposure time or both. Also, the image processing has to guarantee that the most interesting spatial frequency bands are increased, and other less relevant bands are suppressed. For a given object velocity, exposure control has to ensure that exposure time is adequate to have the best compromise between power and motion blur. The image processing can adapt to the average intensity and motion compensation to benefit inter-frame information handling [1, 2]. These region and domain-specific parameters are combined to form a customized organ program.

Today's operator is required to manually switch the organ programs according to the body regions, often also during different stages of the surgical procedure. However, this is complex and time consuming during the surgery as the surgeon has to choose from a

Springer Fachmedien Wiesbaden GmbH, ein Teil von Springer Nature 2022
K. Maier-Hein et al. (Hrsg.), *Bildverarbeitung für die Medizin 2022*,
Informatik aktuell, https://doi.org/10.1007/978-3-658-36932-3_20

list of available organ programs for every imaged anatomy. Hence, it would be desirable that the machine can automatically detect the body regions and set the organ programs accordingly. The classical approach is to use all the position data like angulation and table positions. However, this approach has limitations due to unknown patient position and patient properties like size and weight. To address these challenges, this work investigates a deep learning algorithm for automatic detection of the imaged anatomical region, which aids the machine to therefore switch the organ programs without manual interaction based on the anatomy, facilitating the surgical workflow and reducing the required manual interaction.

We analyse and evaluate our method on interventional radiographs acquired during cardiac interventions. Specifically, the proposed algorithm is optimised to classify the acquired X-ray image into three classes, the left coronary artery (LCA) [3], right coronary artery (RCA) [3], or the left ventricle (LV) [4] shown in (Fig. 1). Each of these structures have unique anatomical characteristics and require an individual organ program. The velocity for the RCA is higher than that of LCA, which requires the motion compensation to be parameterized differently. On the other hand, the LV requires a higher frame rate and regulation stop due to the contrast being filled as seen in (Fig. 1c). However, this has to be done before the injection of the contrast medium as it would be too late to switch the organ program midway through the procedure. Hence, the images we use do not contain any artery information, except for the catheter tip, which makes the process of detection and classification even more challenging (Fig. 2a). Despite these challenges, we can show that our algorithm achieves encouraging results that are comparable to the average performance of human experts.

2 Materials and methods

2.1 Data properties and preparation

The radiographic sequences used for our analysis were obtained during surgical interventions on the cardiac region. Each sequence consists of a variable number of frames

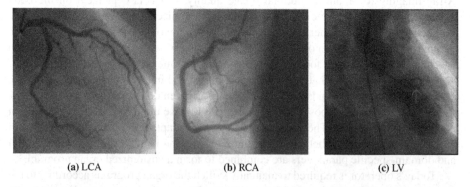

(a) LCA   (b) RCA   (c) LV

Fig. 1. Radiographs with contrast agent acquired during intervention in the instrumented cardiac region. (a), left coronary artery [3]. (b), right coronary artery [3]. (c), left ventricle with pigtail catheter [4]. The individual arrows mark the catheter tips.

and is available in a raw format, which signifies that neither a filtering nor any image processing techniques have been performed on them yet. As discussed in Section 1, the sequences contain information on whether the imaged anatomy shows the LCA, RCA, or LV. For subsequent neural network training, we consider only the first frame of the sequence as it does not contain the contrast medium. To account for the intensity variations and type of acquisitions, a multi-site dataset with a total of 324 images (115 LCA, 104 RCA and 105 LV), were used and split into 247 (0.75%) for training, 28 (0.1%) for validation, and 49 (0.15%) for testing. To further evaluate the generalisation performance of our model, an independent hold-out test set of 79 single-site images were used for final model evaluation which contains 14 images of class LCA, 20 of class RCA, and 45 of class LV. Since the images in the sequences are not pre-processed, they are not corrected for flip or rotation and contain the collimator region. Even though the collimator appears to be a black region that bears no information, it still contains background information which adds noise to the image. To alleviate potential negative effects during optimization of the neural network, the collimator region is removed from the image using certain parameters obtained and stored during acquisitions. Figures (2b, 2c) provide an understanding of the original radiograph with visible collimator blades and the corrected image, respectively. The original images are of variable resolutions, starting with the lowest being 896×896 px and the highest being 1920×2480 px. Because of this, all images within a mini-batch were edge-padded according to the highest image resolution present in the batch. The pre-processed images were provided as input to the network along with the labels.

2.2   Network architecture and training protocol

The neural network training was performed with two different network architectures, MobileNetV2 [7] and ResNet-50 [8]. Both architectures are used as pre-trained models with ImageNet weights. (Fig. 3) describes the proposed method used for training. The MobileNetV2 and Resnet-50 models were used for feature extraction, followed by a fully-connected layer for classification. The heuristically chosen hyperparameters used

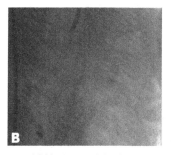 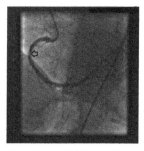 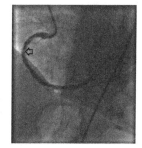
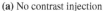

(a) No contrast injection   (b) Noisy collimator area   (c) Collimator-free image

Fig. 2. Challenges on interventional radiographs of the cardiac region. (a), radiograph without contrast injection with no visible artery [5]. (b), collimated area with noisy residual information [6]. (c) automatically removed collimator area [6].

are a batch size of 3 and a learning rate of 0.0001. To account for the multi-class classification scenario, categorical-cross entropy with Softmax activation function was used as loss function with Adam optimzer. We used early stopping on the validation loss with a patience of 10. The training was performed on a 16 GB NVIDIA Quadro P5000 graphics card.

3   Results

The network was evaluated for Precision, Recall, F1-score and the area under the receiver operating characteristic curve (AUC). Two models were evaluated for the task, MobileNetV2 and ResNet-50. From the results in (Tab. 1), we observe the macro (micro) average F1-score of the two models ResNet-50 and MobileNetV2 as 0.79 (0.80) and 0.72 (0.73), respectively. Based on the comparison, it is clear that the ResNet-50 yields superior classification performance compared to the MobileNetV2. Hence, the subsequent experiments were performed using only the Resnet-50 model. To further evaluate the ResNet-50 model, it was tested on the independent hold-out test set (Sec. 2.1) consisting of 79 images (Tab. 2). We observe that the Resnet-50 model still provides plausible predictions on the independent data originating from a different dataset. The model yields an average micro F1-score of 0.80 and macro F1-score of 0.77, which is similar to the results obtained on the original test set.

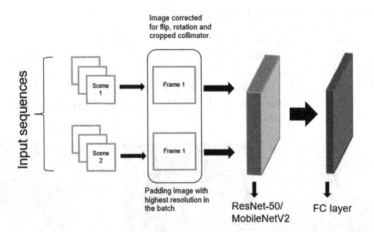

Fig. 3. Proposed method: Network architecture of the ResNet-50 and MobileNetV2 for image classification. A sequence (variable frames) is provided as input, and only the first frame is considered. This image is corrected for flip, rotation and the collimator is cropped. Every image is padded with the highest resolution of the batch. These images and the labels are provided as input to the ResNet-50/MobileNetV2 model for feature extraction. These extracted features are then passed through the fully-connected (FC) layer to predict a class label for the corresponding input image.

Tab. 1. Classification metrics for the ResNet-50 and MobileNetV2 on the test split.

Model	Class label	No. of samples	Precision	Recall	F1-score
ResNet-50	LCA	21	0.86	0.86	0.86
	RCA	13	0.71	0.77	0.74
	LV	15	0.79	0.73	0.76
MobileNetV2	LCA	21	0.78	0.86	0.82
	RCA	13	0.59	0.77	0.67
	LV	15	0.89	0.53	0.67

Tab. 2. Classification metrics for the ResNet-50 on the independent hold-out test set.

Class label	No. of samples	Precision	Recall	F1-score	AUC
LCA	14	0.82	0.64	0.72	0.81
RCA	20	0.59	0.85	0.69	0.82
LV	45	0.97	0.82	0.89	0.90

To evaluate the model further, we compare the model's performance against the performance of expert evaluators. We conducted this experiment using four experts in the field. Similar to the network, the first frame of the scene is presented from the test data to the experts. (Fig. 4) presents the Precision, Recall and F1-scores comparing the performance of the model vs average expert performance for the three classes. We observe that the model performance is close to the average expert performance. For the LCA class (Fig. 4a), we see that the recall of the model is lower than the expert scores, which is caused by a comparatively higher number of false-positives. On contrary, the precision value of the model is higher than the expert score, indicating a low number of false-negatives. This is because the features of RCA and LV are very similar to LCA in some of the images, leading to false negatives. Similar results can be seen for the RCA (Fig. 4b), where the precision values almost match the average rate scores, but where the recall value is again inferior. Interestingly, the model performance for LV is worse than the expert rates in all evaluation metrics (Fig. 4c). This is because LV images typically show instrumentation with a pigtail catheter (Fig. 1c), which is easy to detect by the experts, even without any contrast medium. Further analysis of the relevant features using GradCam [9] visualisation techniques showed that the model is not learning from the catheter but from anatomical references. We argue that this explains the difference between model performance and expert prediction.

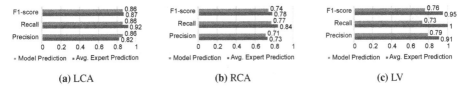

(a) LCA   (b) RCA   (c) LV

Fig. 4. Comparison between the model performance and the average expert prediction for the respective artery classes.

4 Discussion

Organ programs are essential during X-ray interventions. Since the parameters differ for individual anatomies, automatic detection of it enables us to set the right parameters by switching to the right organ program. In this work, we propose an automatic classification algorithm that can reliably detect three different anatomical regions (LCA, RCA and LV) in cardiac applications. Our experiments demonstrate that the classification performance is very close to that of expert raters. However, in the case of LV, the performance is substantially lower than the experts rating, which can be attributed to the networks inability to exploit information about the catheter type and location. We expect that the model can be improved by utilising this information, e.g., by implicit approaches like visual attention, or definitive methods like concurrent catheter localisation. Ultimately, we seek to exploit our approach's universal design to extend it to other complex anatomies like Neurological and Gastrointestinal regions.

Acknowledgement. We would like to thank Siemens Healthcare GmbH (Forchheim) for the financial support and also their assistance on this project.

References

1. Aichinger H, Dierker J, Joite-Barfuß S, Säbel M. Radiation exposure and image quality in X-Ray diagnostic radiology. Springer, 2012.
2. Dobbins III JT. Image quality metrics for digital systems. Handb Med Imaging. 2000;1:161–222.
3. Heart foundation. https://www.heartfoundation.org.nz/your-heart/heart-tests/coronary-angiography. Accessed: 2021-10-29.
4. Joudinaud T, Baron F, Etchegoyen L. Unusual diagnosis of ascending aorta dissection with left ventricular angiogram. Heart. 2006;92(12):1855.
5. Mehrotra S, Sharma PP, Sharma YYP. Very delayed coronary stent fracture presenting as unstable angina: a case report. Int J Case Rep Imag. 2017;8(2):147.
6. Obiagwu C, John J, Mastrine L, Borgen E, Shani J. Acute pulmonary embolism masquerading as acute inferior myocardial infarction. J Med Cases. 2014;5(2).
7. Sandler M, Howard AG, Zhu M, Zhmoginov A, Chen LC. MobileNetV2: inverted residuals and linear bottlenecks. Proc CVPR. 2018:4510–20.
8. He K, Zhang X, Ren S, Sun J. Deep residual learning for image recognition. Proc CVPR. 2016:770–8.
9. Selvaraju RR, Das A, Vedantam R, Cogswell M, Parikh D, Batra D. Grad-CAM: visual explanations from deep networks via gradient-based localization. Int J Comput Vis. 2019;128(2):336–59.

Ermittlung der Geometrie von Amputationsstümpfen mittels Ultraschall

Carina Krosse[1], Rainer Brucher[2], Alfred Franz[3]

[1]Fakultät für Informationstechnik, Hochschule Mannheim
[2]Institut für Medizintechnik und Mechatronik, Technische Hochschule Ulm
[3]Institut für Informatik, Technische Hochschule Ulm
krosse@mail.hs-ulm.de

Zusammenfassung. Die genaue Vermessung der Geometrie von Amputationsstümpfen ist elementar für die Herstellung einer Prothese. Konventionell wird die Geometrie mittels Gipsabdruck oder optischen 3D Scannern ermittelt. Nachteile sind hohe Kosten, Subjektivität und mögliche Ungenauigkeiten durch Patientenbewegungen. In dieser Arbeit wird daher als Alternative der Einsatz von Ultraschall zur Vermessung untersucht. Die Machbarkeit und Genauigkeit wird mit einem klinischen B-Mode Gerät geprüft. In Ergänzung wird getestet, ob dieser Ansatz auch mit A-Mode Scans einer Stiftsonde umsetzbar ist. Der Fokus liegt hierbei besonders auf der Detektion der Hautoberfläche und des Knochens eines Oberschenkelstumpfs. Die Messungen wurden an einem Stumpfphantom aus ballistischer Gelatine mit einem 3D-gedruckten Knochen durchgeführt. Die Oberfläche konnte mittels B-Mode mit einer Genauigkeit von 1,0 mm gemessen und eine 3D Rekonstruktion erstellt werden. Die Messung mittels A-Mode war mit einer Genauigkeit von 0,5 cm möglich.

1 Einleitung

Der prothetische Ersatz amputierter Gliedmaßen sorgt für das Wiedererlangen des Selbstwertgefühls und die Wiederherstellung der Mobilität [1]. In Deutschland leben ca. 150000 Menschen mit einer Beinprothese und ca. 57% dieser Personen leiden unter mäßigen bis starken Schmerzen [2, 3]. Diese Zahlen weisen darauf hin, dass viele Menschen von dem optimierten Herstellungsprozess einer Prothese profitieren würden.

Die Interaktion zwischen dem Stumpf und Prothesenschaft (schalenartige Verbindung zwischen Stumpf und Prothese) bestimmt die Qualität der Passform. Herkömmliche Methoden sind der Gipsabdruck oder die Vermessung mittels optischen 3D Scannern. Ersteres erfolgt händisch und ist subjektiv, der optische Scanner benötigt freie Sicht und Patientenbewegungen können die Bildaufnahme stören [2]. Beide Methoden vermessen ausschließlich die Geometrie des Amputationsstumpfes, um diese Abmessungsdaten für den Prothesenbau zu nutzen. Wünschenswert wäre eine Methode, die zusätzlich zur Geometrie, Details der Stumpfmuskulatur und Inhomogenität des Gewebes in der Modellierung berücksichtigt und ein quantitatives, reproduzierbares Verfahren darstellt [1].

In Forschungsprojekten wurden bereits Ansätze untersucht, die auch innere Strukturen darstellen können. Die Verfahren Computertomographie (CT) und Magnetresonanztomographie (MRT) werden eingesetzt, um Informationen über den Stumpf zu erlangen. Die gute Knochenauflösung beim CT und die Möglichkeit der Unterscheidung von Weichteilen im MRT machen die Verfahren attraktiv. Nachteilig sind jedoch hohe Anschaffungskosten, ionisierende Strahlung beim CT und die Scanaufnahmezeit. Zudem wird die Untersuchung im Liegen durchgeführt wodurch die natürliche Form des Stumpfs verändert wird [1, 2, 4].

Die Erfassung der Stumpfgeometrie mittels Ultraschall wurde bisher noch kaum untersucht, könnte den Messvorgang jedoch vereinfachen, vereinheitlichen und objektivieren sowie die Erkennung innerer Strukturen ermöglichen. In einer verwandten Arbeit konnte die Hautoberfläche bereits mit Ultraschall detektiert werden, allerdings von außen durch die Luft [5]. Auch zur Geometrievermessung wurden bereits einige Forschungsprojekte durchgeführt. In einer weiteren verwandten Arbeit wurde Ultraschall im Wasserbad eingesetzt [1]. Nachteilig sind jedoch die Signalabschwächung im Wasserbad und Gliedmaßenbewegungen, die zu schlechterer Bildauflösung führen.

Im Gegensatz zu den verwandten Studien, sollte in dieser Arbeit die Rekonstruktion mittels einer auf der Haut aufgesetzten Ultraschallsonde mit Messungen durch das Gewebe erfolgen. Ziel war daher der Bau eines Gelatinephantoms und die Erkennung der Hautoberfläche und des Oberschenkelknochens durch das Gewebe mittels Ultraschall. Die Machbarkeit und Genauigkeit soll mit einem klinischen B-Mode Gerät untersucht werden. Zusätzlich wird geprüft mit welcher Genauigkeit diese Messungen mit einem handlichen A-Mode Scanner durchführbar sind, da dieser kostengünstiger und potentiell einfacher anzuwenden ist.

2   Materialien und Methoden

2.1   Phantombau

Die Phantomherstellung mit ballistischer Gelatine (Ballistic 3, GELITA AG, Eberbach, Deutschland) gewährleistet eine möglichst realistische Simulation von Gewebe. Das

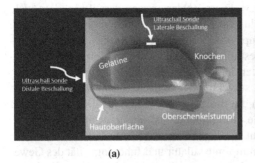
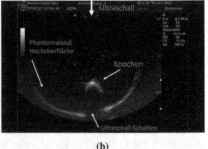

(a)   (b)

Abb. 1. a) Gelatinephantom und Skizze des Versuchsaufbaus b) B-Bild von Hautoberfläche und Phantom per lateraler Beschallung.

Phantom wurde in einer thermoplastischen Form gegossen, die Größe und Geometrie eines typischen Oberschenkelstumpfs widerspiegelt. Der mit eingegossene Oberschenkelknochen wurde per 3D-Druck, im Fused Deposition Modeling (FDM) Verfahren hergestellt, unter Berücksichtigung der stark unterschiedlichen akustischen Impedanz mit ausgeprägter Echogenität. Er wurde in feiner Auflösung und voll gedruckt. Dabei wurde PLA+ Filament verarbeitet. Die Abbildung 1a zeigt das resultierende Phantom.

2.2 B-Mode Messungen

Die B-Mode Messungen wurden mit einem Ultraschallgerät der Firma GE erstellt (GE LOGIQ P5, GE Healthcare GmbH, Deutschland). Hierzu diente die Transvaginalsonde GE E8C, da diese eine Entfernung von bis zu 15 cm schallen kann (Frequenz = 8 MHz) und sich der Konvexschallkopf mit einem Radius von 1 cm gut eignet, um die Stumpfform, die auf Abbildung 1a sichtbar ist, abzubilden. Die laterale und distale Beschallung wurde an dem Oberschenkelphantom durchgeführt und im direkten Kontakt mittels Kopplungsgel realisiert.

Um die Genauigkeit der Stumpfoberflächenvermessung zu ermitteln, wurde ein B-Mode-Bild des distalen Stumpfendes erstellt, wie in Abbildung 2a gezeigt. Hierfür kam ein vereinfachtes Gelatinemodell zum Einsatz, das nur den distalen Teil des Stumpfs simuliert. Als Referenz wurde die Oberfläche an 17 Stellen innerhalb der Schallebene mit einer Nadelspitze abgetastet, die mittels eines elektromagnetischen (EM) Trackingsystem lokalisiert wurde. Hierbei kam das Trackingsystem Aurora® (Northern Digital Inc., Waterloo, Canada) mit dem Tabletop Feldgenerator und der lokalisierbaren Aurora® Needle, 18G/150 mm, Chiba zum Einsatz. Ultraschallbild und Trackingkoordinatensystem wurden zuvor punktbasiert im Wasserbad nach der von März et al. beschriebenen Methode kalibriert [6], wobei die Ultraschallsonde mit einem weiteren EM Sensor (Aurora® 6DOF Cable Tool) lokalisiert wurde. Als Software für Kalibrierung und Messungen kam das open-source Medical Imaging Interaction Toolkit (MITK) [7] mit dem Plugin org.mitk.gui.qt.igt.app.ultrasoundtrackingnavigation zum Einsatz. Als Maß für die Genauigkeit wurde pro Messpunkt der euklidische Abstand zwischen der Referenzmessung und der im US-Bild lokalisierten Hautoberfläche bestimmt und über alle 17 Messpunkte gemittelt [6].

Um durch B-Mode Ultraschall eine 3D-Rekonstruktion des Stumpfphantoms zu erstellen, wurde die Sonde in 30° Grad Schritten um die eigene Achse gedreht, wie die Abbildung 3a zeigt. In jeder Pose wurde ein B-Bild aufgezeichnet und mit Hilfe von MITK [6, 7] in einer virtuellen Szene entsprechend der Aufnahmepose zu den anderen Bildern ausgerichtet. In jedem Bild wurden dann im Abstand von ca. 0,5 cm Punkte auf der gut kontrastierten Hautoberfläche markiert und mit den Oberflächenpunkten der anderen Bilder in der 3D Szene visualisiert.

2.3 A-Mode Messungen

Als A-Mode Ultraschallsonde wurde eine Stiftsonde verwendet, die im Rahmen eines Projektes der Technischen Hochschule Ulm erstellt und programmiert worden ist. Es handelt sich um eine 2 MHz Sonde (Basler Medizintechnik Schweiz). Diese ist im pulsed wave mode betrieben. Ein Piezoelement emittiert einen Schallpuls und schaltet

Tab. 1. Ergebnisse der A-Mode Messungen.

A-Mode Messung	Ultraschallmessung	Referenzmessung	Fehler
Haut-Haut (lateral)	14,1 cm	14,2 cm	0,1 cm
Haut-Haut (distal)	22 cm	21,5 cm	0,5 cm
Haut-Knochen (lateral)	7,9 cm	8 cm	0,1 cm
Haut-Knochen (distal)	23 cm	22,5 cm	0,5 cm

daraufhin zum Empfangen des Echos um. Mittels dieser Sonde wurde die Distanz zwischen dem Aufsatzpunkt der als Hautsimulation dienenden Phantomoberfläche und der gegenüberliegenden Hautseite sowohl in distaler als auch in lateraler Richtung gemessen, wie in Abbildung 3 dargestellt. Außerdem wurde auch die Detektion des simulierten Knochens in beiden Richtungen getestet.

3   Ergebnisse

Das erste Gelatinephantom ist auf Abbildung 1a dargestellt. Die B-Mode Messungen (Abb. 1b) zeigen, dass bei lateraler Beschallung die Hautoberfläche und der Knochen detektierbar sind.

Die Hautoberfläche konnte dabei an 17 Referenzpunkten mit einer mittleren Abweichung von $1,0 \pm 0,5$ mm ($\mu \pm \sigma$) vermessen werden (Abb. 2). Die aus mehreren B-Bild Aufnahmen rekonstruierte 3D-Szene ist in Abbildung 3 dargestellt. Gut sichtbar ist der Ultraschallschatten des Knochens im unteren Teil des Bildes.

Auch mittels A-Mode Stiftsonde konnte an ausgewählten Stellen sowohl der Abstand zum Knochen als auch zur gegenüberliegenden Hautoberfläche bestimmt werden. Ein Beispiel für eine A-Mode Messung, die den Werten aus Tabelle 1 zugrunde liegt, ist in der Abbildung 4 visualisiert.

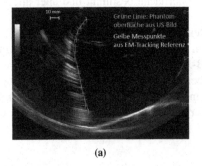   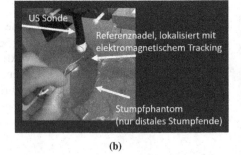

(a)   (b)

Abb. 2. (a) Detektion der Hautoberfläche mit EM Tracking. (b) Phantom für Oberflächenmessung.

4 Diskussion

In dieser Arbeit wurde die Vermessung des Gelatinephantoms eines Oberschenkel-stumpfs mittels Ultraschall beschrieben. In den Ergebnissen ist ersichtlich, dass die Ziele der Hautoberflächen- und Knochendetektion erreicht werden können.

Die initialen Versuche zur 3D Rekonstruktion liefern visuell ein sinnvolles Ergebnis. Erste Vergleichsmessungen mit der Referenzmethodik eines optischen 3D Scanners lieferten eine hohe Genauigkeit bei der Hautoberflächen Erfassung. Um die Genauigkeit zusätzlich für die Vermessung des Knochens zu ermitteln, sind künftig Referenzaufnahmen, beispielsweise mit einem CT notwendig.

Die gut kontrastierte Hautoberfläche wurde von Hand markiert. In Zukunft sollte hierfür ein automatischer Algorithmus entwickelt werden, um die Gesamtmethodik praktisch anwendbar zu machen.

Abbildung 1b zeigt, dass für eine 3D Rekonstruktion des Stumpfs eine einzige Messung nicht ausreichend sein wird (Ultraschallschatten und Artefakte). Es ist denkbar, mehrere Insonierungspositionen festzulegen, um daraus ein 3D Bild zu erstellen und den Ultraschallschatten zu reduzieren.

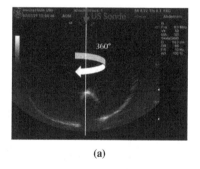

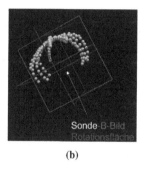

(a)   (b)

Abb. 3. (a) 360° Rotation der Ultraschall B-Bild Sonde bei lateraler Beschallung. (b) 3D Rekonstruktion der lateralen Beschallung der Hautoberfläche mit MITK.

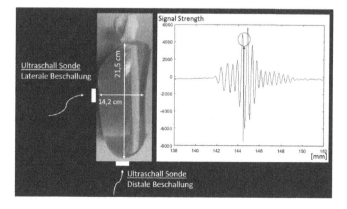

Abb. 4. Laterale Beschallung im A-Mode von Haut- zu Hautoberfläche mit Echomaximum.

Die kostengünstige A-Mode Messmethode sollte weiter geprüft werden. Wünschenswert wäre, dass ein Orthopädietechniker in der Lage ist, die A-Mode Sonde ohne Vorkenntnisse anzusetzen und 3D-Scan-Messungen zu erstellen. Denkbar wäre eine Methode, bei der vorgefertigte Messpunkte in einem Liner (innere Auskleidung einer Prothese) vorhanden sind. Der Liner sorgt dafür, dass durch das Ansetzen der Sonde keine Verformung des Stumpfes stattfindet.

Bei der Phantomerstellung fehlen in dieser Ausarbeitung realistische Aspekte wie verschiedene Haut-, Muskel- und Fettschichten. Diese sollten in Folgearbeiten ebenfalls simuliert werden.

Zusammenfassend konnte in dieser Arbeit gezeigt werden, dass die Vermessung der im Gelatinemodell simulierten Haut und des Knochens in einem Oberschenkelstumpfmodell mittels Ultraschall möglich ist. Die für die Hautvermessung ermittelte Genauigkeit von ca. einem Millimeter ist vielversprechend und sollte bei Folgeversuchen in realistischeren Settings verifiziert werden. Ein weiterer wichtiger Aspekt ist die Erkennung des Oberschenkelknochens, dessen Position durch die vorhandenen Echogenität ermittelt werden konnte. Die Messungen lassen zudem vermuten, dass auch die Kräfteübertragung in den Hüftknochen beurteilt werden kann. Dies ist vielversprechend mit Hinsicht auf die angestrebte Methodik zur Prothesenoptimierung.

Danksagung. Ich bedanke mich bei den Kollegen an der THU, Thomas Sziemeth, Kevin Hörsch, Gerhard Keller, Daniel Jäger und Volker Schilling-Kästle für die Unterstützung beim 3D Druck, der Sonde und dem optischen 3D Scan bedanken. Ebenfalls bedanke ich mich bei Fabian Kramer für die Hilfe bei der Durchführung der Messungen.

References

1. Douglas T, Solomonidis S, Sandham W, Spence W. Ultrasound imaging in lower limb prosthetics. IEEE Trans Neural Syst Rehabil Eng. 2002;10(1):11–21.
2. Ranger BJ, Feigin M, Zhang X, Moerman KM, Herr H, Anthony BW. 3D ultrasound imaging of residual limbs with camera-based motion compensation. IEEE Trans Neural Syst Rehabil Eng. 2019;27(2):207–17.
3. Simone Oehler. Beinprothesen: Langzeittest zu Belastungen. Ed. by Dtsch Arztebl 2010, 107(3): A-97 / B-82 / C-82. 2010.
4. D. Bonacini, C. Corradini, U. Cugini, G. Magrassi. 3D digital models reconstruction: residual limb analysis to improbe prosthesis design. 2007.
5. Yuanming Feng, Ron Allison, Xin-Hua Hu, Helvecio Mota, Todd Jenkins, Melodee L. Wolfe et al. An ultrasonic device for source to skin surface distance measurement in patient setup. Int J Radiat Oncol Biol Phys. 2005;61(5):1587–9.
6. März K, Franz AM, Seitel A, Winterstein A, Bendl R, Zelzer Sea. MITK-US: real-time ultrasound support within MITK. Int J Comput Assist Radiol Surg. 2014;9(3):411–20.
7. Nolden M, Zelzer S, Seitel A, Wald D, Müller M, Franz, A. M. et al. The Medical Imaging Interaction Toolkit: challenges and advances: 10 years of open-source development. Int J Comput Assist Radiol Surg. 2013 Jul;8.

Monte Carlo Dose Simulation for In-Vivo X-Ray Nanoscopy

Fabian Wagner[1], Mareike Thies[1], Marek Karolczak[2], Sabrina Pechmann[3],
Yixing Huang[1], Mingxuan Gu[1], Lasse Kling[3,4], Daniela Weidner[5], Oliver Aust[6],
Georg Schett[5], Silke Christiansen[3,4], Andreas Maier[1]

[1]Pattern Recognition Lab, FAU Erlangen-Nürnberg
[2]Institute of Medical Physics and Microtissue Engineering, FAU Erlangen-Nürnberg
[3]Fraunhofer Institute for Ceramic Technologies and Systems IKTS, Forchheim
[4]Institute for Nanotechnology and Correlative Microscopy e.V. INAM, Forchheim
[5]Department of Internal Medicine 3 - Rheumatology and Immunology, FAU Erlangen-Nürnberg
and University Hospital Erlangen
[6]Leibniz Institute for Analytical Sciences ISAS, Dortmund
fabian.wagner@fau.de

Abstract. In-vivo x-ray microscopy (XRM) studies can help understanding the bone metabolism of living mice to investigate treatments for bone-related diseases like osteoporosis. To adhere to dose limits for living animals and avoid perturbing the cellular bone remodeling processes, knowledge of the tissue-dependent dose distribution during CT acquisition is required. In this work, a Monte Carlo (MC) simulation-based pipeline is presented, estimating the deposited energy in a realistic phantom of a mouse leg during an in-vivo acquisition. That phantom is created using a high-resolution ex-vivo XRM scan to follow the anatomy of a living animal as closely as possible. The simulation is calibrated on dosimeter measurements of the x-ray source to enforce realistic simulation conditions and avoid uncertainties due to an approximation of the present number of x-rays. Eventually, the presented simulation pipeline allows determining maximum exposure times during different scan protocols with the overall goal of in-vivo experiments with few-micrometer isotropic CT resolution.

1 Introduction

X-ray microscopy (XRM) systems are usually employed in materials science due to their high resolution down to 500 nm paired with large photon fluence [1]. Exceptional optical properties and great bone-soft tissue contrast make XRM particularly valuable for imaging bones in the context of osteoporosis research to resolve so-called *Lacunae*, tiny bone cavities containing cells known to be heavily involved in bone metabolism [2]. The overall goal is to repetitively image living mice in a preclinical setting and observe the influence of medication on the bone metabolism. However, radiation dose so far prohibits resolving Lacunae in in-vivo studies, as dose and CT resolution are known to be tightly connected.

In this work we estimate the radiation dose in a potential in-vivo setting, imaging the tibia bone of a mouse. First, a realistic bone phantom is created based on high-resolution ex-vivo bone scans. Second, the radiation dose is estimated in a Monte Carlo simulation obeying x-ray physics and scan geometry. Third, the simulation is calibrated to the XRM system via air kerma measurements from an ionization chamber. Eventually, the developed pipeline can estimate deposited dose in different components of the mouse phantom and scan parameters can be adapted to adhere to radiation limits for different types of scanned tissue. Together with investigations on the data acquisition and image processing [1, 3] this paves the way for in-vivo imaging the bone metabolism and to better understand osteoporosis.

2   Materials and methods

2.1   X-ray physics

An x-ray beam with intensity $I_0(E)$ and spectral energy distribution E is attenuated when penetrating an object of thickness dx and energy-dependent absorption coefficient $\mu(x, E)$ following the Beer-Lambert law

$$I = \int_0^{E_{\max}} I_0(E) \exp\left(-\int \mu(x, E)dx\right) dE \tag{1}$$

The beam intensity is attenuated as x-rays transfer their energy to the imaged object via the photoelectric and Compton effect. The so-called *kerma* K quantifies the kinetic energy dE_{kin} transferred to secondary particles like electrons within an irradiated volume of mass m. It is defined as

$$K = \frac{dE_{kin}}{m} = \frac{dE_{kin}}{\rho V} \tag{2}$$

and properly approximates the deposited energy in volume V of density ρ for the medical CT energy regime. Analogously, the so-called *air kerma* defines the kerma in a given volume of air and is used in this work to calibrate the simulated dose values to the XRM system. The dose can harm living tissue due to stochastic effects [4] and, therefore, is to be minimized in CT imaging.

2.2   Realistic mouse tibia bone phantom

A simulation of the absorbed dose requires knowledge of the material composition and density distribution of the imaged object. To realistically model the composition of the imaged mouse leg, a mouse phantom is created based on an ex-vivo scan of an extracted mouse tibia bone in the following way. The voxel intensities of the CT reconstruction act as the template for the density distribution in the bone region. We derive densities directly from voxel intensities using a linear mapping. The calibration function

$$\rho(I) = \left(2.398 \cdot I + 1.2 \cdot 10^{-3}\right) \frac{g}{cm^3} \tag{3}$$

deriving density ρ from voxel intensities I is estimated using reported density values from literature (air: $0.00120479 \frac{g}{cm^3}$, cortical bone: $1.92 \frac{g}{cm^3}$) [5].

All voxel densities $< 1.0 \frac{g}{cm^3}$ are regarded as background, which yields the segmentation mask of the bone material. Furthermore, a realistic phantom is created by filling the interior of the bone with bone marrow (0.95 $\frac{g}{cm^3}$ [5]) and adding cylinder-shaped soft-tissue around the bone (1.3 $\frac{g}{cm^3}$ [5]). Additionally, the phantom is downsampled to shape $128 \times 128 \times 128$ as the performance of the Monte Carlo dose simulation is strongly dependent on the number of voxels in the phantom. Figure 1 illustrates the phantom generated from an ex-vivo bone scan, which is used in the following.

2.3 Monte Carlo simulation

A Monte Carlo (MC) simulation is performed to accurately estimate the deposited dose distribution in the constructed mouse phantom. The MC framework *GAMOS* [6] based on the simulation toolkit *Geant4* [7] is employed, properly modeling photon-matter interactions in the x-ray energy regime. 30, 40, and 60 kV tungsten anode x-ray spectra with 1, 1, and 2 mm aluminium filtration (*SpekPy* [8]) are investigated as tube configuration, matching conventionally used settings on the XRM system when scanning bones. The mouse phantom is placed $r = 40$ mm away from the cone-beam x-ray source to mimic a realistic animal placement. Subsequently, the simulation is conducted for $N_{phantom} = 7.5 \cdot 10^7$ photons, randomly emitted within the solid angle of the cone Ω, well covering the size of the phantom $A < \Omega r^2$. The respective photon energy is randomly sampled from the filtered source spectrum.

During the simulation, the individual photons are propagated through the system while probabilistically taking into account interactions with matter depending on photon energy and material characteristics. Eventually, deposited energy is recorded in each voxel within the phantom, from which the tissue-dependent dose is calculated. Propagating enough photons in the simulation allows predicting dose accurately in the real-world XRM system, following the MC principle.

2.4 Calibration to the XRM system

To scale the simulated number of photons to the real number of x-rays in the XRM system (ZEISS Xradia 620 Versa), the dose simulation is calibrated with air kerma measurements of the x-ray source [9]. Air kerma is measured exposing an ionization

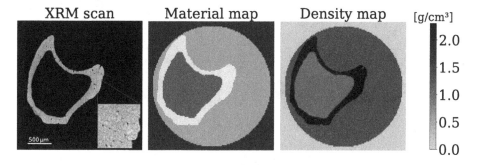

Fig. 1. Left: Ex-vivo XRM scan of a mouse tibia with Lacunae visible in the zoomed region. Middle: Generated material map. Right: Density map of the constructed phantom.

chamber placed in front of the x-ray tube with 30, 40, and 60 kV tube voltage and 2, 3, and 6.5 W power respectively. Subsequently, the result K_{meas} is compared with a MC simulation of the air kerma K_{sim} with source-detector distance equivalent to the tube measurement and source configuration matching the experiment from Section 2.3. The scaling factor for the dose simulation yields

$$\alpha = \frac{K_{meas}}{K_{sim}} \frac{N_{air}}{N_{phantom}} \tag{4}$$

considering the number of propagated photons in the air and phantom simulation. The simulated kerma in the phantom is multiplied with α to match the number of photons during a real XRM acquisition. As K_{meas} is measured in $[\frac{eV}{s}]$, the results are calibrated to one second of exposure. The calibration on a real dosimeter measurement allows determining realistic radiation conditions in the simulation without relying on assumptions on the x-ray generation within the source or estimating the number of emitted photons in the system.

3   Results

The MC simulation stores the deposited 3D energy distribution in the voxelized mouse phantom, which is illustrated in Figure 2. Due to the high bone density compared to the other tissue types, the 3D visualization of the deposited energy emphasizes the bone structure with the knee region on the left side and the tibia part to the right. Using the phantom material map as segmentation mask, the dose D_η for each type of tissue η is derived dividing the accumulated energy in each tissue by its total mass m_η

$$D_\eta = \frac{1}{m_\eta} \sum_{v_i \in V_\eta} E_{v_i} = \frac{1}{\rho_\eta V_\eta} \sum_{v_i \in V_\eta} E_{v_i} \tag{5}$$

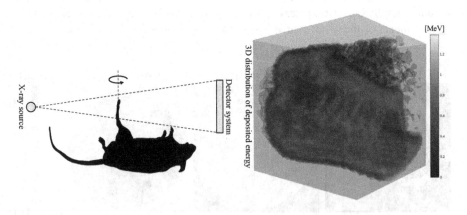

Fig. 2. Left: In-vivo scan setup with the tibia bone placed in the center of rotation. Right: 3D visualization of the simulated accumulated energy distribution in the knee joint/tibia region of the animal.

Tab. 1. Total deposited dose per second exposure for the different types of tissue during full power XRM scans with 30 kV (2 W), 40 kV (3 W), and 60 kV (6.5 W) tube voltage.

Tissue	Dose (30 kV) [$\frac{mGy}{s}$]	Dose (40 kV) [$\frac{mGy}{s}$]	Dose (60 kV) [$\frac{mGy}{s}$]
Bone marrow	70.5	496.1	322.3
Soft-tissue	297.6	1405.2	1239.1
Cortical bone	1283.8	8634.1	5439.4
Air	0.2	0.9	0.6

The resulting dose is summarized in Table 1 for all different materials and source spectra. As the scaling factor α calibrates the simulation to one second of exposure, the unit is [$\frac{mGy}{s}$]. Note, that the simulations approximate the dose in three conventional XRM protocols with different tube voltage and tube power. Hence, the respective exposure time must be chosen individually to achieve a comparable image quality. Due to its high density, the cortical bone absorbs the highest amount of energy with $1.3 - 8.6 \frac{Gy}{s}$ in the respective high-power acquisition. However, it is also the most robust part of the mouse leg in terms of stochastic effects. The bone marrow is much more sensitive to radiation and absorbs $0.07 - 0.5 \frac{Gy}{s}$.

4   Discussion

The dose values for different investigated source spectra presented in Table. 1 can not be directly related. Due to varied source powers ($2 - 6.5$ W), changing source efficiency for different tube voltages, and differing spectral filters (1 mm and 2 mm Al), the photon fluence is not comparable between the simulations. In practice, significantly longer exposure times are required, e.g., for the 30 kV compared to the 60 kV acquisition to achieve an equivalent contrast on the detector. Hence, image quality must be taken into account when deciding on a set of in-vivo minimum-dose acquisition parameters. The total tissue dose is then obtained by multiplying the minimum exposure time required to achieve the desired image quality with the simulated dose per second.

In-vivo mouse measurements require keeping the total body dose < 10 Gy to minimize stochastic effects to the animal and its bone metabolism [4]. Resolving few-micrometer Lacunae requires multiple hours of exposure using the presented XRM settings. Therefore, the extremely high dose values prohibit in-vivo measurements with reasonable exposure times for all of the investigated acquisition protocols so far. However, sophisticated denoising algorithms in combination with low-dose acquisition techniques [3] can significantly reduce dose while maintaining high image quality to push XRM in-vivo studies to the micrometer scale. In future work, a more accurate mouse phantom can be created from an ex-vivo XRM scan of a complete mouse leg, visualizing the soft-tissue extent. Particularly the leg close to the mouse body is only roughly modeled assuming cylinder-shaped tissue in the presented simulations.

Due to the high flexibility of the simulation script, various acquisition, geometry, and object parameters can be investigated without requiring additional costly phantom measurements. Additionally, compared to purely computational dose estimation techniques, estimations on the number of photons and their generation in the source can be avoided by calibrating the simulation to real dosimeter measurements. In summary, the presented MC dose simulation tool allows identifying limiting scan parameters for developing a measurement and data processing pipeline for in-vivo experiments being capable of imaging the bone metabolism.

References

1. Mill L, Kling L, Grüneboom A, Schett G, Christiansen S, Maier A. Towards in-vivo X-ray nanoscopy, acquisition parameters vs. image quality. Proc BVM. 2019:251–6.
2. Grüneboom A, Kling L, Christiansen S, Mill L, Maier A, Engelke K et al. Next-generation imaging of the skeletal system and its blood supply. Nat Rev Rheumatol. 2019;15(9):533–49.
3. Huang Y, Mill L, Stoll R, Kling L, Aust O, Wagner F et al. Semi-permeable filters for interior region of interest dose reduction in X-ray microscopy. Proc BVM. 2021:61–6.
4. Baker JE, Fish BL, Su J, Haworth ST, Strande JL, Komorowski RA et al. 10 gy total body irradiation increases risk of coronary sclerosis, degeneration of heart structure and function in a rat model. Int J Radiat Biol. 2009;85(12):1089–100.
5. NIST standard reference materials. https://www.nist.gov/srm. 2008.
6. Arce P, Rato P, Canadas M, Lagares JI. GAMOS: a geant4-based easy and flexible framework for nuclear medicine applications. IEEE Nucl Sci Symp Conf Rec. IEEE. 2008:3162–8.
7. Agostinelli S, Allison J, Amako Ka, Apostolakis J, Araujo H, Arce P et al. Geant4—a simulation toolkit. Nucl Instrum Methods Phys Res A. 2003;506(3):250–303.
8. Bujila R, Omar A, Poludniowski G. A yalidation of SpekPy: A software toolkit for modelling x-ray tube spectra. Phys Med. 2020;75:44–54.
9. Hupfer M, Kolditz D, Nowak T, Eisa F, Brauweiler R, Kalender WA. Dosimetry concepts for scanner quality assurance and tissue dose assessment in micro-ct. Med Phys. 2012;39(2):658–70.

Abstract: How to Generate Patient Benefit with Surgical Data Science

Results of an International Delphi Process

Matthias Eisenmann[1,2], Minu D. Tizabi[1], Keno März[1], Lena Maier-Hein[1]

[1]Division of Computer Assisted Medical Interventions, German Cancer Research Center
(DKFZ), Heidelberg
[2]For complete author list, please see full publication [1]
m.eisenmann@dkfz.de

An increasing number of data-driven approaches and clinical applications have been studied in the fields of radiological and clinical data science, but translational success stories in surgery are still lacking as revealed by an international poll among experts in the field of Surgical Data Science (SDS) in 2019. To come up with a roadmap for faster clinical translation and exploitation of the full potential of SDS, we conducted a 4-round Delphi process [2] involving a consortium of 50 medical and technical experts from 51 institutions. Four areas essential for moving the field forward were identified. Consensus was derived on a mission statement for each of the four areas along with a set of goals that are necessary to accomplish the respective mission. This process yielded a set of 6–9 consensus goals per mission and the following mission statements: Technical infrastructure: Make the data needed for training, validating, evaluating and applying SDS algorithms accessible to and exchangeable between researchers, healthcare professionals and other stakeholders, both live and retrospectively. Data annotation and sharing: Facilitate data sharing across institutions and establish large-scale, representative and quality-checked annotated databases. Data analytics: Align SDS methods research with clinical objectives and priorities. Clinical translation: Promote a cultural shift toward SDS-driven clinical practice. Finally, the consortium collaboratively compiled a list of relevant stakeholders and then rated their importance for the four missions. The resulting document [1] (accepted for publication in the journal of Medical Image Analysis) forms a detailed roadmap for the research community on how to generate patient benefit with SDS which will be presented at the conference.

References

1. Maier-Hein L, Eisenmann M, Sarikaya D, März K, Collins T, Malpani A et al. Surgical data science: from concepts toward clinical translation. Med Image Anal. 2022;76.
2. Hsu CC, Sandford B. The Delphi technique: making sense of consensus. Pract Assess Res Eval. 2007;12(10):1–8.

Abstract: The Importance of Dataset Choice
Lessons Learned from COVID-19 X-ray Imaging Models

Beatriz Garcia Santa Cruz[1,2], Matias Nicolas Bossa[3], Jan Soelter[2], Frank Hertel[1,2], Andreas Husch[2]

[1]Centre Hospitalier de Luxembourg, Luxembourg
[2]University of Luxembourg, Luxembourg
[3]Vrije Universiteit Brussel, Belgium
garciasantacruz.beatriz@gmail.com

The robust translation of medical imaging-based models from research to real clinical settings opens new challenges. A prominent recent case is the development of models for the prediction of COVID-19 pneumonia from planar X-Ray imaging. Hundreds of models, intended for clinical use, were published within the last months. In a critical appraisal, most published models were characterised for having a high risk of bias, hampering their safe clinical use [1]. One of the main causes for such risks might be the use of rapidly collected and poorly described datasets during the model development. Attempting to address this, we conducted the first systematic review of publicly available COVID-19 X-ray datasets focusing on the datasets characteristics that potentially induce bias and/or uncontrolled confounders into the models [2]. Using PRISMA, we identified 112 unique datasets and only 11 were found suitable for further analysis. We evaluated the risk of bias aspects using adapted CHARMS and BIAS tools. To quantify the impact of such issues, we conducted a dataset frequency analysis of published papers over 12 months. We found that in general, the dataset description was poor calling for better documentation. Also, dataset remixes combining several source datasets might lead to accidental data leakage. Temporal analysis revealed researchers tended to choose the datasets based on their size and availability instead of their quality. These results highlight the necessity of paying more attention to the dataset selection process. Our work concludes with a set of general practical advice for modellers to reduce these common pitfalls. We anticipate our article is not only useful for COVID-19 researchers but a representative case of the current state of the area.

References

1. Wynants L, Van Calster B, Collins GS, Riley RD, Heinze G, Schuit E et al. Prediction models for diagnosis and prognosis of covid-19: systematic review and critical appraisal. bmj. 2020;74.
2. Garcia Santa Cruz B, Bossa MN, Sölter J, Husch AD. Public Covid-19 X-ray datasets and their impact on model bias: a systematic review of a significant problem. Med Image Anal. 2021;74:102225.

© Der/die Autor(en), exklusiv lizenziert durch
Springer Fachmedien Wiesbaden GmbH, ein Teil von Springer Nature 2022
K. Maier-Hein et al. (Hrsg.), *Bildverarbeitung für die Medizin 2022*,
Informatik aktuell, https://doi.org/10.1007/978-3-658-36932-3_24

Analysis of Celiac Disease with Multimodal Deep Learning

David Rauber[1,2], Robert Mendel[1], Markus W. Scheppach[3], Alanna Ebigbo[3], Helmut Messmann[3], Christoph Palm[1,2]

[1]Regensburg Medical Image Computing (ReMIC), Ostbayerische Technische Hochschule Regensburg (OTH Regensburg), Regensburg, Germany
[2]Regensburg Center of Biomedical Engineering (RCBE), OTH Regensburg and Regensburg University
[3]Department of Gastroenterology, Augsburg University Hospital, Augsburg, Germany
david.rauber@oth-regensburg.de

Abstract. Celiac disease is an autoimmune disorder caused by gluten that results in an inflammatory response of the small intestine. We investigated whether celiac disease can be detected using endoscopic images through a deep learning approach. The results show that additional clinical parameters can improve the classification accuracy. In this work, we distinguished between healthy tissue and Marsh III, according to the Marsh score system. We first trained a baseline network to classify endoscopic images of the small bowel into these two classes and then augmented the approach with a multimodality component that took the antibody status into account.

1 Introduction

Celiac disease (CD) is a complex disorder caused by an autoimmune reaction to ingested gluten. The associated microscopic manifestation in the small intestine is usually divided into five histological categories, Marsh 0 - IV, with Marsh 0 representing healthy small intestinal mucosa and Marsh I - IV representing gradually progressive destruction of the intestinal epithelium. Due to its miscellaneous expression and hard to identify endoscopic appearance, CD is often overseen during routine endoscopy and therefore the disease is underreported. Hence, our goal is to use deep learning to identify CD on endoscopic images of the small intestine. In this work, we introduce a deep learning based method to distinguish between healthy tissue and Marsh III. We also compare the results between an image-only baseline and a multimodal approach. Multimodal approach means that in addition to endoscopic images, the antibody status (Transglutaminase, Gliadin) is also used. Multimodal learning is a current topic of growing interest, but to our knowledge there is no work that combines endoscopic images with clinical parameters to classify celiac disease.

2 Materials and methods

This chapter describes the dataset, the preprocessing, the model architecture and finally the training procedure.

© Der/die Autor(en), exklusiv lizenziert durch
Springer Fachmedien Wiesbaden GmbH, ein Teil von Springer Nature 2022
K. Maier-Hein et al. (Hrsg.), *Bildverarbeitung für die Medizin 2022*,
Informatik aktuell, https://doi.org/10.1007/978-3-658-36932-3_25

Tab. 1. Number of study participants and resulting available endoscopic images.

Class	Study Population		Images	
	Count	%	Count	%
Healthy	323	64	846	50
Marsh III	182	36	858	50

2.1 Dataset

The dataset was acquired from Augsburg University Hospital. It consists of endoscopic images of the small bowel and clinical parameters. Because the data were collected retrospectively, not every clinical parameter is necessarily available for each patient. It is also possible that several endoscopic images were acquired from one patient (Tab. 1). In this work, antibody status is used as an additional input parameter in the described methods. The antibody status is positive or negative depending on whether it can be detected in the blood. The images are from daily routine and were not acquired according to a standardized procedure. Therefore, not only white light overview images are included in the dataset, but also indigo, near focus and NB (narrow band) images (Fig. 1). The left side of Table 2 shows that there is a strong correlation between uncollected antibody status and class Healthy as well as positive antibody status and class Marsh III. Considering each uncollected and negative antibody status as Healthy and the positive ones as Marsh III results in an F1 score of 0.9. For this reason, we randomly created a subset of the data in which we attempted to reduce this bias. This subgroup included the same number of samples for Healthy and Marsh III classes when antibody status was not collected. Thus, the information that there is no antibody status available no longer tells us anything about the underlying class. We also equated the significance of positive and negative antibody status to the corresponding class (Tab. 2). After this reduction, the trivial F1 score decreased to 0.75 when calculated in the same way as above. However, by removing the bias in the uncollected samples, a higher trivial F1 score can be obtained by classifying all uncollected and positive samples as Marsh III. In this case, the F1 score was 0.83. This value should be at least reached by any algorithm using the antibody status.

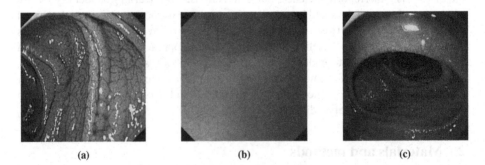

(a)   (b)   (c)

Fig. 1. Different kinds of image modalities: (a) Indigo. (b) Near-Focus. (c) NBI.

Tab. 2. Number of antibody statuses recorded for healthy and pathological cases. Left, the original dataset. On the right, the balanced dataset.

Antibody	Original Healthy		Marsh III		Balanced Healthy		Marsh III	
	Count	%	Count	%	Count	%	Count	%
uncollected	678	80	88	10	88	34	88	34
negative	160	19	51	6	160	63	8	3
positive	8	1	719	84	8	3	160	63

2.2   Preprocessing

In a first step, the data were divided into five folds of equal size to perform 5-fold cross-validation. The samples were chosen in such a manner that all images of a patient were in one of these folds. Care was also taken to ensure that the different antibody states were equally distributed across the different folds. Finally, patients were randomly selected under these constraints, so the recordings are not chronologically ordered. This was necessary because the quality of endoscopic images has improved over time due to technological advances in the development of endoscopes, and therefore there are qualitative differences between early and recent images. This development also leads to an increase of the spatial resolution of the images, therefore all images were resized to a resolution of 500×500 pixels. To obtain reproducible results, a fixed seed was used.

2.3   Model architecture

In general, a classification network consists of an encoder and a classifier. The encoder extracts discriminative features from the input and the classifier attempts to separate the inputs based on these features and assign them to a target class. For image classification, a convolutional neural network (CNN) based on a sequence of convolutional layers and nonlinear activation functions is usually used to extract features. The kernels of the convolutional layers are the parameters learned during training. In the past, it has been shown that some architectures are particularly well suited for image classification. One of these is the widely used ResNet [1], which we used in our experiments with 18 layers. In this work, we focus on the classification of endoscopic images in combination with the antibody status as an additional clinical parameter. There are several strategies for merging information from different sources [2, 3]. We used a joint feature fusion approach, because the dimensions and the informativeness of the inputs are different. This means that the extracted image features were fused with the one-hot encoded antibody status to obtain more discriminative features. We also tried to project the antibody status into a high dimensional feature space by three fully connected layers before merging (Fig. 2). This corresponds to an high dimensional embedding layer. To combine the two feature vectors, we introduced a feature fusion module (FFM). In this module, the feature vectors were merged into a single vector that contains the important information from both input sources to accomplish the classification task. The resulting vector has the same length as the image feature vector. This vector is finally propagated to the classifier (Fig. 2).

2.3.1   Feature fusion module. The core of the feature fusion module is a matrix-vector multiplication, where the matrix is learned during training and the vector is the concatenation of the image and antibody feature vectors. Figure 3 illustrates this functionality. The weights of the matrix determine the influence of the features in the resulting fused feature vector. Here, we suggest three different initialization strategies. In a trivial solution, the matrix is initialized randomly. A second option is to initialize the first (red) block with an identity matrix and the second (blue) with zeros. This would preserve the image features at the beginning of the training. The last variant combines both strategies, where the first part of the matrix is initialized with an identity matrix and the second part randomly. Since antibody status was not always available, a strategy had to be developed to address this in the FFM. The first option was to encode the antibody status into three different states (uncollected, negative, and positive). The second option was to encode only the negative and positive status and bypass the FFM with a skip connection in case of an uncollected antibody status.

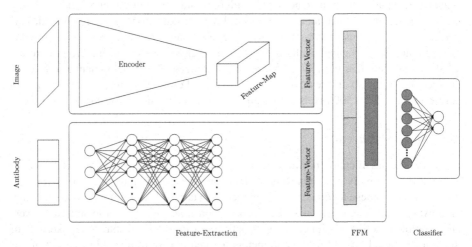

Fig. 2. After separate processing of the image and antibody data, the features are combined by a Feature fusion module (FFM) and classified afterwards.

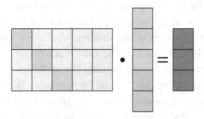

Fig. 3. Illustration of the feature fusion by a matrix-vector multiplication. The learned matrix elements serve as weights of the features from the different modalities.

Tab. 3. Results of image-only baseline and those of the multimodal strategies. The multimodal strategies distinguish between direct concatenation and a previous projection of the one-hot encoded antibody status into a high-dimensional feature space.

	Baseline	One-Hot		Projection			
		2	3	32	64	128	256
F1	0.74	0.93	0.92	0.93	0.94	0.94	0.93
sensitivity	0.78	0.94	0.92	0.95	0.95	0.94	0.93
specificity	0.66	0.93	0.92	0.92	0.92	0.93	0.92

2.4 Training

Due to the fact that medical datasets are usually small, it is common practice to use a model pre-trained on ImageNet [4] and finetune it to the desired application [5]. This is possible due to the hierarchical structure of the features extracted from a CNN. In this work, we used the pre-trained weights from PyTorch for the encoder. All the other layers were randomly initialized following the scheme of He et al. [6]. Another step to deal with the small amount of data is to perform image transformations to increase the size of the dataset. The transformations involved random horizontal and vertical flips as well as random resizing and rotation of the image. The rotation varied between ±45 degrees and the resizing between ±0.1%. In the validation phase, only normalization was performed. The network was trained for 200 epochs with Stochastic Gradient Descent (SGD), a learning rate of 0.001, momentum 0.9 and $1e-4$ weight decay. The chosen batch size was 20. Cosine Annealing was used as a learning rate scheduler. There was also a linear warm-up phase over 10 epochs at the beginning. The cross entropy was used as a loss function.

3 Results

The following reported results are the summarized results of the individual folds. This means that a global confusion matrix was accumulated over all folds, which was then used to calculate the F1-metric. In our image-only baseline, we reached an F1 score of 0.74. This value could be increased by taking the antibody status into account. As mentioned above, there were several possible strategies. Table 3 shows that a direct concatenation of the antibody status results in an F1 score of 0.93 when the FFM is skipped in the absence of an antibody status (One-Hot 2). This value decreased to 0.92 when "uncollected" was coded as a third possible antibody status and the FFM was always applied (One-Hot 3). Furthermore, Table 3 shows the effects of projecting the antibody status into a higher dimensional space. The dimensions 64 and 128 resulted in the highest F1 score of 0.94. We also evaluated the effects of different initialization strategies for the FFM. The simple random initialization led to an F1 result of 0.94. The "image-preserving" initialization reduced the F1 to 0.92. With the combination of both strategies, we achieved an F1 result of 0.94.

4 Discussion

Our goal in this work was to detect celiac disease on endoscopic images of the small intestine using Deep Learning. Table 3 shows that this goal was reached with an F1 score of 0.74. This result is worse than using antibody status alone (F1 0.83), but it does not require extensive analysis of blood values. The results also showed that classification accuracy was improved by combining image features as well as the antibody status (F1 0.94). However, a projection of the antibody status into a higher-dimensional space was not required and did not significantly affect the results compared to one-hot encoding. In addition, the influence of different initialization strategies for the FFM was investigated. This showed that image-preserving initialization of the fusion matrix slightly reduced classification accuracy. The goal of further research is to improve the results of image-only validation by using multimodal inputs only during training. Furthermore, there are several other clinical parameters such as age, gender, and Hb level that should also be investigated. We will also validate the described method with an external data set to demonstrate the generality of our method.

References

1. He K, Zhang X, Ren S, Sun J. Deep residual learning for image recognition. Proc IEEE CVPR. 2016:770–8.
2. Baltrušaitis T, Ahuja C, Morency LP. Multimodal machine learning: a survey and taxonomy. IEEE Trans Pattern Anal Mach Intell. 2019;41(2):423–43.
3. Huang SC, Pareek A, Seyyedi S, Banerjee I, Lungren MP. Fusion of medical imaging and electronic health records using deep learning: a systematic review and implementation guidelines. NPJ Digit Med. 2020;3(1):1–9.
4. Russakovsky O, Deng J, Su H, Krause J, Satheesh S, Ma S et al. Imagenet large scale visual recognition challenge. Int J Comput Vis. 2015;115(3):211–52.
5. Raghu M, Zhang C, Kleinberg J, Bengio S. Transfusion: Understanding transfer learning for medical imaging. Adv Neural Inf Process Syst. 2019;32:3347–57.
6. He K, Zhang X, Ren S, Sun J. Delving deep into rectifiers: Surpassing human-level performance on ImageNet classification. Proc IEEE ICCV. 2015:1026–34.

Form Follows Function

Smart Network Design Enables Zero-shot Network Reuse

Weilin Fu[1,2], Lennart Husvogt[1,4], Katharina Breininger[1], Roman Schaffert[1],
Omar Abu-Qamar[5], James G. Fujimoto[4], Andreas Maier[1,3]

[1]Pattern Recognition Lab, Friedrich-Alexander University
[2]International Max Planck Research School Physics of Light (IMPRS-PL)
[3]Erlangen Graduate School in Advanced Optical Technologies(SAOT)
[4]Biomedical Optical Imaging and Biophotonics Group, MIT, Cambridge, USA
[5]New England Eye Center, Tufts Medical Center, Boston, MA, USA
weilin.fu@fau.de

Abstract. In this work, we construct and train a learning-based neural network pipeline for retinal vessel segmentation on fundus images and transfer the preprocessing module directly onto OCTA en face projections. Without additional fine-tuning, the transferred module retains the edge-preserving denoising functionality, as our smart network design enables zero-shot domain adaptation. Compared to a denoising network trained on OCTA data, the transferred preprocessing module is superior with regard to performance, generalization ability, and numerical stability. In addition, Frangi's vessel segmentation of the preprocessed images outperforms the predictions using pretrained full segmentation networks. The selection of fitting Gaussian scales of the Frangi filter in the target domain can bypass the over/under-segmentation problem caused by the vessel diameter mismatch between the two domains. The contribution of this work is two-fold: we provide an exemplary evidence that smart design of network pipelines allows for flexible functional module reuse across different imaging modalities, i.e. zero-shot domain adaptation; and we discover a deep learning-based vessel segmentation pipeline for OCTA en face images which reaches an AUC score of 0.9418 without additional training.

1 Introduction

Optical Coherence Tomography Angiography (OCTA) and fundus photography are two widely used imaging modalities in ophthalmology [1]. Image quality improvement in both modalities can assist the analysis of many eye-related diseases. In [2], a denoising autoencoder built upon total variational multi-norm loss function minimization is applied on fundus photographs. In [3], a dilated-residual U-Net (DRUNET) [4] is trained to enhance the image quality of OCT B-scans. Both models are trained with corrupted and clean image pairs. Another approach which avoids the requirement of noisy-clean image pairs is built on the idea of known operator learning [5]. In [6], a preprocessing module is embedded into a segmentation pipeline for retinal vessel segmentation from fundus photographs, and is proven to serve as an edge-preserving denoising filter. However, due to the lack of publicly available training data with corresponding vessel annotations, the same method cannot be reproduced on OCTA data.

© Der/die Autor(en), exklusiv lizenziert durch
Springer Fachmedien Wiesbaden GmbH, ein Teil von Springer Nature 2022
K. Maier-Hein et al. (Hrsg.), *Bildverarbeitung für die Medizin 2022*,
Informatik aktuell, https://doi.org/10.1007/978-3-658-36932-3_26

Domain adaptation [7] provides a promising direction for cross-modality knowledge transfer. In this work, we investigate on zero-shot domain adaptation across the source fundus and the target OCTA domains. To do so, we require network modules with specific functions, such that they would be transferable and reusable without further tuning and could be engineered into pipelines for alternative tasks as known operations [5]. To achieve this, we define a preprocessing interface using a custom loss function. The preprocessing quality of the module is compared against the classical bilateral filter and a denoising DRUNET. As figure of merit, we compare the resulting vessel maps with the ground truth created from an expensive 30-fold OCTA repeat scan. Analysis of the evaluation metrics shows that the transferred module achieves superior preprocessing performance comparing to the bilateral filter and the DRUNET. Additionally, it is proved that the proposed pipeline outperforms the one-shot transferred full segmentation network pipeline [6] as for avoiding over/under-segmentation of vessels with mismatched diameters.

2   Methods and material

2.1   Proposed methods

The proposed vessel preprocessing module (VP) is a three-level U-Net with 16 filters in the initial convolutional layer. The module is trained within a fundus retinal vessel segmentation pipeline following the approach in [6]. It is constrained by an ℓ_2-regularizer, aiming to generate enhanced images that resemble the inputs, i.e., we design an interface in the output layer of the VP module that will restrict its function to preprocessing according to the definition of Niemann [8]. On fundus images, the pretrained VP module serves as a denoising filter which preserves and enhances vessel information. The module is then directly transferred onto OCTA en face projections.

Two baseline preprocessing methods are implemented for comparison. The bilateral filter is utilized. The parameters are set to $\sigma_{spatial} = 1.0, \sigma_{intensity} = 0.2$ according to a preliminary grid search. The DRUNET [4] is modified as followings: the transpose convolutional (Conv) layer is replaced with an upsampling followed by 1×1 Conv layer to avoid checkerboard artifacts, and the activation functions are switched from ELU to ReLU to save computational power.

A quantitative evaluation of the preprocessing step is performed. The Frangi vesselness responses of the preprocessed images are compared against a manually annotated vessel map, which is validated by an OCTA expert. In order to create OCTA data of maximal quality, the subject was scanned 30 times to enable averaging. The Gaussian scales of the Frangi filter are set from 0.5 to 1.4 with a step size of 0.3. To validate the necessity of modularized network block transfer, the segmentation performance of two full segmentation pipelines [6], which are pretrained on fundus data and directly applied on OCTA data, are also reported. One model is the three-level U-Net, the other is the VP module + Frangi-Net pipeline, which has eight Gaussian scales ranging from $\sigma = 0.5$ to $\sigma = 4.0$. Common evaluation metrics for pixel-wise segmentation, such as the AUC score, F1 score, accuracy, sensitivity, specificity and SSIM are analyzed for various pipelines: DFF, short for Direct Frangi Filter without preprocessing; BFF, short for Bilateral Filter + Frangi Filter; DRF, short for DRUNET + Frangi Filter; VFF, short for VP module + Frangi Filter; DUN, short for pretrained U-Net transfer without preprocessing; and VFN, short for VP module + Frangi-Net.

2.2 Data

2.2.1 Fundus database. The DRIVE [9] database is used to train the VP + Frangi-Net segmentation pipeline. DRIVE contains 20 training and 20 testing RGB fundus photographs of 565×584 pixels. Four images are randomly selected as the validation set. The preparation procedure follows that in [6].

2.2.2 OCTA database. Two databases of 2-D OCTA en face projections are utilized. The single-scan OCTA volumes of both databases are acquired with a prototype ultrahigh speed swept source OCT at the Massachusetts Institute of Technology [10].

For testing purposes, we utilize 30 registered en face projections of OCTA volumes acquired from a healthy 28-year-old male volunteer. The OCTA volumes are 500 A-scans by 100 B-scans by 250 pixels in the axial direction, and the en face projections measure 100×500 pixels. The projection images are accumulatively averaged in ten random sequences, achieving ten slightly different testing sets of 30 images with gradually enhanced image quality for standard deviation computation. To train the DRUNET, a second dataset of 9 registered OCTA en face projections of shape 400×400 is used. The projections are generated from volumes with 400 A-scans by 400 B-scans by 700 pixels in the axial direction.

To roughly align the intensity range of the vessel regions of interest in the source and target domains, testing images (I) are firstly normalized to $(0, 1)$, then the transform $I = 1 - 3 \cdot \Gamma_{0.8}(I)$ is applied, where $\Gamma_{0.8}(\cdot)$ represents a gamma transform with $\gamma = 0.8$.

3 Results

The mean and standard deviation of different experiment pipelines over the ten testing sets are reported. Quantitative results for the average images of 1, 5, 10, 15, 20, 25, 30 single scans are presented in Tables 1 and 2. Preprocessed testing image patches using the VP module and the denoising DRUNET are presented in Figure 1. Both methods can visibly reduce the noise level, yet the VP module is more competent in preserving and enhancing the vessel connectivity. It can be observed that with the VP module, the 10-scan-average image approaches the quality of the 30-scan-average image. To compare the segmentation performance of all employed pipelines, the binarized segmentation maps from a 10-scan-average image are displayed in Figure 2. Direct visual inspection indicates that the differences between DFF and BFF pipelines are marginal, while VFF achieves considerably improved segmentation masks. The pretrained full segmentation pipelines, namely DUN and VFN, as well as the DRUNET tend to ignore tiny vessel while over-segment thick ones. Quantitative evaluation confirm that VFF achieves the best performance w.r.t. almost all metrics, reaching an AUC score of 0.9132 with 10 scans, and 0.9418 with 30 scans.

Tab. 1. Quantitative evaluation of all experiment pipelines over the average image of different numbers of single scan projections. (Part 1)

	DFF	BFF	DRF	VFF	VFN	DUN
			SSIM			
1	.3821±.0630	.3639±.0614	.4493±.0670	.3206±.0473	.2829±.0367	.2391±.0307
5	.5761±.0243	.5535±.0251	.6422±.0069	.5843±.0371	.4500±.0285	.4767±.0298
10	.6440±.0092	.6289±.0095	.6528±.0088	.6768±.0099	.5189±.0108	.5535±.0103
15	.6658±.0037	.6525±.0063	.6586±.0051	.7092±.0041	.5431±.0070	.5766±.0052
20	.6787±.0029	.6683±.0048	.6560±.0110	.7331±.0033	.5583±.0063	.5918±.0045
25	.6869±.0026	.6792±.0027	.5942±.0199	.7493±.0038	.5659±.0041	.5999±.0051
30	.6907±.0000	.6832±.0000	.6334±.0099	.7591±.0000	.5673±.0000	.6072±.0000
			AUC			
1	.7600±.0414	.7596±.0413	.7770±.0390	.7349±.0375	.7225±.0292	.7651±.0267
5	.8665±.0078	.8667±.0081	.8884±.0042	.8761±.0133	.8258±.0191	.8629±.0136
10	.8921±.0036	.8929±.0036	.8940±.0041	.9132±.0041	.8633±.0057	.8933±.0039
15	.9014±.0010	.9022±.0011	.8972±.0027	.9260±.0019	.8753±.0042	.9027±.0017
20	.9067±.0017	.9073±.0018	.8991±.0026	.9340±.0014	.8835±.0026	.9085±.0017
25	.9104±.0007	.9113±.0009	.8609±.0110	.9389±.0010	.8881±.0020	.9125±.0009
30	.9128±.0000	.9135±.0000	.8829±.0048	.9418±.0000	.8894±.0000	.9144±.0000
			F1 score			
1	.5888±.0644	.5841±.0617	.6290±.0619	.5324±.0647	.3951±.0656	.3272±.0738
5	.7477±.0114	.7440±.0140	.7839±.0052	.7566±.0212	.6203±.0326	.6593±.0292
10	.7864±.0060	.7813±.0047	.7918±.0058	.8097±.0051	.6901±.0114	.7260±.0089
15	.7984±.0041	.7952±.0040	.7956±.0037	.8299±.0030	.7129±.0065	.7434±.0055
20	.8069±.0026	.8024±.0034	.7961±.0048	.8453±.0022	.7267±.0054	.7551±.0040
25	.8120±.0020	.8093±.0023	.7506±.0158	.8553±.0019	.7338±.0035	.7613±.0055
30	.8140±.0000	.8111±.0000	.7786±.0071	.8622±.0000	.7349±.0000	.7673±.0000
			Accuracy			
1	.7647±.0269	.7625±.0265	.7759±.0276	.7454±.0208	.7213±.0153	.7088±.0140
5	.8381±.0062	.8353±.0065	.8542±.0026	.8404±.0097	.7909±.0105	.7998±.0104
10	.8579±.0027	.8554±.0027	.8584±.0025	.8707±.0028	.8175±.0032	.8287±.0038
15	.8650±.0014	.8622±.0018	.8613±.0016	.8830±.0023	.8274±.0024	.8374±.0016
20	.8695±.0012	.8670±.0016	.8622±.0020	.8924±.0014	.8333±.0019	.8427±.0014
25	.8725±.0008	.8704±.0011	.8348±.0086	.8988±.0012	.8367±.0015	.8458±.0014
30	.8736±.0000	.8718±.0000	.8507±.0039	.9033±.0000	.8377±.0000	.8480±.0000
			Sensitivity			
1	.5014±.0734	.4957±.0695	.5661±.0806	.4326±.0721	.2720±.0590	.2125±.0564
5	.7071±.0174	.7064±.0257	.7798±.0158	.7333±.0404	.5058±.0448	.5736±.0465
10	.7712±.0158	.7617±.0097	.7942±.0180	.8114±.0115	.5998±.0221	.6693±.0167
15	.7884±.0163	.7887±.0114	.7962±.0137	.8410±.0050	.6318±.0124	.6948±.0151
20	.8040±.0114	.7964±.0113	.7932±.0152	.8665±.0076	.6534±.0109	.7152±.0123
25	.8120±.0085	.8106±.0092	.7337±.0268	.8815±.0060	.6635±.0063	.7252±.0161
30	.8152±.0000	.8111±.0000	.7738±.0138	.8920±.0000	.6632±.0000	.7391±.0000

Tab. 2. Quantitative evaluation of all experiment pipelines over the average image of different numbers of single scan projections. (Part 2)

	DFF	BFF	DRF	VFF	VFN	DUN
			Specificity			
1	.8998±.0086	.8994±.0105	.8835±.0120	.9060±.0194	.9520±.0160	.9636±.0161
5	.9054±.0052	.9015±.0062	.8924±.0080	.8954±.0085	.9372±.0086	.9159±.0102
10	.9024±.0065	.9035±.0043	.8914±.0081	.9011±.0043	.9292±.0079	.9105±.0055
15	.9043±.0080	.9000±.0047	.8947±.0070	.9046±.0042	.9278±.0041	.9106±.0067
20	.9031±.0061	.9033±.0054	.8976±.0066	.9058±.0041	.9257±.0036	.9081±.0060
25	.9035±.0042	.9012±.0048	.8867±.0085	.9077±.0033	.9256±.0021	.9076±.0067
30	.9037±.0000	.9030±.0000	.8902±.0048	.9091±.0000	.9273±.0000	.9038±.0000

4 Discussion

In this work, we explore a preprocessing interface to create a vessel preprocessing module that is directly transferred from source fundus data to target OCTA en face data without further need for fine-tuning. It is observed that DRUNET remarkably enhances the image quality, especially for the more noise-corrupted input images. Interestingly, input images of the DRUNET with enhanced quality do not coincide with improved segmentation performance. Besides, both ignorance of small vessels and over-emphasis on thick ones are observed independent of the number of averaged scan projections. In contrast, the quality of the processed image improves stably with better quality of the input for the VP module. This indicates that the DRUNET is overfitted to noisy input and thick vessels, while VP module generalizes well on varied data distributions. As for model stability, DRUNET is also inferior to the VP module. Numerical differences between the 10 30-scan average images, which are at the magnitude of 10^{-7}, cause non-zero standard deviations in all evaluation metrics in DRUNET. Comparing the vessel segmentation results of the VFF with the pretrained full segmentation pipelines, we

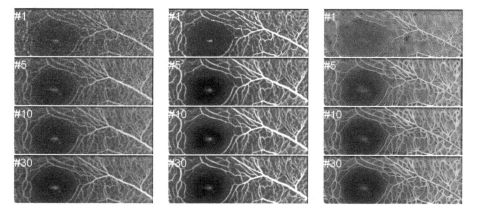

Fig. 1. Preprocessed average images of different numbers of single projections. From left to right columns: original, DRUNET processed and VP module processed patches.

Fig. 2. Overlay (yellow) of the vessel segmentation map of a 10-scan-average image from different experiments (green) with the ground truth (red).

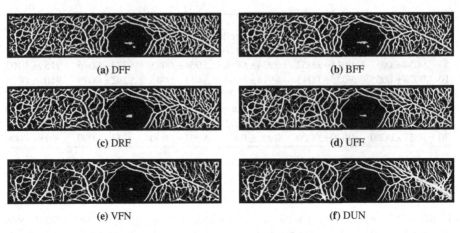

(a) DFF

(b) BFF

(c) DRF

(d) UFF

(e) VFN

(f) DUN

conclude that the re-selection of fitting Frangi filter scales circumvents the problem of vessel diameter mismatch between the two modalities.

References

1. Skalet AH, Li Y, Lu CD et al. Optical coherence tomography angiography characteristics of iris melanocytic tumors. Ophthalmol. 2017.
2. Biswas B, Ghosh SK, Ghosh A. DVAE: deep variational auto-encoders for denoising retinal fundus image. Hybrid Machine Intelligence for Medical Image Analysis. 2020:257–73.
3. Devalla SK, Chin KS, Mari JM, Tun TA, Strouthidis NG, Aung T et al. A deep learning approach to digitally stain optical coherence tomography images of the optic nerve head. Invest Ophthalmol Vis Sci. 2018.
4. Ronneberger O, Fischer P, Brox T. U-Net: convolutional networks for biomedical image segmentation. MICCAI. 2015.
5. Maier AK, Syben C, Stimpel B, Würfl T, Hoffmann M, Schebesch F et al. Learning with known operators reduces maximum error bounds. Nat Mach Intell. 2019.
6. Fu W, Breininger K, Schaffert R, Ravikumar N, Maier AK. A divide-and-conquer approach towards understanding deep networks. MICCAI. 2019.
7. Wilson G, Cook DJ. A survey of unsupervised deep domain adaptation. arXiv preprint arXiv:1812.02849. 2018.
8. Niemann H. Pattern analysis. Vol. 4. Springer Science & Business Media, 2012.
9. Staal J, Abràmoff MD, Niemeijer M, Viergever MA, Van Ginneken B. Ridge-based vessel segmentation in color images of the retina. IEEE Trans Med Imaging. 2004;23(4):501–9.
10. Choi W, Moult EM, Waheed NK et al. Ultrahigh-speed, swept-source optical coherence tomography angiography in nonexudative age-related macular degeneration with geographic atrophy. Ophthalmol. 2015.

Abstract: C-arm Positioning for Spinal Standard Projections in Different Intra-operative Settings

Lisa Kausch[1,2], Sarina Thomas[1], Holger Kunze[3], Tobias Norajitra[1], André Klein[1,2], Jan El Barbari[4], Maxim Privalov[4], Sven Vetter[4], Andreas Mahnken[5], Lena Maier-Hein[1], Klaus Maier-Hein[1]

[1]CAMIC, German Cancer Research Center, Heidelberg
[2]Medical Faculty, Heidelberg University
[3]Advanced Therapy Systems Division, Siemens Healthineers, Erlangen
[4]MINTOS Research Group, Trauma Surgery Clinic Ludwigshafen
[5]Division of Diagnostic and Interventional Radiology, University Hospital Marburg
l.kausch@dkfz-heidelberg.de

Trauma and orthopedic surgeries that involve fluoroscopic guidance crucially depend on the acquisition of correct anatomy-specific standard projections for monitoring and evaluating the surgical result. This implies repeated acquisitions or even continuous fluoroscopy. To reduce radiation exposure and time, we propose to automate this procedure and estimate the C-arm pose update directly from a first X-ray without the need for a pre-operative computed tomography scan (CT) or additional technical equipment. Our method is trained on digitally reconstructed radiographs (DRRs) which uniquely provide ground truth labels for arbitrary many training examples. The simulated images are complemented with automatically generated segmentations, landmarks, as well as a k-wire and screw simulation. To successfully achieve a transfer from simulated to real X-rays, and also to increase the interpretability of results, the pipeline was designed by closely reflecting on the actual clinical decision-making of spinal neurosurgeons. It explicitly incorporates steps like region-of-interest (ROI) localization, detection of relevant and view-independent landmarks, and subsequent pose regression. To validate the method on real X-rays, we performed a large specimen study with and without implants (i.e. k-wires and screws). The proposed procedure obtained superior C-arm positioning accuracy ($p_{\mathrm{Wilcoxon}} \ll 0.01$), robustness, and generalization capabilities compared to the state-of-the-art direct pose regression framework. This work was first presented at MICCAI 2021 [1].

References

1. Kausch L, Thomas S, Kunze H, Norajitra T, Klein A, El Barbari J et al. C-arm positioning for spinal standard projections in different intra-operative setting. International Conference on Med Image Comput Comput Assist Interv. 2021:352–62.

© Der/die Autor(en), exklusiv lizenziert durch
Springer Fachmedien Wiesbaden GmbH, ein Teil von Springer Nature 2022
K. Maier-Hein et al. (Hrsg.), *Bildverarbeitung für die Medizin 2022*,
Informatik aktuell, https://doi.org/10.1007/978-3-658-36932-3_27

Abstract: Verbesserung des 2D U-Nets für die 3D Mikrotomographie mit Synchrotronstrahlung mittels Multi-Axes Fusing

Ivo M. Baltruschat[1], Hanna Ćwieka[2], Diana Krüger[2], Berit Zeller-Plumhoff[2], Frank Schlünzen[1], Regine Willumeit-Römer[2], Julian Moosmann[3], Philipp Heuser[1,4]

[1]Deutsches Elektronen-Synchrotron DESY, Notkestr. 85, 22607 Hamburg, Germany
[2]Institute of Metallic Biomaterials, Helmholtz-Zentrum hereon, Geesthacht, Germany
[3]Institute of Materials Physics, Helmholtz-Zentrum hereon, Geesthacht, Germany
[4]Helmholtz Imaging, Deutsches Elektronen-Synchrotron DESY, Germany
ivo.baltruschat@desy.de

Die genaue Segmentierung großer 3D-Volumina ist eine sehr zeitaufwendige und für die Analyse und Interpretation unabdingbare Aufgabe. Die am Synchrotron gemessene Mikrotomogramme (SRµCT) zu segmentieren, ist besonders anspruchsvoll, sowohl für algorithmische Lösungen, als auch für die Experten, da sich die Daten durch geringen Kontrast, hohe räumliche Variabilität und Messartefakte auszeichnen. Am Beispiel von 3D Tomogrammen zu Biodegradationsprozessen von Knochenimplantaten untersuchten wir die Skalierung des 2D U-Nets für hochaufgelöste Graustufenvolumina unter Verwendung von drei wichtigen Modellhyperparametern (d. h. Modellbreite, -tiefe und Eingabegröße) [1]. Um die 3D-Informationen der SRµCTs zu nutzen, wird die Vorhersage der Segmentierung aus drei orthogonalen Blickrichtungen gemacht und anschließendem Fusionieren derselben. Wir haben diese Fusionierung erweitert und den Effekt der Nutzung von mehr als drei Achsen untersucht. In der Auswertung vergleichen wir die Ergebnisse der Skalierung des U-Nets durch Intersection over Union (IoU) und quantitative Messungen von Osseointegrations- und Degradationsparametern. Zusammenfassend lässt sich feststellen, dass eine kombinierte Skalierung des U-Netzes (d.h. alle drei Modellparameter werden gemeinsam geändert) und eine Mehrachsenvorhersage, die mit Soft Voting fusioniert wird, den höchsten IoU für die Klasse „Degradationsschicht" von 0.813 gegenüber der Baseline von 0.801 ergibt. Abschließend zeigte die quantitative Analyse, dass die auf der Grundlage der Modellsegmentierung berechneten Parameter weniger von den Ground-Truth-Ergebnissen abwichen als die auf der Grundlage der halbautomatischen Segmentierungsmethode berechneten.

References

1. Baltruschat IM, Ćwieka H, Krüger D, Zeller-Plumhoff B, Schlünzen F, Willumeit-Römer R et al. Scaling the U-Net: segmentation of biodegradable bone implants in high-resolution synchrotron radiation microtomograms. Sci Rep. 2021;11(1):24237.

© Der/die Autor(en), exklusiv lizenziert durch
Springer Fachmedien Wiesbaden GmbH, ein Teil von Springer Nature 2022
K. Maier-Hein et al. (Hrsg.), *Bildverarbeitung für die Medizin 2022*,
Informatik aktuell, https://doi.org/10.1007/978-3-658-36932-3_28

Efficient Patient Orientation Detection in Videofluoroscopy Swallowing Studies

Luisa Neubig[1], René Groh[1], Melda Kunduk[2], Deirdre Larsen[2], Rebecca Leonard[3], Andreas M. Kist[1]

[1]Department Artificial Intelligence in Biomedical Engineering, Friedrich-Alexander-University Erlangen-Nürnberg, Germany
[2]Department of Communication Sciences and Disorders, Louisiana State University, USA
[3]University of California, Davis, USA
andreas.kist@fau.de

Abstract. Swallowing disorders are commonly examined using videofluoroscopy swallowing studies (VFSS). To comprehensively evaluate the swallowing process, a typical VFSS contains different patient orientations. In order to quantify the swallowing physiology, a VFSS is systematically and temporally segmented for different patient orientations. However, no fully automatic temporal segmentation tool is available. Here, we show that in general multiple deep neural networks (DNNs) are suitable for this task. We found that a variety of optimization algorithms result in generalizing DNNs. Using a systematic architectural scaling approach, we found that an efficient ResNet18 variant is sufficient to classify a full VFSS recording of about 1800 frames in less than 14 s on conventional CPUs. In the future, our findings allow a successful clinical implementation.

1 Introduction

Swallowing disorders are commonly investigated via fiberoptic endoscopy or VFSS [1]. During a VFSS, the patient swallows multiple Barium-containing boluses of varying texture and size [2]. This swallowing process is recorded at 30 frames per second (fps) with single X-ray images [3]. To visualize different aspects of the swallowing behavior,

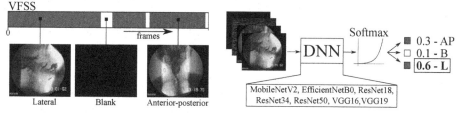

Fig. 1. Workflow of patient orientation detection. Image classes are lateral (blue), anterior-posterior (red) and blank (white). Each recording frame is classified independently using a deep neural network (DNN) into one of the three classes.

© Der/die Autor(en), exklusiv lizenziert durch
Springer Fachmedien Wiesbaden GmbH, ein Teil von Springer Nature 2022
K. Maier-Hein et al. (Hrsg.), *Bildverarbeitung für die Medizin 2022*,
Informatik aktuell, https://doi.org/10.1007/978-3-658-36932-3_29

different patient orientations are recorded, namely in a lateral and anterior-posterior view [3]. One recording consists of concatenated swallows of different patient orientations interspaced with blank or noisy images, summarized with the term blank. These three VFSS image classes are shown in Figure 1. The sequence of patient orientations and their duration in VFSS is strongly dependent on the patient and the examination. As a result, the temporal distribution of single VFSS events can hardly be known a-priori.

In the clinic, VFSS are visually graded and interpreted by the examiner. However, deep learning approaches that rely on the application of DNNs are emerging. DNNs are used to extract quantitative information, such as bolus location and hyoid bone trajectories [4, 5], but are mostly trained for a single patient orientation. These DNNs could be used to leverage the potential of finding patterns in VFSS [6] or to extract quantitative measures to identify dysphagia risk [7]. Patient orientation detection is therefore crucial to allow a fully automatic data analysis of a VFSS. This includes categorizing individual swallows dependent on patient orientation and selecting the most appropriate downstream DNN for further image analysis. However, to our knowledge, this issue has not been addressed in literature. We hypothesized that DNNs for image classification are good candidates for fully automatic patient orientation detection.

In this work, we mined a selection of established DNNs to classify single images if they were acquired in lateral or anterior-posterior patient orientation, or if these images only contain artifacts. We found that multiple DNNs are able to tackle this task, where ResNet18 is not only among the most accurate techniques, but also the fastest. We further optimized the ResNet18 architecture to minimize the computational costs while maintaining high classification accuracy.

2   Materials and methods

We were provided 8 and 136 VFSS recordings by Louisiana State University (LSU) and the University of California, Davis (UC Davis), respectively, resulting in a dataset containing 144 VFSS recordings in total. These recordings were performed in agreement with the respective ethical review committees. Each VFSS was labeled by LN, in consultation with our medical cooperation partner of LSU and UC Davis, in sections from one of the three image classes (lateral, anterior-posterior and blank) using a custom written annotation tool.

Next, we generated a database of single images. First, we split the dataset in 124 videos (87 %) for training and 20 videos (13 %) for testing. In addition, 10 % of training data was used for validation to regularize the training process, e.g., avoid overfitting. For each video, class and annotated event, we extracted up to 20 individual frames. As there was no common resolution among the VFSS recordings, we resized all images to 224 × 224 px. Prior to training, images were normalized to the range of 0 to 1. To increase the variation among the training dataset, we incorporated data augmentation. We used horizontal flip because this transformation was already present in the data due to the different acquisition orientations of the recordings. The sequences predominantly consisted of images classified as lateral, as it represents the main patient orientation in a typical VFSS. This resulted in an imbalance for the three classes. In detail, the training set consisted of 5334 images for lateral and 1409 images for anterior-posterior patient orientation. 1266 images were classified as blank.

DNNs were setup, trained and evaluated using TensorFlow/Keras (version 2.1.0/2.3.1). For this study, we used the following DNN architectures in their default configuration as core model: MobileNetV2, ResNet50, VGG16, VGG19, EfficientNetB0, ResNet34, ResNet18. After this core model, we added a GlobalAveragePooling2D layer and a Dense layer with three units and softmax activation comprising the full model. We trained every full model with a variety of optimizers, namely Adam, Nadam, Adadelta, Adagrad, Adamax, RMSprop and SGD(momentum = 0.9). Training was performed for 40 epochs with a learning rate of 1×10^{-4} optimizing the categorical cross-entropy loss. We trained and measured model inference on an RTX 2080 Ti GPU. For proving the applicability of the patient orientation detection in clinics, we additionally measured the inference time on a user-grade CPU (Intel(R) Xeon(R) Silver 4110 CPU).

3   Results

We selected seven established architectures and seven optimization algorithms to estimate which combination is the most suitable for our data. Therefore, we trained and evaluated each combination in terms of validation and test accuracy. The validation accuracy, shown in Figure 2a, showed in most of the combinations more than 90 % accuracy

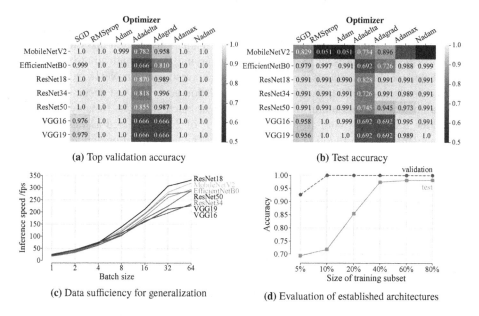

(a) Top validation accuracy

(b) Test accuracy

(c) Data sufficiency for generalization

(d) Evaluation of established architectures

Fig. 2. Evaluation of the performance on validation data (a) and test data (b) of established architectures with respect to the accuracy. (c) Visualization of the inference speed over the batch size of the established architectures in. (d) covers how much data is needed to achieve generalization along training.

on the validation data. Only training with Adadelta or Adagrad showed insufficient classification accuracy leading only to chance-level estimations in some configurations. The evaluation of the test accuracy shown in Figure 2b, shows that most of the DNNs achieve a test accuracy close to 100 %. MobileNetV2 is the only architecture that does not generalize and performs worse on novel data.

As inference time is a crucial factor for clinical application, we investigated the inference speed for each neural network. We found that only with a batch size greater or equal to eight, the inference speed across DNN architectures differ (Fig. 2c). Our analysis shows that ResNet18 outperforms all other architectures and is capable of processing more than 300 fps at a batch size of 64. ResNet18 has nearly identical performance on unseen data as the competing architectures, but it is significantly faster. Therefore, we chose ResNet18 as the basis for subsequent experiments. The reliability of DNNs is key for its applicability in clinical practice. Hence, we considered if the amount of provided VFSS data is sufficient to make reliable predictions, i.e. the test accuracy was higher than 95 %. In the following the term prediction covers the prognosis on the patient orientation in the regarding frame of the VFSS. We systematically varied the amount of training data (5 %, 10 %, 20 %, 40 %, 60 % and 80 %), while keeping the size and the data of the test set constant. Using 10-fold cross validation, we found that with 40 % of the total data, we gain a reliable and robust model (Fig. 2d), indicating that our data pool is sufficiently large enough for clinical applications.

As DNNs are often overparameterized for a given problem, we mined the ResNet18 architecture (Fig. 3a). The ResNet18 architecture relies on the hyperparameter regarding the initial filter size F that scales the channels throughout the architecture. By default, F is set to 64, resulting in a model with around 11M parameters (Tab. 1). We hypothesized that a lower F value is still sufficient for patient orientation classification. We therefore trained the ResNet18 architecture by varying F systematically to 2, 4, 8, 16, 32, 48 and 64. Table 1 shows the evaluation of the investigated ResNet18 variants (with respect to the initial filter sizes) regarding validation accuracy, test accuracy, number of parameters and prediction time (CPU, GPU at batch size 64). Notably, we found that even a ResNet18 with an initial filter size F of 2 (abbreviated as ResNet18-2F) has more than 95 % validation and test accuracy. The best validation and test accuracy

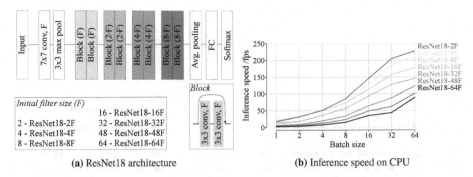

(a) ResNet18 architecture

(b) Inference speed on CPU

Fig. 3. (a) General ResNet18 architecture for varying initial filter size F. (b) Inference speed on CPU for varying initial filter size F over different batch size for multiple ResNet18 configurations.

Tab. 1. Comparing metrics of different ResNet18 configurations with varying initial filter size F.

ResNet18 Initial filter size	Validation accuracy	Test accuracy	Number of parameters	Prediction time /s CPU (batch size 64)	Prediction time /s GPU (batch size 64)
2F	1.000	0.992	11,298	13.66	10.64
4F	1.000	0.994	44,392	14.41	10.18
8F	1.000	1.000	175,98	16.25	10.07
16F	1.000	0.991	700,756	18.14	10.46
32F	1.000	0.991	2,796,708	25.04	10.53
48F	1.000	0.984	6,287,860	33.63	11.13
64F	1.000	0.992	11,174,212	44.98	12.21

of 100 % was represented by the ResNet18 architecture with an initial filter size F of 8 (ResNet18-8F). The model parameters across F configurations varied significantly. ResNet18 architectures with an initial filter size F of 2, 4 or 8 only contained 0.1% - 2% of the parameters of the original ResNet18 model.

We next were interested in the effect of F on the inference speed. We investigated how inference speed is dependent on F and the batch size (Fig. 3b). As we aim for a clinical implementation, we tested the inference speed on a CPU. We found that ResNet18-2F outperforms every other architecture, and has more than twice the frame rate as the ResNet18-64F implementation while keeping the same test accuracy (Fig. 3b).

The image classification is, however, only a small part of the detection workflow. Consequently, we investigated the total processing time including the prediction of the patient orientation in each frame and the preprocessing of the VFSS data itself. We analyzed an entire VFSS recording consisting of ca. 1800 frames using CPU or GPU. Figure 4a shows that there is a negligible difference between the prediction time of the ResNet18-2F and ResNet18-64F on the GPU. However, we observe an enormous difference between the two implementations when using CPU for inference. While the ResNet18-64F needs 200 s for loading, preprocessing and predicting the patient orientation of an entire VFSS using a batch size of one, the ResNet18-2F

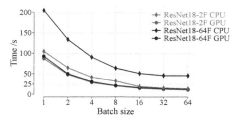

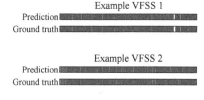

(a) Prediction time including loading and preprocessing of the VFSS

(b) Exemplary qualitative assessment on two entire VFSS

Fig. 4. (a) shows the decreasing of required time of the DNNs for predicting the patient orientation in each frame of a VFSS based on the batch size. (b) compares the prediction of each frame against the corresponding ground truth.

is able to complete this process in only half of the time. Finally, the ResNet18-2F can also compete with the prediction time on the GPU, showing that all three test cases (ResNet18-2F(GPU), ResNet18-2F(CPU) and ResNet18-64F(GPU)) require the same time with a batch size of equal to or greater than 16. This indicates that using a ResNet18-2F with a batch size of 16 and larger creates the opportunity of a hardware independent efficient usage of the DNN. This configuration needs less than 25 seconds to process an entire VFSS recording of about ca. 1800 frames.

In addition to the characteristics of the ResNet18-2F architecture being fast and very efficient on several metrics, we were interested on the qualitative output of the ResNet18-2F. We compared the temporal VFSS segmentation of the ResNet18-2F against our manually labelled view class labels, which define our ground truth. Figure 4b shows a qualitatively high overlap of prediction and ground truth in both example VFSS recordings. This confirms that ResNet18-2F is both reliable and efficient in its predictions for clinical implementation.

4 Discussion

In this work, we showed that the ResNet18 DNN architecture with an initial filter size $F = 2$ is sufficient for efficient patient orientation detection in VFSS.

It is important to note that we relied in this study on the data of two independent institutions. However, it still remains to be seen how our findings perform on VFSS generated with different scanners and paradigms. Nevertheless, we believe that our findings will be a good starting point for downstream DNN selection and quantitative measure extractions.

References

1. Espitalier F, Fanous A, Aviv J, Bassiouny S, Desuter G, Nerurkar N et al. International consensus (ICON) on assessment of oropharyngeal dysphagia. Eur Ann Otorhinolaryngol Head Neck Dis. 2018;135(1):S17–S21.
2. Bonilha HS, Blair J, Carnes B, Huda W, Humphries K, McGrattan K et al. Preliminary investigation of the effect of pulse rate on judgments of swallowing impairment and treatment recommendations. Dysphagia. 2013;28(4):528–38.
3. Ingleby HR, Bonilha HS, Steele CM. A tutorial on diagnostic benefit and radiation risk in videofluoroscopic swallowing studies. Dysphagia. 2021.
4. Caliskan H, Mahoney AS, Coyle JL, Sejdić E. Automated bolus detection in videofluoroscopic images of swallowing using Mask-RCNN. 2020 42nd Annual International Conference of the IEEE Engineering in Medicine Biology Society (EMBC). 2020:2173–7.
5. Kim HI, Kim Y, Kim B, Shin DY, Lee SJ, Choi SI. Hyoid bone tracking in a videofluoroscopic swallowing study using a deep-learning-based segmentation network. Diagnostics. 2021;11(7).
6. Leonard R. Swallowing in the elderly: evidence from fluoroscopy. Perspectives on Swallowing and Swallowing Disorders (Dysphagia). 2010;19(4):103–14.
7. Vansant MB, Parker LA, McWhorter AJ, Bluoin D, Kunduk M. Predicting swallowing outcomes from objective videofluoroscopic timing and displacement measures in head and neck cancer patients. Dysphagia. 2020;35(5):853–63.

Towards Weakly Supervised Segmentation of Orthopaedic X-ray Images Using Constrained-CNN Losses

Nikolaus Arbogast[1,2], Holger Kunze[2,3], Florian Kordon[2,3,4], Benedict Swartman[5], Jan S. El Barbari[5], Katharina Breininger[1]

[1]Department Artificial Intelligence in Biomedical Engineering, FAU Erlangen-Nürnberg
[2]Siemens Healthineers AG
[3]Pattern Recognition Lab, FAU Erlangen-Nürnberg
[4]Erlangen Graduate School in Advanced Optical Technologies (SAOT), FAU Erlangen-Nürnberg
[5]BG Trauma Center Ludwigshafen
nikolaus.arbogast@fau.de

Abstract. In the past decade, deep neural networks have gained much attention in medical imaging applications. Especially fully supervised methods have received a lot of interest as medical decision making relies on robust predictions. The ability to be more flexible and adaptive to individual anatomical differences gives them an advantage compared to unsupervised methods. However, generating high-quality labels requires expert knowledge, attention to detail and is time-consuming. Replacing such high-quality labels with simpler annotations, such as scribbles, bounding boxes, and points, requires a network to fill in the missing information required to perform at full-supervision-like performance. This work investigates a constrained loss function integrated in a weakly supervised training of a convolutional neural network (CNN) to obtain segmentations of four different bones on lateral X-ray images of the knee. The evaluation of the different trained models with respect to the Dice coefficient shows that the proposed loss function can improve the mean Dice score across all bones from 0.262 to 0.759 by adding a size loss to the cross entropy function while using weak labels.

1 Introduction

Convolutional neural networks (CNNs) have revolutionized the segmentation of medical images [1]. While they outperform alternative approaches like thresholding techniques or adaptive contouring across a variety of tasks, large representative data sets are needed to train these networks. In medical applications, full supervision for the training of CNNs is typically applied to achieve high and robust segmentation performance. The downside of full supervision is the necessity of laborious data annotation for segmentation. Different strategies have been proposed to reduce the efforts when developing a CNN-based approach for a new task. A commonly employed technique is transfer learning, during which a network that was originally trained on a general or related task is fine-tuned for the task of interest [2]. While this can reduce the amount of training data needed and increase robustness, it typically still uses a fully annotated data set for fine-tuning. One alternative way to overcome this limitation is using weak labels [3]. Here, the annotated information does not cover the entire or the exact region of interest. Instead,

© Der/die Autor(en), exklusiv lizenziert durch
Springer Fachmedien Wiesbaden GmbH, ein Teil von Springer Nature 2022
K. Maier-Hein et al. (Hrsg.), *Bildverarbeitung für die Medizin 2022*,
Informatik aktuell, https://doi.org/10.1007/978-3-658-36932-3_30

the annotation may consist of only local annotations encompassing a limited number of pixels (e.g., point annotations, scribbles) or labels with reduced complexity (e.g., coarse polygonal annotations). Incorporating these weak labels in the training of a CNN is challenging since the resulting cost function tends to have multiple local minima [3], and inequality constraints can help to improve the training result as shown by Pathak et al. [4].

Kervadec et al. proposed a computationally more efficient cost function that directly incorporates an inequality constraint to integrate prior knowledge related to the size of the segmentation object [5]. They tested this approach on left ventricle, vertebral body, and prostate segmentation of magnetic resonance images (MRIs). In this paper, we study this constraint for the segmentation of more complex objects, namely femur, patella, tibia, and fibula, on lateral knee X-ray images. The bones have been selected to feature different sizes and height-width ratios. Furthermore, varying proportions of the bone are shown on the X-ray images. While bony structures often have comparatively well-defined boundaries in X-ray images, the transmissive nature of X-rays and overlapping structures represent unique challenges for weakly supervised learning. At the same time, the high volume of acquired X-ray images make them an ideal candidate to leverage the possibility of these approaches.

2 Materials and methods

In this section, we define how we incorporate the size constraint into the training, provide details on the data and describe the experiments conducted in this study.

2.1 Size loss

In the remainder of this work, we will refer to the defined inequality constraint as the *size loss*. Following Kervadec et al. [5], it can be expressed as

$$C(V_S) = \begin{cases} (V_S - a)^2, & \text{if } V_S < a \\ (V_S - b)^2, & \text{if } V_S > b \\ 0, & \text{otherwise} \end{cases} \quad (1)$$

where V_S is the sum over the per-pixel softmax predictions S for an input image, and a refers to the lower and b the upper size boundary for the object of interest. This means if the sum over the predictions lies in between the two size boundaries, no loss is added. Otherwise, the difference to the size boundary is penalized quadratically. For the selection of boundaries a and b different strategies are applicable:

2.1.1 Loose. All structures' lower and upper boundaries are set to 1 % and 25 % of the image size, respectively. This represents a case with almost no prior knowledge about the anatomical size of the objects of interest.

2.1.2 Equal. The lower and upper boundaries for all bone structures (femur, patella, tibia, and fibula) are set equally. The lower and upper boundaries are set as the smallest and largest bone size in the whole data set computed from the fully annotated ground truth labels.

2.1.3 Precise.

Individual lower and upper boundaries for each of the four bone structures are set, computed with a 10 % buffer from the individual smallest and largest size of the full mask labels, representing the case with more detailed prior knowledge about the size of the object of interest.

For the CNN training with weakly labeled data sets, the size loss can be added to the partial cross entropy H_{pCE} with a weighting factor λ [5]

$$L(S) = H_{pCE}(S) + \lambda C(V_S) \tag{2}$$

thereby penalizing both wrong predictions in image regions for which a (partial) label is available and a deviation from the expected size.

2.2 Data

For the study, 251 diagnostic lateral X-Ray images of the knee are used. Each image originates from a different subject and was manually annotated with full mask labels for the femur, fibula, patella, and tibia as a baseline for this work. Based on the weak label creation by Kervadec et al. [5], weak labels are created by eroding the original segmentation masks with a rectangular kernel of size 2 px×3 px ten times or fewer if the mask would be deleted. Furthermore, we create "spot" labels by randomly selecting a random foreground pixel in the ground truth mask as a weak annotation label in each training epoch. An example image with ground truth and corresponding weak labels is shown in Figure 1.

The data set is split randomly into a train, validation, and test set containing 163 (65 %), 38 (15 %), and 50 (20 %) images, respectively. Offline data augmentation was used to increase the training data by a factor of 10 with one of the following augmentations applied to each added image: Gaussian blur with random kernel size [5, 15], random brightening by ±50 %, random contrast scaling by ±75 %, horizontal

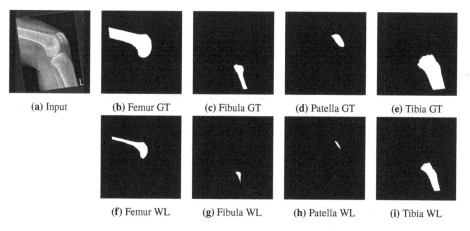

(a) Input	(b) Femur GT	(c) Fibula GT	(d) Patella GT	(e) Tibia GT
	(f) Femur WL	(g) Fibula WL	(h) Patella WL	(i) Tibia WL

Fig. 1. Example image with corresponding ground truth (GT) in the top row and eroded weak labels (WL) masks in the bottom row for femur, fibula, patella, and tibia.

Tab. 1. Dice coefficient on the test set for model settings full supervision (FS), partial cross entropy only (pCE only), loose size boundaries (Loose), equal size boundaries (Equal), precise size boundaries (Precise), and random spot label (Spot).

Bone	FS	pCE only	Loose	Equal	Precise	Spot
Femur	0.946	0.451	0.677	0.704	0.797	0.596
Fibula	0.915	0.178	0.220	0.495	0.691	0.815
Patella	0.916	0.118	0.181	0.717	0.827	0.914
Tibia	0.885	0.301	0.573	0.631	0.820	0.623

flip, vertical flip, random Poisson noise, random rotation by up to $\pm 179°$, sharpening with a random factor between $[1.0, 2.0]$, and random translation in x-/y-direction by up to ± 100 pixels. The images were down-sampled to 512×512 from their original resolution of 1024×1024. Afterwards, the images were normalized to a range between $[0, 1]$.

2.3 Experiments

To study the inequality constraints, we compare the CNN training with weak labels to a fully supervised training. For the training with weak labels a cost function with *no*, *loose*, *equal*, and *precise* size loss is performed. For the spot label, the *precise* size loss is applied. Following Kervadec et al.[5], we chose the efficiency net (ENet) [6] as the segmentation network. For the fully supervised training, cross entropy is chosen as cost function. Equation (2) is used as cost function for the training with weak labels to compare the different strategies to define the boundaries presented in Section 2.1. For all training runs, Adam optimizer with learning rate $5e^{-4}$ is chosen. For each configuration and each bone separately, a network is trained for 25 epochs (100 epochs for the training using spot label), ensuring convergence of the training. Finally, we determine the Dice score for each configuration on the test set for each of the four bone structures. The weighting factor λ of the size loss was set to 0.01.

3 Results

The results for all models selected based on the highest Dice coefficient on the validation set can be seen in Table 1. From the quantitative results, a clear trend can be observed. While the fully supervised approach yields an expected high performance between 0.945 and 0.885, the performance of the weakly supervised approaches increases with increasingly restrictive size boundaries. Furthermore, we see that the drop in performance strongly depends on the structure of interest, which likely relates to the size and shape of the bone. We see a strong relationship between segmentation performance and bone size for the spot label, with performance for the patella almost on par with the fully supervised setting. However, this observation is likely biased by the fact that the spot labels were generated randomly for each epoch separately. Qualitative segmentation masks of the femur and patella in comparison to full supervision are depicted in Figure 2 to juxtapose the performance on the largest and smallest bone.

4 Discussion

This work shows that for weakly supervised X-ray images, enforcing inequality constraints via the loss function of CNNs proposed in [5] can improve the results of weakly supervised training. As demonstrated in the experiments, a considerable improvement in segmentation performance can already be shown given only rough estimates of the object of interest's size and can therefore be used to explore anatomical regions for which no fully labeled data is available. Since the *precise* model, which uses structure-specific size boundaries, demonstrated the highest Dice score in our evaluation, a bootstrapping approach to refine structure-wise boundaries is an interesting direction for future research.

When looking at the segmentation results in more detail, errors can be found especially in more complex parts close to the border of the bone like notches or bulges. This is especially apparent for the femur, which often shows a more complex morphology in X-ray images. For the eroded weak labels, these boundary regions are typically not

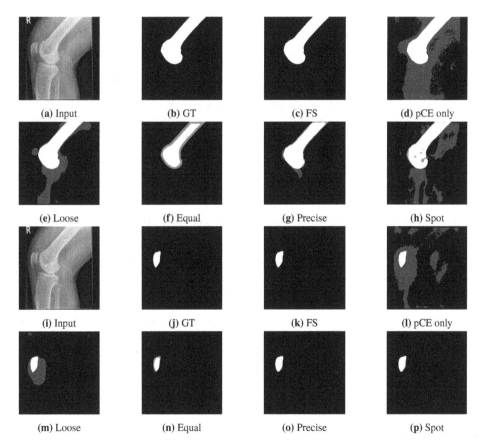

Fig. 2. Qualitative results of all models for femur (b-h) and patella (i-p) bone on an example image. Green: false positive pixels. Lilac: false negative pixels.

included in the supervised part of the cost function. Here, the performance of the spot-based annotations points toward an interesting remedy. Instead of using comparatively large static weak labels, the use of multiple smaller annotations that specifically include boundary regions seems to provide a superior coverage of the structures' variability. However, given that the spot labels were created randomly for this setting, the trade-off between the number of spot annotations and annotation time has to be further investigated. As a further limitation, it should be noted that the generation of weak labels using erosion is somewhat artificial. We expect that a similar annotation and training effect can be obtained by using a brush with a bone-specific size for weak annotations in a scribble-like fashion.

The investigated variants provide promising results for label-efficient training of CNN-based segmentation of X-ray images. Our experiments show that the performance is robust also for bones with large fluctuations in the part of structures visible in the X-ray images. Specifically, a small amount of fully labeled data enriched with scribble- or spot-like weak labels will allow to both define appropriate size boundaries and robustly learn segmentation tasks for X-ray images with limited annotation efforts.

Disclaimer. The methods and information presented here are based on research and are not commercially available.

Acknowledgement. The authors gratefully acknowledge funding of the Erlangen Graduate School in Advanced Optical Technologies (SAOT) by the Bavarian State Ministry for Science and Art. K. Breininger gratefully acknowledges the support of Siemens Healthineers within her endowed professorship program.

References

1. Hesamian MH, Jia W, He X, Kennedy P. Deep learning techniques for medical image segmentation: achievements and challenges. J Digit Imaging. 2019;32(4):582–96.
2. Dutta P, Upadhyay P, De M, Khalkar R. Medical image analysis using deep convolutional neural networks: CNN architectures and transfer learning. Proc ICICT. 2020:175–80.
3. Tajbakhsh N, Jeyaseelan L, Li Q, Chiang JN, Wu Z, Ding X. Embracing imperfect datasets: a review of deep learning solutions for medical image segmentation. Med Image Anal. 2020;63:101693.
4. Pathak D, Krähenbühl P, Darrell T. Constrained convolutional neural networks for weakly supervised segmentation. Proc ICCV. IEEE Computer Society, 2015:1796–804.
5. Kervadec H, Dolz J, Tang M, Granger E, Boykov Y, Ayed IB. Constrained-CNN losses for weakly supervised segmentation. Med Image Anal. 2019;54:88–99.
6. Paszke A, Chaurasia A, Kim S, Culurciello E. ENet: a deep neural network architecture for real-time semantic segmentation. CoRR. 2016;abs/1606.02147.

3D Reconstruction of the Colon from Monocular Sequences

Evaluation by 3D-printed Phantom Data

Ralf Hackner[1], Thomas Eixelberger[1], Milan Schmidle[1], Volker Bruns[1],
Edgar Lehmann[2], Udo Geissler[2], Thomas Wittenberg[1]

[1]Fraunhofer Institute for Integrated Circuits IIS, Erlangen
[2]E&L Medical Systems, Erlangen
ralf.hackner@iis.fraunhofer.de

Abstract. Image based documentation of diagnostic findings in screening colonoscopy is currently achieved by capturing single images. Nevertheless, these lack precise information about their location in the colon. Creating a panorama map of the lumen of the colon during the examination, which shows detected lesion in their context, can support the endoscopist during the documentation process. Moreover, such a panoramic map also provides information about the completeness of an examination. An important step towards such a panoramic model is a robust 3D reconstruction of the colon in a first step. Nevertheless, as colonoscopy provides only monocular image data, 3D reconstruction of the colon is challenging. Therefore, we created a 3D reconstruction pipeline, consisting of a DCNN to estimate the depth for a single video frame and the concatenation and fusion of the depth maps to a 3D model based on feature consensus. As with real colonoscopic data, ground truth information regarding the exact extension and geometry of the colon is not available, we produced a modular 3D printed phantom of the colon to evaluate the proposed reconstruction method. The phantom was examined with standard withdrawal motions using two different colonoscopes resulting in endoscopic video streams. From these sequences the 3D reconstruction was computed, and the results were aligned and compared with the ground truth obtained from CAD-blueprint of the phantoms. In all cases, the achieved quality was highly sufficient.

1 Introduction

A common challenge in the field of diagnostic gastroscopy and especially colonoscopy is the limited field of view during an examination of the gastrointestinal tract. Thus, the image-based documentation of diagnostic findings of lesions during screening colonoscopy is currently archived by digitally capturing and storing single images in combination with the approximation of a rough value, how many centimeters the endoscope has been inserted into the patient. However, due to the ego-motion and variability of the colon and its unknown compression and extension during the insertion and withdrawal process of the colonoscope, this value is often not precise. Hence, creating a *panoramic map* of the examined lumen of the colon during the endoscopic examination, depicting the detected lesion in their anatomical context, can support the endoscopist during the documentation process. Ideally, the computation and creation of such a map should happen in real-time directly during the colonoscopic examination as such a map can additionally provide immediate visual feedback to the physician, reflecting whether the lumen has been inspected completely.

An important step towards such a panoramic model is a robust 3D reconstruction of the colon in a first step. Nevertheless, as colonoscopy provides only monocular image data, the 3D reconstruction of the colon is challenging.

1.1 Challenges

3D reconstruction from of a complex hollow organ such as the colon monocular video streams presents us with several challenges. First, the spatial depth of the individual two–dimensional images must be determined. Since no other sources of information (such as CT scans, active illumination or stereo images) are available, this information must be estimated solely from the 2D images of the endoscope. The illumination by the colonoscope, the reflective tissue structure and motion of the endoscope can provide valuable clues for this process. It must also be considered that individual areas of the colon may not be completely captured, either because they are hidden behind the haustrae or are covered by fluid or impurities. Furthermore, the large intestine is not a rigid object, but always in strong motion, so that images taken at different times can possibly not be merged accurately with each other.

1.2 Related work

Early attempts for the three-dimensional reconstruction of the colon or (closely related) the stomach make use of the light intensity and the fact, that the only light source in the colon is coaxially bundled with the endoscope [1, 2] to approximate the depth within the examined lumen. A similar approach using the average light density has been proposed for the reconstruction of the esophagus [3]. However, these approaches are quite sensitive to changes in the reflective behavior of the tissue surface. To utilize information other than the endoscopic illumination, current approaches make use of deep neural networks of the approximation of the depth. Thus, *Freeman et al.* [4] as well as *Recasens et al.* [5] were recently able to perform 3D-reconstructions of large intestines.

2   Methods and material

2.1   Methods

Within the scope of generating panoramic maps from monocular video data a 3D model of the examined colon must be achieved as central step Therefore, we created a 3D-reconstruction pipeline, consisting of (a) a frame selection and pre-processing step, (b) a deep convolutional neural network (DCNN) to estimate the depth for each single video frame and (c) the concatenation and fusion of the depth maps to a 3D model based on feature consensus.

2.1.1 Preprocessing. As first step, this pipeline removes blurred, underexposed or otherwise unusable frames from the video stream. Therefor we trained a random forest, with features including the variance of Laplacian, a color histogram in the HSV color space with 32 bins and the ratio of pixels belonging to an edge, detected with a Canny edge detector. To compensate the barrel distortion of the fish-eye camera of the video colonoscope, previously acquired calibration information is used to undistort the image frames. During the calibration we also obtained the field of view of the camera, which is needed for a correct depth estimation.

2.1.2 Depth-map approximation. To estimate the 3D geometry of the colon at a certain point t from the intensity and structures depicted a single video frame $I(t)$ and its predecessor $I(t-1)$, we apply a DCNN.

More specifically, a modified U-Net with a ResNet encoder [6] is used for this purpose. Such a modified U-Net has previously been trained from 12000 image pairs. Each such image pair $(I(t), I(t-1))$ has a known spatial relationship, and has been simulated from a digital colon model whose inside has been covered with real and artificial textures of the colon [7]. During the production state, the DCNN receives a successive pair of frames $I(t)$ and $I(t-1)$ from a colonoscopic video sequence, and in return provides an approximated depth map $D(I(t))$ of this frame. From this depth map the corresponding 3D-point cloud $P(I(t))$ can be computed for each frame.

2.1.3 Point-cloud fusion. In the next step a subset of the successively computed point clouds $P(t), P(t+1), P(t+2), \dots$ is concatenated and fused with each other in the 3D-space. Therefore, we extract feature points by the SURF [8] and AKAZE [9] feature extraction methods. To compensate the changes in the illumination an adaptive contrast correction is applied before. The thus extracted features are matched by using a fast library to approximate nearest neighbors (FLANN) based heuristic [10]. Based on the depth map obtained from the neuronal network described above, the 3D coordinates of the features are calculated. The final transformation for the registration step is esti-

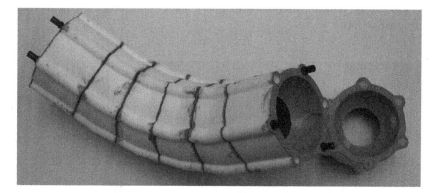

Fig. 1. A modular 3D-printed colon phantom with seven parts which can be varied with respect to their order and their rotation.

mated by using the Levenberg–Marquardt method. To avoid incorrect registrations, the transformation is checked for plausibility. Specifically no extreme sheering or sudden changes in size are allowed, and the reprojection error or the feature points is expected to be below a certain average threshold.

If the proposed transformation for registration is sufficient, the new fragment is added to the resulting cloud.

2.2   Material

2.2.1   3D-printed colon phantom. As for real colonoscopic image data, ground truth information regarding the exact extension and geometry of the colon is not available, and commercially available colon phantoms lack an adequate surface texture (which is needed for depth estimation), a modular, 3D-printed and stackable phantom of the colon was designed and produced. This phantom has a known geometry and an inner luminal surface mimicking as closely as possible a real colon regarding texture and reflection. Each single 3D-printed module represents one haustra (Fig. 1). The individual modules can be combined with different order and rotation, and thus are able to represent different curvatures and flexures of the colon and even include lesions such as adenomas or polyps.

The inner luminal surface features depict a hand-painted vascularization structure and has been coated with a glossy lining to mimic the reflective behavior of the mucosa. Since all modules are 3D-printed, an exact ground truth for the complete object is available (Fig. 2). The additive manufactured phantom as used in our experiment has a total length of about 28 centimeters. The inner diameter is in the range between 3 cm and 5 cm. There exist straight segments and slightly bent segments with an angle of 16 degrees each. In the examined configuration of the modules, we have a total angle of 48 degrees.

2.2.2   Recordings. To evaluate the proposed 3D-construction algorithm of the colon, we created four video sequences of the phantom using two different colonoscopes (*Storz Gastropack 2504* and *Olympus Excera* II XCF H160). The obtained image sequences were achieved on typical insertion, withdrawal, and examination movements common during colonoscopy.

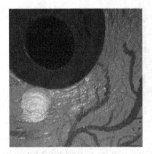 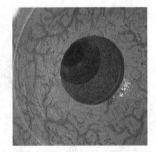 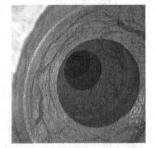

Fig. 2. Examples of the inner surface of the 3D-printed phantom with a round lumen.

3   Results

Based on the four acquired colonoscopic video streams, depicting the intraluminal texture of the colon phantom, 3D reconstructions were computed. An example (recorded with the Storz Gastropack system) is shown in Figure 3. For the evaluation, we aligned the reconstructed 3D models with the ground truth obtained from 3D print templates by comparing the distance between the model and the ground truth. In the example depicted in Figure 3, a planar section of the ground truth can be seen as overlay. Gaps, as they appear between the first and second segment, as well as in the last segment, indicate, that the corresponding region has not been seen captured during the withdrawal and recording process. A comparison between the aligned models and the ground truth has shown, that the position of the reconstructed surface points is up to 7 mm away from the expected position. The reconstructed models consist of 273 to 321 single fragments. For the angle spanned between the outermost segments, we measured values between 46 degree and 49 degree for our samples, close to the expected value of 48 degree.

4   Discussion

In principle, the reconstruction of the phantom was successful in all four tests. The basic tubular shape was essentially correctly recognized in all cases and the fragments were correctly arranged. So far noted weaknesses in the process were the correct determination of distance between the outer wall and the central axis of the tubular reconstruction. In some cases, the extensions of the haustrae were estimated to be up to an error $E_{max} = 7$ mm. These errors are caused by the depth estimation DCNN. However, this error will not necessarily provide problem for the intended use of a flat panorama since a back projection into the plane along the central axis will be carried out here anyway. Thus, the achieved results are sufficient for our purpose. The pairwise registration of the individual depth fragments was rather robust, despite changing perspectives during the

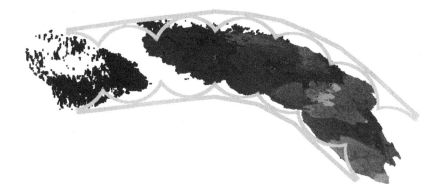

Fig. 3. 3D reconstruction and concatenation of successive 3D point clouds from the colon phantom overlayed with a planar section of its CAD blueprint.

recording. To achieve a practical image map, a comprehensive shading correction will also be necessary to deal with the strong illuminance changes (Fig. 3). What we could not demonstrate with the described experiment is to what extent the method is robust against the intrinsic movement of the colon. Thus, further experiments with real patient data will be addressed next.

Acknowledgement. Parts of the research has been funded by the Bavarian Research Society (BFS) under the project GastroMapper (AZ-1349-18).

References

1. Trinh DH, Daul C, Blondel W, Lamarque D. Mosaicing of images with few textures and strong illumination changes: application to gastroscopic scenes. 2018 25th IEEE International Conference on Image Processing (ICIP). 2018:1263–7.
2. Hong D, Tavanapong W, Wong J, Oh J, De Groen PC. 3D reconstruction of colon segments from colonoscopy images. 2009 Ninth IEEE International Conference on Bioinformatics and BioEngineering. IEEE. 2009:53–60.
3. Prinzen M, Raithel M, Bergen T, Mühldorfer S, Nowack S, Wilhelm D et al. Panorama mapping of the esophagus from gastroscopic video. Bildverarbeitung für die Medizin 2015. Springer, 2015:455–60.
4. Freedman D, Blau Y, Katzir L, Aides A, Shimshoni I, Veikherman D et al. Detecting deficient coverage in colonoscopies. IEEE Trans Med Imaging. 2020;PP:1–1.
5. Recasens D, Lamarca J, Fácil JM, Montiel JMM, Civera J. Endo-depth-and-motion: reconstruction and tracking in endoscopic videos using depth networks and photometric constraints. 2021.
6. Walluscheck S, Wittenberg T, Bruns V, Eixelberger T, Hackner R. Partial 3D-reconstruction of the colon from monoscopic colonoscopy videos using shape-from-motion and deep learning. Current Directions in Biomedical Engineering. 2021;7(2):pp. 335–338.
7. Hackner R, Walluscheck S, Lehmann E, Eixelberger T, Bruns V, Wittenberg T. A geometric and textural model of the colon as ground truth for deep learning-based 3D-re-construction. 2021:298–303.
8. Bay H, Tuytelaars T, Van Gool L. Surf: speeded up robust features. Vol. 3951. 2006:404–17.
9. Alcantarilla PF, Solutions T. Fast explicit diffusion for accelerated features in nonlinear scale spaces. IEEE Trans Pattern Anal Mach Intell. 2011;34(7):1281–98.
10. Muja M, Lowe DG. Fast approximate nearest neighbors with automatic algorithm configuration. VISAPP. 2009.

Diffusion MRI Specific Pretraining by Self-supervision on an Auxiliary Dataset

Leon Weninger[1], Jarek Ecke[1], Chuh-Hyoun Na[2], Kerstin Jütten[2], Dorit Merhof[1]

[1]Institute of Imaging & Computer Vision, RWTH Aachen University
[2]Department of Neurosurgery, University Hospital RWTH Aachen
leon.weninger@lfb.rwth-aachen.de

Abstract. Training deep learning networks is very data intensive. Especially in fields with a very limited number of annotated datasets, such as diffusion MRI, it is of great importance to develop approaches that can cope with a limited amount of data. It was previously shown that transfer learning can lead to better results and more stable training in various medical applications. However, the use of off-the-shelf transfer learning tools in high angular resolution diffusion MRI is not straightforward, as such 3D approaches are commonly designed for scalar data. Here, an extension of self-supervised pretraining to diffusion MRI data is presented, and enhanced with a modality-specific procedure, where artifacts encountered in diffusion MRI need to be removed. We pretrained on publicly available data from the Human Connectome Project and evaluated the success on data from a local hospital with three modality-related experiments: segmentation of brain microstructure, detection of fiber crossings, and regression of nerve fiber spatial orientation. The results were compared against a setting without pretraining, and against classical autoencoder pretraining. We find that it is possible to achieve both improved metrics and a more stable training with the proposed diffusion MRI specific pretraining procedure.

1 Introduction

Magnetic Resonance Imaging is used to obtain insights into the anatomy and the physiological processes of the body. Specifically, high angular diffusion MRI (dMRI) can reveal microscopic details about brain tissue architecture. This procedure allows to separate brain components, detect diseases and study white matter connectivity [1]. These technical advances have become indispensable in medicine and are therefore of great importance for research and clinical applications.

However, analysis of a three-dimensional image is time-consuming and tedious for trained medical professionals. Computer-aided methods can speed up this process and provide results fast and with high quality even for large datasets. Artificial neural networks are particularly suited to recognize the underlying structures and have achieved outstanding results in recent years. However, in order to train neural networks for specific applications, the training data needs to be annotated, a task which often demands domain expert knowledge. Thus, such annotated data is only available to a limited extent. It is

© Der/die Autor(en), exklusiv lizenziert durch
Springer Fachmedien Wiesbaden GmbH, ein Teil von Springer Nature 2022
K. Maier-Hein et al. (Hrsg.), *Bildverarbeitung für die Medizin 2022*,
Informatik aktuell, https://doi.org/10.1007/978-3-658-36932-3_32

hence beneficial to develop methods that obtain optimal and generalizable results from small amounts of annotated data. Pretraining already led to improved results on datasets of various imaging modalities [2, 3]. In dMRI, pretraining was heretofore carried out by training the network two times for the exact same task, first on an auxiliary dataset, and then fine-tuning on the target dataset [4].

We propose a self-supervised domain-specific pretraining approach for dMRI data that uses an auxiliary dataset but does not rely on annotated data. A publicly available high-resolution dRMI dataset from the Human Connectome Project (HCP) [5] was used for pretraining, and lower quality data from a local hospital for the target applications. First, the HCP data was spatially downsampled and interpolated in q-space to the resolution of the local data (Sec. 2.1). Then, the HCP dataset was artificially distorted with diffusion-MRI specific artifacts, namely eddy current, ghosting, motion and biasfield simulations, and Gaussian noise (Sec. 2.3). A U-Net [6] was trained to remove these artifacts from the dataset (Sec. 2.2). This pretrained U-Net was finally re-trained on the local dataset for three different domain typical applications: brain microstructure segmentation, detection of fiber crossings, and fiber direction estimation (Sec. 2.4). This pretraining scheme was evaluated against a random initialization of neural network weights and against autoencoder pretraining (Sec. 3).

2   Materials and methods

2.1   Data

The actual dataset of interest comprises 28 healthy subjects from the hospital University Hospital Aachen. All subjects have given written informed consent prior to study enrolment. The study was approved by the local ethics committee (EC 294/15). Each dataset consists of a T1 and a dMRI scan. The dMRI images were acquired on a Siemens 3T Prisma scanner with 64 single-shell gradient directions (b-value = $1000 \frac{s}{mm^2}$, same gradient directions for every acquisition, one b0 acquisition), TE=81 ms, TR=6300 ms, anterior-posterior phase encoding, and an isotropic voxel size of 2.4 mm. For all experiments, the 64 gradient direction acquisitions were divided by the b0 acquisition, resulting in directed diffusion-attenuated images with values between 0 and 1. For each experiment, this dataset was randomly divided into 15 train, 5 validation and 8 test subjects.

The pretraining was conducted with a dataset from the HCP [5], which provides high-resolution multi-shell 3T dMRI data. Three spherical shells (b=1000, 2000 and $3000 \frac{s}{mm^2}$) with 90 gradient directions each were acquired in an isotropic resolution of 1.25 mm (for more details on acquisition parameters see Ref. [5]). From this database, the first 50 subjects of the 100 unrelated subjects release were selected, which were divided into 45 train and 5 validation subjects. To make the data comparable to the clinical data, only the b=$1000 \frac{s}{mm^2}$ shell was selected. This data was spatially downsampled to an isotropic voxel size of 2.4 mm, and the gradient directions were interpolated to the directions of the local data by using 8th order spherical harmonics.

2.2 Network architecture and training details

For all experiments, a network structure following the U-Net architecture [6] in a 3D version with 64 input channels was used. The number of feature maps was reduced to 16 in the first 3×3 convolution, and then doubled in each of the following two downsampling steps. The contracting and the expansive path thus consisted of three steps. All trainings were carried out with an ADAM optimizer and a learning rate of 0.001 on an Nvidia RTX 2080 Ti GPU. When switching from pretraining to the final application, only the output layer was exchanged an re-initialized, using an appropriate amount of outputs depending on the experiment. All experiments were implemented using PyTorch Lightning, the code is available under www.github.com/JarekE/PretrainingForDiffusionMRI.

2.3 Diffusion-MRI specific pretraining procedure

For pretraining on the HCP dataset, a self-supervised procedure was implemented, where the U-Net is trained to remove diffusion-MRI specific artifacts. For this purpose, we artificially modified the input images by randomly selected distortions (motion, ghosting, bias field and Gaussian noise) as implemented in TorchIO [7] (number of ghosting artifacts = 2, otherwise default parameters), and to eddy current distortion simulations [8] with random stretching factors between 0.9 and 1.1 in direction of the phase encoding of the clinical data (Fig. 1). These distortions appear more often and with stronger intensities in acquisitions of everyday clinical practice (i.e. also in our local dataset) than in the HCP dataset, as hospital data are acquired under stricter time constraints. Thus, pretraining to recognize and remove those artifacts on an auxiliary dataset should lead to better and more robust results during the final applications on the local dataset. To test this hypothesis, a second vanilla autoencoder pretraining was carried out. Here, the input images needed to be reproduced by the network without any previously applied distortions.

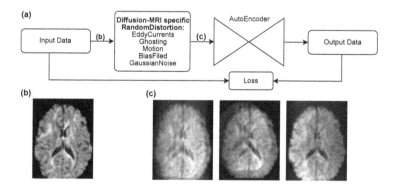

Fig. 1. *(a)* Schematic structure of pretraining using diffusion MRI specific distortions. *(b)* A slice of an exemplary input image. *(c)* Three exemplary distorted images of the input slice. Training and distortions were carried out in 3D.

2.4   Experiments for evaluation

Three experiments that relate to different fundamental use cases of dMRI and form a comprehensive basis for evaluating the effects of pretraining were performed on the local dataset. They comprise a segmentation, a classification, and a regression task. The differently pretrained models were retrained to reproduce a groundtruth generated with classical methods as described below.

2.4.1   Segmentation. To create a tissue map, the accompanying T1 image was segmented into white matter, gray matter, and cerebrospinal fluid with FSL Fast [9]. It was then transformed to the individual diffusion space through an affine registration of the T1 and the diffusion image. The neural networks were then trained to determine the segmentation map from the dMRI data.

2.4.2   Fiber direction. Using Constrained Spherical Deconvolution [10], the fiber orientation distribution function (fODF) of white matter was obtained. For this purpose, the response function of a single fiber was estimated, and the diffusion signal was deconvolved to obtain the fODF. Then, the largest peak from this fODF was extracted for all white matter voxels, its orientation mapped to a hemisphere, the polar and azimuthal angle were determined, and normalized to values between 0 and 1.

2.4.3   Fiber crossings. To obtain a crossing fiber groundtruth, the same fODF estimation as for the fiber direction was used. From the fODF, the number of peaks in white matter voxels was determined, whereby a local maximum must have had at least half the amplitude of the largest peak and be separated by more than 25° from other peaks to be considered a separate fiber bundle. The maximum number of fiber tracts per voxel was set to three.

3   Results

With regard to the paucity of training data, two aspects were evaluated: The impact of pretraining on prediction accuracy, and on possible overfitting on training data, which can quickly occur when a small number of training samples is used.

Training the U-Net for identifying a fiber direction, overfitting behavior was observed. This overfitting effect was strongest if pretraining is omitted, whereas significantly less overfitting was observed when autoencoder pretraining was used (Fig. 2a). Thus, a more consistent and sustainable learning success was achieved with pretraining. For the segmentation and fiber crossing tasks, no overfitting was observed, independent of pretraining.

When evaluating final performance on the test set, task-specific scores — multiclass F1 score for segmentation, accuracy for detection of fiber crossings, mean squared error for fiber direction — were utilized. The final scores were determined with four different training runs, each with eight test images. Random initialization of the network was outperformed by the proposed pretraining in all experiments (Fig. 2b). For segmentation, the improvement was 1.4 % (one-sided paired sample t-test: p<0.005), for fiber crossings 0.3 % (p<0.05) and 0.67 % for the fiber direction (p<0.05). However, vanilla autoencoder pretraining outperformed the proposed approach in the fiber direction task. Thus, while pretraining on the auxiliary dataset was beneficial in every task, adding the domain-specific distortions to the pretraining improved the final score only in two of three experiments.

4 Discussion

We have shown that — if domain-specific distortions are used — self-supervised pre-training on auxiliary data stabilizes the training process and improves performance of deep learning in dMRI tasks. However, the magnitude of the pretraining effect is dependent on the specific task. Of particular interest is the disparate behavior of the regression problem in relation to the other two experiments, where vanilla autoencoder pretraining on the auxiliary data outperformed the proposed diffusion-MRI specific pretraining scheme. An explanation of this effect could be that pretraining without distortions provides a basis for the network to learn detailed structures, making it possible to avoid overfitting and to achieve improvements in a noise-prone task such as regression of the fiber direction. In contrast, the U-Net was able to achieve good results in the other exper-

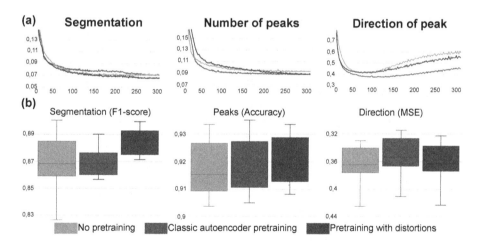

Fig. 2. (a) Validation loss of the three experiments, 300 epochs, averaged over four training runs. After the initial phase characterized by rapid improvements, the segmentation (left) and classification (middle) experiments showed stable learning behavior, with slightly better validation scores for pretraining. In the regression problem (right), less overfitting behavior was obtained by pretraining. (b) Test set results for the segmentation task (F1-score), the number of peaks (accuracy) and for the direction of the largest peak (mean squared error, inverted scale). For the segmentation and the number of peaks, pretraining of the neural network with distortions showed the best results, for the direction the setting with classic autoencoder pretraining had the smallest error.

iments even without pretraining. Here, understanding and correcting possible distortions is more important for further improvements.

In this paper, a self-supervised pretraining scheme for deep learning on diffusion MRI was proposed. Given the focus on the benefit of pretraining, reported absolute values need to be taken with a grain of salt. Choices of network architecture and optimizer parameters were equally set for all experiments to reasonable default parameters. While this choice makes the different pretraining approaches comparable, a computationally expensive exhaustive hyperparameter search could have led to better absolute results. Further, the application of the pretrained network to further datasets is not straightforward: As the number of input features of the network depends on the diffusion acquisition scheme, the network cannot be directly applied to other diffusion acquisitions. Instead, the number and directionality of diffusion weighted images of auxiliary and main dataset need to be matched before pretraining. A q-space interpolation of the auxiliary dataset, and even of the main dataset, if different acquisitions have different acquisition directions, would thus be necessary.

Acknowledgement. This work was funded by the German Research Foundation (Deutsche Forschungsgemeinschaft, DFG) under project number 269953372 (IRTG 2150) and project number 417063796.

References

1. Descoteaux M. High angular resolution diffusion imaging (HARDI). Wiley Encyclopedia of Electrical and Electronics Engineering. American Cancer Society, 2015:1–25.
2. Zhou Z, Sodha V, Pang J, Gotway MB, Liang J. Models genesis. Med Image Anal. 2021;67:101840.
3. Taleb A, Loetzsch W, Danz N, Severin J, Gaertner T, Bergner B et al. 3D self-supervised methods for medical imaging. NeurIPS. Vol. 33. Curran Associates, Inc., 2020:18158–72.
4. Li Y, Qin Y, Liu Z, Ye C. Pretraining improves deep learning based tissue microstructure estimation. MICCAI CDMRI. Springer, 2021:173–85.
5. van Essen DC, Smith SM, Barch DM, Behrens TEJ, Yacoub E, Ugurbil K. The WU-Minn human connectome project: an overview. NeuroImage. 2013;80:62–79.
6. Ronneberger O, Fischer P, Brox T. U-Net: convolutional networks for biomedical image segmentation. MICCAI. Springer, 2015:234–41.
7. Pérez-García F, Sparks R, Ourselin S. TorchIO: a python library for efficient loading, pre-processing, augmentation and patch-based sampling of medical images in deep learning. Comput Methods Programs Biomed. 2021;208:106236.
8. Andersson JL. Chapter 4 - geometric distortions in diffusion MRI. Diffusion MRI (Second Edition). Ed. by Johansen-Berg H, Behrens TE. Second Edition. Academic Press, 2014:63–85.
9. Zhang Y, Brady M, Smith S. Segmentation of brain MR images through a hidden Markov random field model and the expectation-maximization algorithm. IEEE Trans Med Imaging. 2001;20(1):45–57.
10. Tournier JD, Calamante F, Connelly A. Robust determination of the fibre orientation distribution in diffusion MRI: non-negativity constrained super-resolved spherical deconvolution. NeuroImage. 2007;35(4):1459–72.

Thrombus Detection in Non-contrast Head CT Using Graph Deep Learning

Antonia Popp[1,2], Oliver Taubmann[2], Florian Thamm[1,2], Hendrik Ditt[2],
Andreas Maier[1], Katharina Breininger[3]

[1]Pattern Recognition Lab, Friedrich-Alexander-Universität, Erlangen-Nürnberg, Germany
[2]Computed Tomography, Siemens Healthineers AG, Forchheim, Germany
[3]Department Artificial Intelligence in Biomedical Engineering, Friedrich-Alexander-Universität,
Erlangen-Nürnberg, Germany
antonia.popp@fau.de

Abstract. In case of an acute ischemic stroke, rapid diagnosis and removal of
the occluding thrombus (blood clot) are crucial for a successful recovery. We
present an automated thrombus detection system for non-contrast computed tomography (NCCT) images to improve the clinical workflow, where NCCT is
typically acquired as a first-line imaging tool to identify the type of the stroke.
The system consists of a candidate detection model and a subsequent classification
model. The detection model generates a volumetric heatmap from the NCCT and
extracts multiple potential clot candidates, sorted by their likeliness in descending order. The classification model performs reprioritization of these candidates
using graph-based deep learning methods, where the candidates are no longer
considered independently, but in a global context. It was optimized to classify the
candidates as clot or no clot. The candidate detection model, which also serves as
the main baseline, yields a ROC AUC of 79.8%, which is improved to 85.2% by
the proposed graph-based classification model.

1 Introduction

Stroke is a severe cerebrovascular disease which causes cell death as a result of low
blood flow in the affected brain area [1]. Two main types can be differentiated: ischemic
stroke develops as a consequence of blood vessel obstruction, i.e. after occlusion of a
cerebral vessel by a blood clot, whereas hemorrhagic stroke results from a bleeding. In
patients suffering from acute ischemic stroke, urgent detection, localization and removal
of the occluding clot is crucial for successful recovery. In clinical routine, non-contrast
computed tomography (NCCT) is typically acquired as a first-line imaging tool in case of
unspecific neurological symptoms or specific signs of stroke, and enables the detection
of ischemic or hemorrhagic stroke.

Several approaches have been published to identify the presence of large vessel
occlusions (LVOs) in CT angiography (CTA) images [2] or NCCT images [3]. In
recent years, a growing number of methods for automated thrombus detection and
localization in NCCT scans have been proposed as well. Earlier detection algorithms
extract potential clot candidates through segmentation in preprocessing and classify them
using statistical machine learning techniques [4, 5]. More recent work predominantly

employs convolutional neural networks (CNNs) for clot segmentation on patches of the NCCT volume prior to classification [6, 7].

The proposed method makes no prior assumptions regarding the location of the clot, i.e. it is not limited to cases of LVO, and considers the entire cerebrovascular system. It relies on a graph neural network (GNN) model to classify previously detected clot candidates jointly and in a patient-global context.

2   Materials and methods

The proposed system is composed of two parts. First, a detection model extracts 15 positions likely to show a clot as candidates and sorts them based on their output probabilities as preliminary likelihood scores. Subsequently, a classification model reorders these candidates by updating their likelihoods. To this end, relations between individual candidates as well as between candidates and their opposite-hemisphere counterparts are modeled as graphs and fed to a GNN.

2.1   Input data

The input of the detection model consists of five channels with intensity-based, geometrical and location-based features. The first channel contains the skull-stripped and cropped, but otherwise unmodified NCCT. The second channel only shows intensities between 56 and 110 Hounsfield units, which is assumed to be the relevant range for clotted blood. The third channel is a vessel probability map in which larger values indicate a higher likelihood of a blood vessel being located at this position. This information is derived from a brain atlas [8] which is non-rigidly registered to the patient scan. The fourth channel visualizes the left-right difference between the two hemispheres and is obtained by mirroring the brain at the mid-sagittal plane and non-rigidly registering it to the unmirrored image, followed by a voxel-wise subtraction. For the fifth channel, a histogram-equalized version of the first channel is computed to increase the contrast.

2.2   Candidate detection model

The target of the detection model is to predict a heatmap with high values for potential clot regions in order to extract potential clot candidates. The heatmap is the output of a 2D U-Net [9] with six levels applied to the slices of the volumetric input channels. The number of feature maps is 32 in the top level and is doubled in each successive level, resulting in 1024 feature maps at the bottom. Stacking the output images results in a volumetric heatmap for each brain scan. The locations of the 15 local maxima with the highest scores (local maximum values) in the heatmap are considered as clot candidates. This number of candidates was chosen empirically as a conservative upper limit; further increasing it did not increase the number of true clots among candidates in our data. The ranking of these candidates by their scores in descending order is the final output of the first model. Seeing as this approach based on a 2D U-Net can be considered fairly standard, the results of this model will also serve as our first baseline. The preprocessing described in section 2.1 was determined to be beneficial by ablation during earlier development of the detection method. Keeping it consistent between the compared approaches allows us to more accurately assess the benefits of the proposed graph model described below.

2.3   Candidate classification model

The classification model aims to reprioritize the clot candidates based on a global assessment and reclassifies them. To this end, the model comprehensively considers the 15 candidates and their respective positions mirrored along the mid-sagittal plane, i.e. the mirrored locations on the opposite hemisphere. This is considered crucial since the hyperdense artery sign indicating a clot appears only on one side of the brain, whereas a healthy brain is assumed to be close to symmetric. In order to create feature representations of the candidates, a region of interest (ROI) of $64 \times 64 \times 32$ voxels is extracted around the position of each candidate and its position mirrored along the mid-sagittal plane, and downsampled by a factor of two in each dimension (Fig. 1). The 30 ROIs, which form the input to the classification model, are extracted from the five input channels given to the first model and from the resulting heatmap (Fig. 1).

The architecture of the classification model is composed of a feature encoder, a reprioritization network and an optional decoder (Fig. 2). The encoder computes feature vectors from each ROI and consists of three stages of alternating 3D convolution, batch normalization, leaky ReLU activation, 3D maximum pooling and dropout layers. After flattening the feature map to a vector in the contracting path, the coordinates of each candidate are appended to its respective feature vector before passing it to a fully connected (FC) layer.

As a second baseline approach we reclassify with a candidate-wise fully connected network (FCN) trained specifically for classification. This model computed one output

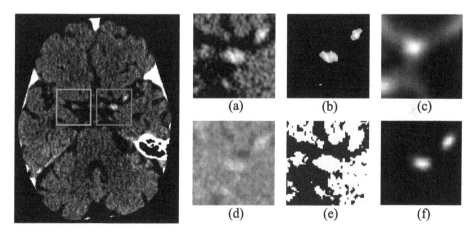

Fig. 1. Segmented slice of the NCCT scan (left) with the ROI around the clot candidate (blue rectangle) and its mirrored position (green rectangle). The six channels of the clot candidate ROI: (a) segmented image, (b) clot intensities, (c) vessel map, (d) left-right difference, (e) histogram-equalized image, (f) heatmap from detection model.

for each individual candidate and consists of five FC layers with a gradually decreasing number of features. It thereby has the same target as our proposed GNN method, but foregoes an evaluation of the global context possible with a GNN, described next.

Each location can be considered a node where the connections to other nodes form a graph which describes the potential relations among each other. The ensuing (partial) node classification task is approached by replacing the FCN with a GNN (Fig. 2), where graph convolutions update the features of the candidates, depending on information exchange with their respective candidate neighborhood. In this work we used the SAGEConv layer [10] with a neighborhood sampling rate of 0.1 and using the mean function for aggregation. Two graph topologies model the links between the locations. A candidate-comparison graph mutually connects all 15 candidates and a bipartite mirror-comparison graph connects each candidate to its corresponding mirrored location to enable the comparison of suspicious regions in both hemispheres. The GNN architecture is a sequence of 8 graph convolutions, of which the first two receive the candidate-comparison graph and the second two receive the mirror-comparison graph topology for feature exchange (Fig. 2). This layer arrangement is repeated once again before each feature vector is passed to an FC layer prior to the final classification. Some additional links are inserted as skip connections between the layers. The output of the classification model consists of updated scores for all candidates which are then sorted (reprioritized) again in descending order.

As a further variant, since reference clot masks were available, we investigated if adding a second, auxiliary task for clot segmentation could further improve the classification performance. For this purpose, a decoder extracts feature vectors after the fourth convolution layer in the FCN or the sixth SAGEConv layer in the GNN, respectively, to generate a tensor with the size of the input ROI. It is an expanding path and consists of alternating 3D upsampling, 3D convolution, batch normalization and leaky ReLU activation functions. In the end, a final 3D convolution creates a volumetric heatmap for each clot.

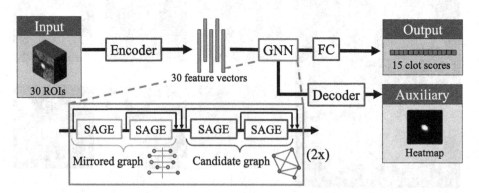

Fig. 2. The architecture of the proposed classification model consists of three parts: an encoder to generate a feature vector from each candidate ROI, a GNN to compute one feature per candidate based on global assessment using SAGEConv layers [10] and a decoder to create a heatmap for clot segmentation as auxiliary task.

3   Results

Both models were trained and evaluated using a dataset of 634 thin-slice NCCT scans of patients suffering from acute ischemic stroke and corresponding reference clot masks obtained by manual segmentation. For the evaluation of the model performances, the data was subdivided into five equally sized subsets for cross-validation with a 3-1-1 split ratio for training, validation and test, respectively. The candidate classification task can be considered a binary classification problem with two classes: clot (positive) and no clot (negative). While each patient had exactly one real clot which ideally matches one candidate, in practice any number of candidates may coincide with (parts of) this clot and is considered a true positive if it does. Binary cross-entropy served as the training loss for both targets, i.e. classification and segmentation. The model is optimized using the Adam optimizer with a learning rate of 0.001. Early stopping is used based on the area under the receiver operating characteristic curve (ROC AUC) for the candidates of all validation set patients. The final evaluation employs the same metric on the candidates of all test set patients.

The cross-validation results of all investigated models are shown in Figure 3. The classification performance of the detection model (first baseline) is given by an AUC of 0.798 ± 0.017. The classification model using only an FCN achieved an AUC of 0.829 ± 0.011, while the GNN classification model performed best with an AUC of 0.852 ± 0.010. Adding the auxiliary segmentation task to the proposed models did not improve the AUC further ($0.825 \pm 0.018, 0.850 \pm 0.015$).

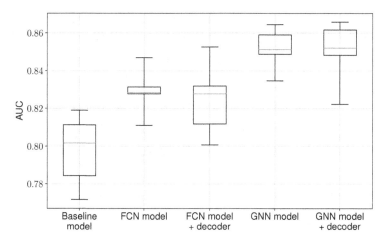

Fig. 3. Classification performance of the candidate detection model and the subsequent models using FCN or GNN. The two whiskers of the box plot indicate the minimum and maximum AUC of the 5 test sets, the lower and upper border of the box show the second and fourth highest result and the orange line is the median.

4 Discussion

The goal of this work was to improve the detection of occluding blood clots in the brain by building upon a detection model which extracts a set of clot candidates from a brain scan and classifies them based on their respective likelihoods. We developed a reclassification model with either a candidate-wise FCN as a second baseline, or a GNN to jointly reclassify the candidates. The GNN model clearly outperformed both baselines, the candidate detection model and the FCN model. Adding a segmentation output as an auxiliary task did not further improve the classification results. In clinical routine, approaches for automated clot detection can enable faster workflows or avoid the risk of missing a clot in a brain scan. Used as a second reader to support radiologists, our system may be a helpful tool in diagnostics and help to ensure more reliable outcomes.

Acknowledgement. KB gratefully acknowledges the support of Siemens Healthineers within her endowed professorship program.

References

1. Campbell BCV, Silva DA de, Macleod MR, Coutts SB, Schwamm LH, Davis SM et al. Ischaemic stroke. Nat Rev Dis Primers. 2019;5(1):70.
2. Murray NM, Unberath M, Hager GD, Hui FK. Artificial intelligence to diagnose ischemic stroke and identify large vessel occlusions: a systematic review. J Neurointerv Surg. 2020;12(2):156–64.
3. Olive-Gadea M, Crespo C, Granes C, Hernandez-Perez M, La Pérez de Ossa, Natalia, Laredo C et al. Deep learning based software to identify large vessel occlusion on noncontrast computed tomography. Stroke. 2020;51(10):3133–7.
4. Takahashi N, Lee Y, Tsai DY, Matsuyama E, Kinoshita T, Ishii K. An automated detection method for the MCA dot sign of acute stroke in unenhanced CT. Radiol Phys Technol. 2014;7(1):79–88.
5. Loeber P, Stimpel B, Syben C, Maier A, Ditt H, Schramm P et al. Automatic thrombus detection in non-enhanced computed tomography images in patients with acute ischemic stroke. Visual Computing for Biology and Medicine. 2017.
6. Shinohara Y, Takahashi N, Lee Y, Ohmura T, Kinoshita T. Development of a deep learning model to identify hyperdense MCA sign in patients with acute ischemic stroke. Jpn J Radiol. 2020;38(2):112–7.
7. Tolhuisen ML, Ponomareva E, Boers AMM, Jansen IGH, Koopman MS, Sales Barros R et al. A convolutional neural network for anterior intra-arterial thrombus detection and segmentation on non-contrast computed tomography of patients with acute ischemic stroke. Appl Sci. 2020;10(14):4861.
8. Kemmling A, Wersching H, Berger K, Knecht S, Groden C, Nölte I. Decomposing the hounsfield unit: probabilistic segmentation of brain tissue in computed tomography. Clin Neuroradiol. 2012;22(1):79–91.
9. Ronneberger O, Fischer P, Brox T. U-Net: convolutional networks for biomedical image segmentation. Med Image Comput Comput Assist Interv. 2015.
10. Hamilton WL, Ying R, Leskovec J. Inductive representation learning on large graphs. arXiv:1706.02216. 2017.

Abstract: A Database and Neural Network for Highly Accurate Classification of Single Bone Marrow Cells

Christian Matek[1,2], Sebastian Krappe[3,4], Christian Münzenmayer[3], Torsten Haferlach[5], Carsten Marr[1]

[1]Institute of Computational Biology, Helmholtz Zentrum München, Munich, Germany
[2]Department of Internal Medicine III, University Hospital Munich,
Ludwig-Maximilians-Universität München, Munich, Germany
[3]Image Processing and Medical Engineering Department, Fraunhofer Institute for Integrated
Circuits IIS, Erlangen, Germany
[4]Department of Computer Science, University of Koblenz-Landau, Koblenz, Germany
[5]MLL Munich Leukemia Laboratory, Munich, Germany
christian.matek@helmholtz-muenchen.de

Fast and accurate morphological classification of cells in bone marrow samples is a key step in the diagnostic workup of many disorders of the hematopoietic system such as leukemias. In spite of its long-established key position, morphological examination of bone marrow samples has been difficult to automatise, and is still mainly performed manually by trained cytologists on light microscopes. In our contribution [1], we present a neural network for classification of light microscopy images of bone marrow samples. The network was developed using what to the authors' knowledge is the most extensive publically available image dataset of bone marrow cells, containing over 170,000 images from the samples of 945 patients diagnosed with a variety of hematological disorders, reflecting the sample entry of a center specialised in hematological diagnostics [2]. The network is shown to be highly accurate for most key cell classes, outperforming previous approaches in single-cell bone marrow examination. We test different network architectures to show our results are robust with respect to the details of network structure. The results are validated on a smaller, external dataset published previously by Choi et al. [3]. We also analyse the network's predictions using recently developed methods of explainable AI, specifically SmoothGrad and GradCAM. These methods suggest that the network has learned to focus on relevant structural features of the bone marrow cells shown.

References

1. Matek C, Krappe S, Münzenmayer C, Haferlach T, Marr C. Highly accurate differentiation of bone marrow cell morphologies using deep neural networks on a large image data set. Blood. 2021;138(20):1917–27.
2. Matek C, Krappe S, Münzenmayer C, Haferlach T, Marr C. An expert-annotated reference dataset for bone marrow cytomorphology. The Cancer Imaging Archive (TCIA). 2021.
3. Choi JW, Ku Y, Yoo BW, Kim JA, Lee DS, Chai YJ et al. White blood cell differential count of maturation stages in bone marrow smear using dual-stage convolutional neural networks. PloS One. 2017;12:e0189259.

© Der/die Autor(en), exklusiv lizenziert durch
Springer Fachmedien Wiesbaden GmbH, ein Teil von Springer Nature 2022
K. Maier-Hein et al. (Hrsg.), *Bildverarbeitung für die Medizin 2022*,
Informatik aktuell, https://doi.org/10.1007/978-3-658-36932-3_34

Comparison of Depth Estimation Setups from Stereo Endoscopy and Optical Tracking for Point Measurements

Lukas Burger[1], Lalith Sharan[1,4], Samantha Fischer[1], Julian Brand[1],
Maximillian Hehl[1], Gabriele Romano[2], Matthias Karck[2], Raffaele De Simone[2],
Ivo Wolf[3], Sandy Engelhardt[1,4]

[1]Group Artificial Intelligence in Cardiovascular Medicine (AICM),
Department of Internal Medicine III, Heidelberg University Hospital, Heidelberg
[2]Department of Cardiac Surgery, Heidelberg University Hospital, Heidelberg
[3]Mannheim University of Applied Sciences, Mannheim
[4]DZHK (German Centre for Cardiovascular Research), partner site Heidelberg/Mannheim
sandy.engelhardt@med.uni-heidelberg.de

Abstract. To support minimally-invasive intraoperative mitral valve repair, quantitative measurements from the valve can be obtained using an infra-red tracked stylus. It is desirable to view such manually measured points together with the endoscopic image for further assistance. Therefore, hand-eye calibration is required that links both coordinate systems and is a prerequisite to project the points onto the image plane. A complementary approach to this is to use a vision-based endoscopic stereo-setup to detect and triangulate points of interest, to obtain the 3D coordinates. In this paper, we aim to compare both approaches on a rigid phantom and two patient-individual silicone replica which resemble the intraoperative scenario. The preliminary results indicate that 3D landmark estimation, either labeled manually or through partly automated detection with a deep learning approach, provides more accurate triangulated depth measurements when performed with a tailored image-based method than with stylus measurements.

1 Introduction

In mitral valve repair (MVR), sutures are placed around the mitral valve annulus, and a ring prosthesis is placed through the sutures on the annulus, to perform *annuloplasty*. MVR is increasingly performed in a minimally invasive setup [1], enabled through endoscopic video display. In this context, $3D$ endoscopes are used more frequently since they facilitate better depth perception. Furthermore, patient-specific physical simulators have been developed for the purpose of surgical training and pre-operative planning [2, 3]. During surgery, the valvular pathomorphology is traditionally assessed by visual intraoperative exploration *in-situ* [4]. However, this approach lacks a quantitative base and is therefore not easily comparable between surgeons. In order to increase reproducibility and for intraoperative decision support, Engelhardt et al. [4] proposed the use of an assistance system for measuring dimensions of the mitral valve geometry (e.g. length of the chordae tendineae, width and shape of the annulus). The system incorporates infra-red based optical stereo tracking of customized instruments that are equipped with spherical markers. It has been successfully applied in 9 patients during surgery [5]. A systematic accuracy investigation [4] revealed that phantom experiments conducted in

© Der/die Autor(en), exklusiv lizenziert durch
Springer Fachmedien Wiesbaden GmbH, ein Teil von Springer Nature 2022
K. Maier-Hein et al. (Hrsg.), *Bildverarbeitung für die Medizin 2022*,
Informatik aktuell, https://doi.org/10.1007/978-3-658-36932-3_35

the actual application environment (OR) deliver a high system accuracy (mean precision 0.12 ± 0.093 mm, mean trueness 0.77 ± 0.39 mm) and a low user error (mean precision 0.18 ± 0.10 mm, mean trueness 0.81 ± 0.36 mm). However, it is cumbersome to setup the system before the surgery. Moreover, the measurements are performed manually, meaning that the user needs to be experienced with the system. Furthermore, in the current setup, the information stream gained from the optical tracking system is not registered to the endoscopic system, which was criticized by the end users. They prefer to have the measurements displayed in the endoscopic image as a "quality check" potentially together with additional information using augmented reality [6].

In this work, we perform a hand-eye calibration of the stereo-endoscopic camera to display the measured points in the endoscopic frames. This introduces additional sources of error caused by hand-eye calibration, which includes estimation of intrinsic and extrinsic camera calibration parameters. We investigate the errors produced by this setup on a rigid phantom and two patient-specific silicone valves mounted on a simulator. Since errors in systems that include an optical tracking device also relate to the individual instrument design, they need to be assessed in an application-related setup [4].

A complementary approach to optical tracking, which does not rely on additional hardware but on the same camera calibration parameters, is to exploit the stereo relation between left and right endoscopic camera frames directly and to detect points which are of interest for distance computation. In particular, the use of deep learning-based models were previously demonstrated for detecting the entry and exit points of annulus sutures in simulation and surgery [7], using a heatmap based multi-instance point detection approach.

The aim of this work is to compare two different setups for recovering depth to support surgical valve repair. Firstly, we use the previously proposed optical tracking based surgical assistance system [4] together with hand-eye calibration (Fig.1 (II)a). Secondly, we use a deep learning based method to detect relevant points from the left and right stereo-endoscopic images [7]; subsequently, the depth at these points from the image pair is estimated (Fig.1 (II)b). Finally, both the methods are compared to manually labeled suture points on the stereo frames, which provides a ground-truth for image-based point detection and a weak ground truth for depth estimation (Fig.1 (II)c).

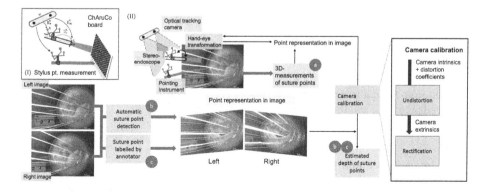

Fig. 1. Overview of the depth estimation setups that are compared in this work.

2   Materials and methods

2.1   Dataset

Mitral valve annuloplasty procedures performed on a surgical simulator with patient-specific valve replica are captured as a video stream in a resolution of 1080×1920 at 25 fps. The *Image1S* stereo-endoscope with 30° degree optics (Karl Storz SE & Co. KG, Tuttlingen, Germany) is used. Two different data sets $data_1$ with 29 frames and $data_2$ with 32 frames was selected from the video streams. Furthermore, 12 frames of a rigid phantom, same as in [4], are used to test the depth measured with the optical tracking system (NDI Polaris Spectra, Northern Digital Inc., Waterloo, Canada). A mean annulus curve computed over manual segmentations from 42 patients served as a base for the phantom. Twelve approximately equidistant small holes on the surface of the phantom serve as a surrogate for the annuloplasty sutures (Fig. 2a-b).

2.2   Optical tracking and hand-eye calibration

To obtain depth measurements from the frame of the optical tracking system, referred to here as the world origin W, the transformation to the camera frame C is required. To track the relative position of the camera, we attach a fixed reference marker R, through which we can determine the unknown transformation D_R^C (Fig. 1(I)). To compute this, we first estimate the transformation of the camera E_W^C from the 2D image points obtained from images of a calibration pattern, and further measure the corresponding 3D points with a stylus tool. The stylus tool is tracked by the optical tracking system, and is calibrated by pivoting the tool around a pin to calculate the offset from the tracked markers. The pivot calibration was performed with 500 images of the tracking tool. We used a custom precision machined *ChArUco* calibration board (calib.io, Svendborg, Denmark) to avoid printing and planarity errors, together with the OpenCV calibration library.

The *EPnP* pose estimation algorithm [8] implementation from OpenCV is then used to calculate the extrinsic camera parameters from the 2D and 3D points. The transformation between the camera C and the rigid marker R can be calculated with

$$D_R^C = E_W^C \cdot (R_W^R)^{-1} \tag{1}$$

A change in the camera position, can be accordingly calculated with the tracked transformation R_W^R

$$E_W^C = D_R^C \cdot R_W^R \tag{2}$$

By measuring the image points with a tracked stylus tool, we can compute the transformation from the camera position. The points that are reprojected using this method are denoted by p_{reproj}, and the depth measurements are denoted by d_{he}. All transformations are computed using a 4x4 affine transformation matrix with $R|t$.

2.3   Image-based point detection

2.3.1   Ground truth. The suture points p_{gt} and point correspondences were manually labeled on the stereo frames by an annotator. Only sutures that can be seen on both the images of the stereo-pair are considered. The labeled points p_{gt} were used for point triangulation to estimate the respective depth $d_{p_{gt}}$ (Fig.1c). Note that due to occlusions, some points which could be measured by the tracked stylus could not be labeled in the images.

2.3.2 Deep learning. The deep learning based heatmap multi-instance point detection method was developed in previous work [7] and is based on the U-Net [9]. A Gaussian distribution of $\sigma = 2$ was applied to the masks of the training dataset, which has a size of 2800 images and an image resolution of 288×512. The model takes as input left or right endoscopic images independently from each other and outputs the locations of the suture points as predictions. Then, two filter steps are applied: Points that lie within a threshold of 6 px radius are considered as *true positives*; point correspondence between left and right image were then determined according to the ground truth. Only the points that are present in both the left and the right images are used for further depth computation d_{p_m}. This leads us to a total of 148 point matches from 327 left and 257 right predicted image points in data$_1$ and in data$_2$ is a total of 156 point matches from 275 left and 239 right predicted image points.

2.4 Evaluation

To evaluate the depth values obtained from the two setups, and their respective comparisons with the labeled suture points, we use three kinds of error, namely: 2D point error in px, 3D point error in mm and the distance between the suture points in 3D in mm. The Euclidean distance is computed to measure the 2D point error for each suture point in the frame. In case of the measured suture point with the optical tracking system, we first project the 3D object points to the image coordinate system, and then compute the Euclidean distance to show the 2D error per suture point per frame (differences between p_{reproj}, p_{gt}, and p_m). Additionally we show the error in 3D space from the left endoscopic camera, to get a better understanding of the performance of depth-estimation (differences between $d_{p_{gt}}$, d_{p_m}, and d_{he}). Since we are also interested in the correct 3D relationship of the suture points, we compare the distance between neighboring suture points to a manually measured distance with a caliper. It is to be noted that the errors introduced by camera calibration is the same for all the three methods compared in the following.

3 Results and discussion

The error of pivot calibration of the short and long styli is reported in Table 1. Furthermore, 12 points were measured using two different stylus tools, on a mitral valve rigid phantom, to compare the re-projection error (Fig. 2). Using the short stylus resulted in a re-projection error of 10.2 px, and the long stylus in 13.73 px. For the simulator datasets, the hand-eye calibration is computed on three different camera poses with multiple point sets comprising approximately 50 points, which result in a re-projection error of 1.49 ± 0.44 px. The resulting depth computation has a mean deviation of 0.8 mm. The calibration with the least error is used for results computation. Table 2 shows the

Tab. 1. Pivot calibration error.

	Default NDI req.	Short stylus tool	Long stylus tool
3D RMS Error	0.4 mm	0.36 mm	0.58 mm
Mean Error	-	0.34 mm	0.51 mm
Maximum 3D Error	0.5 mm	0.48 mm	1.78 mm
Major Angle	45°	60.82°	55.19°
Minor Angle	45°	54.92°	47.39°

Tab. 2. 2D error computed for the suture points in px.

	$p_{gt} - p_{\text{reproj}}$		$p_m - p_{\text{reproj}}$		$p_m - p_{gt}$	
	Left	Right	Left	Right	Left	Right
data$_1$	11.74 ± 7.98	11.55 ± 7.63	11.23 ± 7.07	10.91 ± 7.16	2.09 ± 1.06	2.2 ± 1.19
data$_2$	10.64 ± 8.29	10.22 ± 8.2	13.86 ± 9.72	13.82 ± 9.8	2.29 ± 1.32	2.37 ± 1.27

error in 2D space, for the left and right images, for each of the three methods that were used to triangulate the points and compute the depth. The error was computed over 26 and 30 image points. In comparison with the ground-truth points, the model points p_m produced a lower error of 10.91 px compared to the reprojected points p_{reproj} (Table 2), while the error between the model points and the reprojected points was the highest with 13.86 px. In the 3D error computation (Table 3), the error between the ground truth points and the points measure from the stylus from data$_2$ was the highest with 4.21 ± 2.86 mm, and the error between the predicted points d_{p_m} from the model and the labelled points $d_{p_{gt}}$ from data$_1$ was the least with 1.47 ± 2.08 mm. The depth between the measured points d_{he} and the depth from the reprojected points are similar, with a difference of 0.0035 ± 0.00745 mm and 0.0074 ± 0.015 mm between each other.

To sum up, when compared to the labelled points, the error measured in 2D and 3D space is least for the points predicted from the deep learning model in comparison

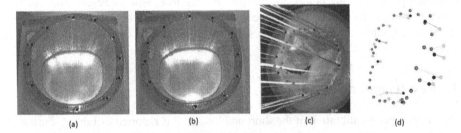

Fig. 2. The left two images show the reprojected 3D points p_{reproj} measured by the stylus tools (red) and manually labeled 2D points p_{gt} (blue). (a) Measurement with short stylus tool on rigid phantom results in a mean re-projection error of 10.2 px; (b) with a long stylus tool a mean re-projection error of 13.73 px to the labeled points is achieved. (c) 2D image points on the left stereo image and (d) corresponding 3D points with back projection stylus points (green), label points d_{gt} (turquoise), model points d_m (black) and 3D stylus measurement d_{he} (orange).

Tab. 3. 3D error computed for the suture points in mm.

	$d_{p_{gt}} - d_{he}$	$d_{p_m} - d_{p_{gt}}$	$d_{p_m} - d_{he}$
data$_1$	3.77 ± 2.83	1.47 ± 2.08	4.14 ± 5.45
data$_2$	2.97 ± 1.89	2.01 ± 2.79	3.06 ± 2.74

with the optical tracking system. Compared to distances measured with a caliper, the error in d_{he} is the highest with 2.1 ± 1.28 mm, while d_{p_m} performed the best with an error of 0.46 ± 0.44 mm and $d_{p_{gt}}$ with an error of 0.7 ± 0.62 mm. However, note in this work, only the *True Positive* predictions from the model are taken into consideration and those which have a corresponding point in the other image. Automatic matching was not considered so far. In conclusion, our preliminary results demonstrate the advantages in accuracy when considering the correctly identified points in endoscope-based image point reconstruction over optically tracked stylus measurements.

Acknowledgement. The research was supported by Informatics for Life project funded by the Klaus Tschira Foundation and the DFG through grant INST 35/1314-1 FUGG, INST 35/1503-1 FUGG, DE 2131/2-1, and EN 1197/2-1.

References

1. Casselman Filip P., Van Slycke Sam, Wellens Francis, De Geest Raphael, Degrieck Ivan, Van Praet Frank et al. Mitral valve surgery can now routinely be performed endoscopically. Circulation. 2003;108:II–48.
2. Boone N, Moore J, Ginty OK, Bainbridge D, Eskandari M, Peters TM. A dynamic mitral valve simulator for surgical training and patient specific preoperative planning. SPIE, 2019.
3. Engelhardt S, Sauerzapf S, Preim B, Karck M, Wolf I, De Simone R. Flexible and comprehensive patient-specific mitral valve silicone models with chordae tendinae made from 3D-printable molds. Int J Comput Assist Radiol Surg. 2019;14(7):1177–86.
4. Engelhardt S, De Simone R, Al-Maisary S, Kolb S, Karck M, Meinzer HP et al. Accuracy evaluation of a mitral valve surgery assistance system based on optical tracking. Int J Comput Assist Radiol Surg. 2016;11(10):1891–904.
5. Engelhardt S, Wolf I, Al-Maisary S, Schmidt H, Meinzer H, Karck M et al. Intraoperative quantitative mitral valve analysis using optical tracking technology. Ann Thorac Surg. 2016;5:1950–6.
6. Engelhardt S, De Simone R, Zimmermann N, Al-Maisary S, Nabers D, Karck M et al. Augmented reality-enhanced endoscopic images for annuloplasty ring sizing. Augmented Environments for Computer-Assisted Interventions. Springer International Publishing, 2014:128–37.
7. Sharan L, Romano G, Brand J, Kelm H, Karck M, De Simone R et al. Point detection through multi-instance deep heatmap regression for sutures in endoscopy. Int J Comput Assist Radiol Surg. 2021.
8. Lepetit V, Moreno-Noguer F, Fua P. EPnP: an accurate O(n) solution to the PnP problem. Int J Comput Vis. 2009;81(2):155.
9. Ronneberger O, Fischer P, Brox T. U-Net: convolutional networks for biomedical image segmentation. MICCAI 2015. Springer International Publishing.

Abstract: M²aia: Mass Spectrometry Imaging Applications for Interactive Analysis in MITK

Jonas Cordes[1,2], Thomas Enzlein[3], Christian Marsching[3], Marven Hinze[1], Sandy Engelhardt[4], Carsten Hopf[3], Ivo Wolf[1]

[1]Faculty of Computer Science, Mannheim University of Applied Sciences, Germany
[2]Medical Faculty Mannheim, University Heidelberg, Germany
[3]Center for Mass Spectrometry and Optical Spectroscopy (CeMOS), Mannheim University of Applied Sciences, Germany
[4]Working Group "Artificial Intelligence in Cardiovascular Medicine" (AICM), University Hospital Heidelberg, Germany
j.cordes@hs-mannheim.de

Mass spectrometry imaging (MSI) is a label-free analysis method for resolving biomolecules or pharmaceuticals in the spatial domain. It offers unique perspectives for the examination of entire organs or other tissue specimens. Owing to increasing capabilities of modern MSI devices, the use of 3D and multi-modal MSI becomes feasible in routine applications — resulting in hundreds of gigabytes of data. To fully leverage such MSI acquisitions, interactive tools for 3D image reconstruction, visualization, and analysis are required, which preferably should be open-source to allow scientists to develop custom extensions. We introduce M²aia (MSI applications for interactive analysis in MITK), a software tool providing interactive and memory-efficient data access and signal processing of multiple large MSI datasets stored in imzML format. M²aia extends MITK, a popular open-source tool in medical image processing. Besides the steps of a typical signal processing workflow, M²aia offers fast visual interaction, image segmentation, deformable 3D image reconstruction, and multi-modal registration. A unique feature is that fused data with individual mass axes can be visualized in a shared coordinate system. We demonstrate features of M²aia by reanalyzing an N-glycan mouse kidney dataset and 3D reconstruction and multi-modal image registration of a lipid and peptide dataset of a mouse brain, which we make publicly available. To our knowledge, M²aia is the first extensible open-source application that enables a fast, user-friendly, and interactive exploration of large datasets. M²aia is applicable to a wide range of MSI analysis tasks. The work was published in GigaScience 2021 [1].

References

1. Cordes J, Enzlein T, Marsching C, Hinze M, Engelhardt S, Hopf C et al. M²aia: interactive, fast, and memory-efficient analysis of 2D and 3D multi-modal mass spectrometry imaging data. GigaScience. 2021;10(7):giab049.

© Der/die Autor(en), exklusiv lizenziert durch
Springer Fachmedien Wiesbaden GmbH, ein Teil von Springer Nature 2022
K. Maier-Hein et al. (Hrsg.), *Bildverarbeitung für die Medizin 2022*,
Informatik aktuell, https://doi.org/10.1007/978-3-658-36932-3_36

Learning Features via Transformer Networks for Cardiomyocyte Profiling

Jan Plier[2,3], Matthias Zisler[3], Jennifer Furkel[1], Maximilian Knoll[1], Alexander Marx[1], Alena Fischer[1], Kai Polsterer[2], Mathias H. Konstandin[1], Stefania Petra[3]

[1]Cardiology, Angiology and Pneumology, Heidelberg University Hospital
[2]Heidelberg Institute for Theoretical Studies, Heidelberg
[3]Mathematical Imaging Group, Heidelberg University
zisler@math.uni-heidelberg.de

Abstract. We introduce an image-based strategy that builds on morphological cell profiling with the purpose of predicting canonical hypertrophy stimulators as proxies for pathomechanisms in cardiology. The traditional approach relies on extracting handcrafted morphological features from unlabeled cell image data in order to reason about cell biology. In this work we employ transformer networks that automatically learn features that help identify which hypertrophy stimulator has been applied on imaged cardiomyocytes. Numerical results illustrate the high predictive performance of this type of neural networks.

1 Introduction

Morphological cell profiling [1] has proven to be a useful and successful technique in creating from microscopy images signatures of cells, also known as cell phenotypes. Typically, one wants to identify these cells which show interesting phenotypes and their sub-populations. Such exploratory data analysis approaches usually involve dimensionality reduction followed by clustering, in the hope that cluster representations of phenotypes emerge. Such an approach applied to images of cardiomyocytes has been presented in [2]. The workflow in [2] involves several nontrivial data analysis steps which include cell segmentation and feature extraction by CellProfiler [3]. However, cardiomyocytes exhibit heterogeneous morphology rendering cell segmentation a nontrivial task that requires manual adjustments for each new experimental setup. Features extracted by CellProfiler capture characteristics related to the size, intensity, shape, texture and neighbourhood information of cells and produce very high dimensional vectors (>1600). While these feature vectors have interpretable entries, this interpretability is lost once they are subjected to (nonlinear) dimensionality reduction. In fact 60-80% of morphological cell profiling studies end up using only 1 or 2 cellular features [4].

Motivated by the fact that features extracted via CellProfiler are not expected to capture aspects of cardiomyocytes useful in identifying hypertrophy stimulators, we advocate the use of learnable features, that do not rely on a-priori cell segmentation. As transformers networks [5] achieve state-of-the-art performance in many tasks including classification, we propose to extract features by transformer networks for classifying

© Der/die Autor(en), exklusiv lizenziert durch
Springer Fachmedien Wiesbaden GmbH, ein Teil von Springer Nature 2022
K. Maier-Hein et al. (Hrsg.), *Bildverarbeitung für die Medizin 2022*,
Informatik aktuell, https://doi.org/10.1007/978-3-658-36932-3_37

cropped cardiomyocytes images. The classes are the 8 canonical hypertrophy simulators, that mimick neurohumoral activation in vitro, (plus control) applied on the imaged cardiomyocytes: Epinephrine/adrenaline (A), angiotensin II (AT), dobutamin (Dob), endothelin-1 (ET), insulin (Ins), isoproterenol (ISO), norepinephrine (NOR) and phenylephrine (PE). The goal of our work is to learn cell profiles and identify pathomechanisms in cardiomyocytes for predicting cardiac disease states.

2   Materials and methods

We consider the classification problem of assigning a label y_k^i to an entire sequence x^i of image patches centred on cell nuclei. The labels stand for the K number of treatment conditions. We design a multilayered artificial neural network $F : \mathbb{R}^D \rightarrow \mathbb{R}^K$ and determine its parameters by minimizing the cross entropy loss

$$\text{loss} = -\sum_{i,k} y_k^i \log(\text{softmax}(F(x^i)))$$

where y_k^i is the label, and $\text{softmax}(F(x^i))$ is the predicted class probability. The rest of the section is organized as follows: we give details on our data set, on the network architecture underlying F and on performed experiments.

2.1   Cell preparation and imaging

Following the established procedure in [2], neonatal rat cardiomyocytes (NRCMs) are treated with 8 canonical hypertrophy simulators under cell culture conditions at a particular concentration. These substances that stimulate the NRCMs were selected from the group of catecholamines as they are known to play a role in pathologic hypertrophy with differences in specificity for α- and β-adrenoreceptors (Phenyleprhine, Noradrenaline, Adrenaline, Dobutamin). In addition, a strong inductor of cell growth not implicated in pathologic hypertrophy - Insulin - is chosen. Microscopy images of treated cells are acquired by immunofluorescence after using fluorescent dyes.

2.2   Image prepossessing

The raw microscopy images, from which we later extract features, are corrected for inhomogeneous background illumination and defocus artifacts. Our pipeline extends the workflow from [2] by integrating: a) an illumination correction similar to [6], b) the choice of the focal plane by z-stacking using a wavelet based approach [7]. This step guarantees a consistent image quality for subsequent feature extraction.

2.3   Data set

We used raw data derived from NRCMs. The latter were transformed to express a GFP fusion protein acting as a marker. Each well in a 94 well plate contained such a cell population that was either subsequently perturbed using one of 8 substances

Tab. 1. Number of image patches for each set and substance. These substances used for incubating the NRCMs are: Epinephrine/adrenaline (A), angiotensin II (AT), dobutamin (Dob), endothelin-1 (ET), insulin (Ins), isoproterenol (ISO), norepinephrine (NOR) and phenylephrine (PE). In the case of control (Ctrl) no substance is applied.

	A	AT	Dob	ET	Ins	Iso	NOR	PE	Ctrl
Train	20431	25367	18600	29621	18605	25982	30192	23617	176140
Valid	6957	8261	6303	9883	6269	8777	11033	7821	58726
Test	6558	8177	5678	10406	6850	8292	10079	7426	59179

(hypertrophic stimuli or inhibitors) or used as control. After adding fluorescent dyes, 5×5 field of view images per well were captured, each containing several hundred cells. For each field of view three channels (DNA – DAPI, desmin – TexasRed, F-actin – Phalloidin) were imaged using the IN Cell Analyzer 2200. After detecting cell nuclei using [8], we extracted for each channel a 128×128 image patch, centered in each nucleus. We used these three channel image patches for subsequent feature extraction and classification. Each image patch was assigned a label according to its treatment condition. We note that for each substance, activation of numerous signaling pathways have been described, to a varying extend. For additional details we refer to [2]. As these signaling pathways are still subject of current research we chose hypertrophy simulators as class labels.

We performed 3 trials, each involving 4 well plates. We extract from each well plate image patches, ensuring that each class has roughly the same number of image patches. However, we withhold a larger number of image patches for control (Tab. 1).

2.4 Network architecture

Our network F has two components: one extracts learnable features for each image patch and one aggregates these features. We refer to Figure 1 for an illustration.

2.5 Feature extraction

To extract learnable features from every image patch, we used the vision transformer (ViT) [9], that uses the transformer model in [5], known from the field of natural language processing. It builds on a multi-head self attention layer and learns global attention over the elements in the sequence to draw global dependencies between input and output. We subdivide each 128×128 image patch into 16 non-overlapping 32×32 images constituting the input sequence for the ViT. The output of the ViT is a sequence of feature vectors. We set their dimension to 10. The output sequence of ViT is augmented by a learnable classification token that we exploit in the next step.

2.6 Feature aggregation

Learnable features are combined using different aggregation methods (Fig. 1):

1. The feature vector extracted via ViT from each image patch is mapped via the softmax function to a vector of length K of class probabilities. These vectors of probabilities are aggregated via majority voting, followed by the final classfier.
2. We take the mean or median of the features extracted from each image patch and obtain a single feature vector that is subsequently used in the final classification.
3. Using the transformer layer, we learn weights that produce a data dependent aggregation. This transformer layer receives as input a sequence of feature vectors (classification tokens), each extracted via ViT from an image patch; it outputs a new sequence of features and again a special classification token that is subsequently used in the final classification.

2.7 Experiments

We performed two experiments. In the first one we determine the optimal sequence length of image patches used for classification. In the second we evaluate the feature aggregation methods. During training we used a batch size equal to 64, set the learning rate to 10^{-4} and used ADAM to optimize the parameters of the network.

3 Results

Figure 2 shows the results of our two experiments: the first evaluates the optimal sequence length of cell crops, the second the performance of our four network architectures. See the image caption for more details. Figure 3 details the second experiment and shows the per label test accuracy of each classifier.

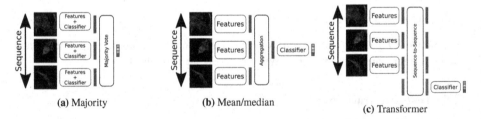

(a) Majority   (b) Mean/median   (c) Transformer

Fig. 1. Illustration of transformer based network architectures. The block tagged "classifier " is a placeholder for a normalization layer followed by a linear layer. The block tagged "features" refers to feature extraction by the ViT architecture. Top left: The first variant (tagged majority) appends to each ViT learnable feature vector a "classifier" layer yielding a sequence of logits. We then use a majority vote lifting these logits for each image patch on the simplex with softmax and then take the geometric mean over the simplex variables for the final decision. Top right: The second variant (tagged either mean or median) uses the mean or median to merge the ViT learnable features into a single feature vector. Bottom: The third variant (tagged transformer), first extracts learnable ViT learnable features appended by a learnable classification token. Then an additional transformer layer is applied (tagged "Sequence-to-Sequence") obtaining a new sequence of features and a new classification token. A layer normalization followed by a linear layer is applied to this new classification token.

4 Discussion

Inspecting Figure 2 (left), we observe that by using only one cell crop for classification, i.e. sequence length equal to 1, we achieve a significantly lower performance than aggregating over more cells. On the other hand, for a sequence length of 25, we see a saturation in performance. Our results imply that a relatively small number of cell patches centred at nuclei suffices for accurate classification and leads to expressive cell profiles without the need of discarding cells that died or have not responded to treatment. In [2] such cells are discarded and single cell features are aggregated per well.

According Figure 2 (right), the median aggregation exhibits the lowest performance. The reason lies most likely in its non-smooth nature. The other three methods are almost performing on par, with the (soft) majority voting over the single cell classification performing best. Note, that the transformer aggregation is the only method with learnable parameters. According to Figure 3, cells treated with dobutamin (Dob) and isoproterenol (Iso) are the most difficult to classify for any aggregation method. In particular median aggregation performs very poor on Dob. This could be due to the fact that Dob and Iso both have a similar agonistic effect on β-adrenergic receptors and thereby trigger the same cellular pathways. In contrast, adrenaline (A) is known to have an agonistic effect on α- and β adrenergic receptors, and norepinephrine (NOR) primarily has an agonistic effect on α adrenergic receptors. We hypothesize that treatments with similar efficacy profiles will exhibit more similar morphological profiles, making them more difficult to distinguish from each other.

In the immediate future we aim to demonstrate the potential of learned features using patient blood treated NRCMs choosing as case study aortic valve stenosis, a cardiac disease with high prevalence in elderly patients.

Acknowledgement. The authors gratefully acknowledge the generous and invaluable support of the Klaus Tschira Foundation.

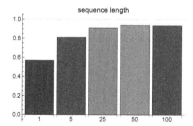
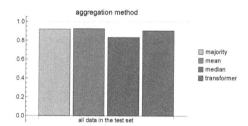

Fig. 2. Left: Influence of sequence length on test accuracy. We show results for the transformer aggregation method only. Alternatives perform similarly. Bars show the test accuracy averaged over 10 runs for sequence length $\in \{1, 5, 25, 50, 100\}$. Right: Test accuracy for each variant of the classifier network. Bars show the accuracy on the test set averaged over 10 runs.

Fig. 3. Inter class test accuracy for each variant of the classifier network. Each bar represents the accuracy on the test set averaged over 10 runs for each label and aggregation method.

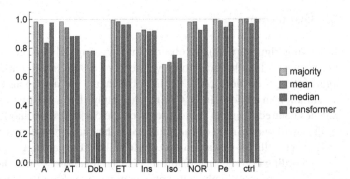

References

1. Caicedo J, Cooper S, Heigwer F, Warchal S, Qiu P, Molnar C et al. Data-analysis strategies for image-based cell profiling. Nat Methods. 2017;14(9):849–63.
2. Furkel J, Knoll M, Din S, Bogert N, Seeger T, Frey N et al. C-MORE: a high content single cell morphology assay for cardiovascular medicine. Cell Rep Med (accepted). 2021.
3. Carpenter A, Jones T, Lamprecht M, Clarke C, Kang I, Friman O et al. CellProfiler: image analysis software for identifying and quantifying cell phenotypes. Genome Biol. 2006;10(7):849–63.
4. Singh S Carpenter AE GA. Increasing the content of high-content screening: an overview. J Biomol Screen. 2014;19(5):640–650.
5. Vaswani A, Shazeer N, Parmar N, Uszkoreit J, Jones L, Gomez AN et al. Attention is all you need. Adv Neural Inf Process Syst. 2017;30.
6. Peng T, Thorn K, Schroeder T, Wang L, Theis FJ, Marr C et al. A BaSiC tool for background and shading correction of optical microscopy images. Nat Commun. 2017;8:14836.
7. Forster B, Van De Ville D, Berent J, Sage D, Unser M. Complex wavelets for extended depth-of-field: a new method for the fusion of multichannel microscopy images. Microsc Res Tech. 2004;65(1-2):33–42.
8. Schmidt U, Weigert M, Broaddus C, Myers G. Cell detection with star-convex polygons. MICCAI 2018. Ed. by Frangi AF, Schnabel JA, Davatzikos C, Alberola-López C, Fichtinger G. Vol. 11071. (LNCS). Springer, 2018:265–73.
9. Dosovitskiy A, Beyer L, Kolesnikov A, Weissenborn D, Zhai X, Unterthiner T et al. An image is worth 16x16 words: transformers for image recognition at scale. ICLR. 2021.

Effect of Random Histogram Equalization on Breast Calcification Analysis Using Deep Learning

Adarsh Bhandary Panambur[1,2], Prathmesh Madhu[2], Andreas Maier[2]

[1]Technology and Innovation Management, Siemens Healthineers, Erlangen, Germany
[2]Pattern Recognition Lab, FAU Erlangen-Nürnberg, Erlangen, Germany
adarsh.bhandary.panambur@fau.de

Abstract. Early detection and analysis of calcifications in mammogram images is crucial in a breast cancer diagnosis workflow. Management of calcifications that require immediate follow-up and further analyzing its benignancy or malignancy can result in a better prognosis. Recent studies have shown that deep learning-based algorithms can learn robust representations to analyze suspicious calcifications in mammography. In this work, we demonstrate that randomly equalizing the histograms of calcification patches as a data augmentation technique can significantly improve the classification performance for analyzing suspicious calcifications. We validate our approach by using the CBIS-DDSM dataset for two classification tasks. The results on both the tasks show that the proposed methodology gains more than 1% mean accuracy and F1-score when equalizing the data with a probability of 0.4 when compared to not using histogram equalization. This is further supported by the t-tests, where we obtain a p-value of $p<0.0001$, thus showing the statistical significance of our approach.

1 Introduction

With an estimated 2.26 million new cases in 2020, breast cancer is the leading cause of malignancy incidence worldwide [1]. Periodic screening of women based on their age groups using mammography has proven to reduce the late-stage incidence and mortality rates [1]. Breast Imaging Reporting and Database System (BI-RADS) is a scoring system used by radiologists to assign categories to the suspicious region of interest on screening mammography based on the type, density, morphology, and distribution of the findings [2]. In addition to observing essential findings such as mass, density, architectural distortions, and asymmetries in the breast, the clinicians also search for bright well-circumscribed findings known as calcification. Calcifications are calcium deposits, generally found inside the ducts, lobules, connective stroma tissue, and vessels of the breast [3]. The analysis of calcification on mammograms is of high importance as its morphology and distribution can be representative of precancerous or malignant cells [3]. As the sensitivity of calcification detection during the initial mammography screening is low [4], computer-aided diagnosis (CAD) methods can potentially support clinicians for better decision making for early detection and analysis of calcifications.

Springer Fachmedien Wiesbaden GmbH, ein Teil von Springer Nature 2022
K. Maier-Hein et al. (Hrsg.), *Bildverarbeitung für die Medizin 2022*,
Informatik aktuell, https://doi.org/10.1007/978-3-658-36932-3_38

Deep learning (DL)-based CAD algorithms have proven to provide effective and robust solutions for automated breast cancer analysis in mammography [5], with many recent approaches showing promising results in calcification analysis tasks [6, 7].

Contrast enhancement techniques have been vastly studied as a pre-processing image technique in whole mammogram image analysis [8]. However, applying these techniques to smaller calcification patches might lead to a loss of class-specific information. This is evident due to the appearance of calcification which generally appears as a bright spot or as a group of scattered bright spots, and equalizing the histograms of such patches might lead to noisy images. Adding noise to the input data is one of the data augmentation techniques used for training DL networks [9]. Data augmentation is the most commonly used strategy in DL to increase the quality of the training data by applying transformations to the input enforcing the network to learn meaningful, class-specific representations [10]. In this work, we investigate the usage of random histogram equalization (RHE) as a data augmentation technique for calcification analysis. Histogram equalization (HE) is a contrast enhancement technique that non-linearly scales the input to a uniform distribution of intensities based on the image's histogram.

The main contributions of our research are: a) We present that using RHE as a data augmentation technique with a probability value of 0.4 can lead to a significant performance gain compared to not using RHE; b) We also present and compare Gradient-weighted Class Activation Mapping (Grad-CAM) [10] for models that were trained using no HE and full HE to show that RHE outperforms both of them in localizing class-specific calcification features.

The remaining organization of the paper is as follows: Section 2 provides a brief description of the data and methods used in our work. Next, we present the quantitative and qualitative results for two and three-class classification tasks in Section 3. Finally, in Section 4, we provide a brief discussion on the results.

2   Materials and methods

2.1   Data

Curated Breast Imaging Subset of Digital Database for Screening Mammography (CBIS-DDSM) is a public dataset consisting of scanned film mammography from multiple institutions across the United States of America [11]. In this research, we utilize a small subset of the dataset consisting of cropped regions of calcifications observed on craniocaudal and/or mediolateral oblique views in the mammogram images.

In Table 1, we show the distribution of the class samples in the training, validation, and test dataset. The dataset consists of 1,546 images divided into training and validation datasets with an 80:20 ratio. In addition, we use an independent test dataset from CBIS-DDSM with 326 images as the test dataset. The verified pathology information available in this dataset is used as the labels for the two classification tasks. The first task involves the binary classification of "Follow-up" versus "No follow-up" calcification patches. The calcifications labeled as "malignant" and "benign" are used for the "Follow-up" class as these patches would require additional clinical investigations. "No follow-up" class consists of "benign without callback" calcifications indicating the lesions are worth tracking but does not require further investigations. Finally, we use the

Tab. 1. The distribution of class samples in the CBIS-DDSM dataset for the two-class (Follow-up versus No follow-up) and three-class problems (Malignant, benign and benign without callback).

	Follow-up	No follow-up	Malignant	Benign	Benign w/o callback
Training	855	382	445	410	382
Validation	217	92	99	118	92
Test	259	67	129	130	67
Total	1331	541	673	658	541

original "malignant", "benign", and "benign without callback" labels for the three-class classification.

2.2 Experimental setup

Based on our initial experiments with various state-of-the-art convolutional neural networks (CNN), we chose a pre-trained ResNet50 [12] as the standard CNN architecture for all the experiments conducted in this research. The final fully connected layer (head) in the CNN is refactored to represent the number of classes, i.e., 2 and 3, respectively. The input images are resized with bilinear interpolation into 224 x 224 pixels, and the pixel values are normalized to the range *[0,1]*. Four fixed data augmentations are used to enhance the quality and size of the training data. Random horizontal flip, random vertical flip, random rotations are used with a probability value of 0.5, and random erasing is used with a probability value of 0.1. The probability value indicates the possibility of the current image being transformed. As this research aims to investigate the effect of RHE as a data augmentation technique in calcification analysis, different experiments with probability values (P) of 0, 0.2, 0.4, 0.6, 0.8, and 1 are conducted. All the CNNs are trained for 30 epochs with a batch size of 16. A weighted binary cross-entropy loss function is optimized using a standard Adam optimizer with a learning rate of $3.2e^{-6}$ and a weight decay of $1e^{-4}$.

Accuracy and F1-score are the two performance evaluation metrics used for the classification task. We further utilize a two-tailed unpaired t-test in order to determine the statistical significance of the classification performances. Finally, the qualitative performance of the CNN is analyzed by localizing the regions in the calcification patch that influenced the model's decision by using the Grad-CAM approach [10]. The entire DL pipeline was developed using PyTorch.

3   Results

In Table 2, we summarize the performance of the trained CNNs on the test dataset for both the two-class and three-class classification tasks. The different values of P in the results denote the probability of a calcification patch being equalized during the training (Tab. 2). The probability value of 0 (P=0) indicates that no HE is used during training or testing, whereas a value of 1 (P=1) indicates all the images are equalized during both training and testing phases. For all the other intermediate values (P=0.2, 0.4, 0.6, 0.8), RHE is used only during training. Each experiment for each probability value

Tab. 2. Classification performance of the trained CNN on the test dataset. Different values of P indicate the probability of RHE on a patch during training. The best results are in *italics*.

	Two-class task		Three-class task	
	Accuracy	F1-Score	Accuracy	F1-Score
$P=0$	0.9215 (0.0066)	0.8838 (0.0078)	0.6632 (0.0126)	0.6855 (0.0131)
$P=0.2$	0.9159 (0.0117)	0.8759 (0.0117)	0.6755 (0.0191)	0.6985 (0.0221)
$P=0.4$	*0.9325 (0.0085)*	*0.8973 (0.0124)*	*0.6840 (0.0193)*	*0.7071 (0.0189)*
$P=0.6$	0.9196 (0.0092)	0.8770 (0.0119)	0.6687 (0.0058)	0.6969 (0.0036)
$P=0.8$	0.9252 (0.0074)	0.8869 (0.0109)	0.6601 (0.015)	0.6839 (0.0159)
$P=1$	0.8724 (0.0179)	0.8103 (0.0111)	0.6252 (0.017)	0.6322 (0.0228)

was run five times to ensure stability in the final reported results. The mean accuracy and F1-score with the standard deviation over five validation runs are reported on the test dataset. In Figure 1, the Grad-CAM visualizations comparing the network outputs for best-performing models for $P=0$ and $P=0.4$ are shown for both the tasks. Figure 2 shows the Grad-CAM visualizations when all the input training calcification patches are histogram equalized.

4   Discussion

As observed in the results summarized in Table 2, the network learns better representations for both the classification tasks using RHE during training with a probability of 0.4 compared to not using HE ($P=0$). For the two-class task, i.e., Follow-up vs. No follow-up, we achieve a mean accuracy and F1-score of 0.9215 and 0.8838, respectively, on the test dataset, when no HE is applied during training. When we increase the probability to a value of 0.4, we reach a mean accuracy of 0.9325 and a mean F1-score of 0.8973. A performance boost of more than 1% is observed in both the mean accuracy and F1-score. The results are then tested for statistical significance of accuracy and F1-score using a t-test, where a two-tailed p-value of $p<0.0001$ is obtained. This clearly shows that using RHE with a probability of 0.4 results in a statistically significant performance. A similar trend is observed in malignant, benign, and benign without callback classification. In this case, we achieve more than 2% gain in both the metrics by using the

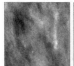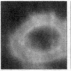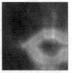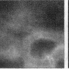

(a) Malignant, Benign, Malignant   (b) Follow-up, No follow-up, Follow-up

Fig. 1. Input image with true class label, Grad-CAM image for $P=0$ and $P=0.4$ with the predicted class labels. The localized regions responsible for misclassifications can be observed while using $P=0$. However, using $P=0.4$, the network is able to learn robust class-discriminative features.

Fig. 2. Input image with true class label, histogram equalized image and the Grad-CAM image with the predicted class label for $P=1$. The network is not able to extract the class-relevant features even though the it is able to localize the suspicious region of calcification.

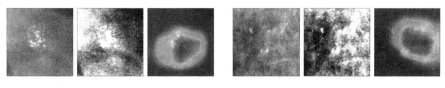

(a) Malignant, Benign　　　　　　　　　　(b) Follow-up, No follow-up

probability value of 0.4, with mean accuracy increasing from 0.6632 to 0.6840 and the F1-score increasing from 0.6855 to 0.7071. A p-value of $p<0.0001$ is obtained, showing a statistically significant classification performance during the t-test.

The increase in performance can be attributed to the randomly injected noise in the form of RHE during training, forcing the network to concentrate on the calcification regions rather than the surrounding anatomical structures. This behavior can be observed using Grad-CAM visualizations in Figure 1. The models trained with random probability of $P=0.4$ are inherently more robust and tend to focus more towards the high-intensity spots indicative of calcifications. The results in Table 2 also show a significant reduction in the performance while using $P=1$, i.e., equalizing the histograms of all images during training and testing. This is due to the enhancement of the contrast in the brighter parts of the image leading to corruption of the class-specific features in the data. In Figure 2, we can observe that the essential features such as the morphology and the distribution of the calcifications are corrupted due to the equalization of the histogram values in the image. Even though the attention of the network is focused towards the region of calcifications, we observe misclassifications.

As the current work involves calcification patches detected on scanned film mammography, we plan to validate the proposed technique using digital mammography images as a part of future work. None of the research involving patch-level calcification analysis has exclusively explored the effect of data augmentations on model performance. However, a systematic evaluation of the individual and composition of different data augmentations would be beneficial to provide insights into the right set of augmentation settings that might contribute to the overall performance of the model. Therefore, we aim to perform additional ablation studies to examine the impact of other data augmentation techniques paired with RHE on calcification analysis.

References

1. Sung H, Ferlay J, Siegel RL, Laversanne M, Soerjomataram I, Jemal A et al. Global cancer statistics 2020: GLOBOCAN estimates of incidence and mortality worldwide for 36 cancers in 185 countries. CA Cancer J Clin. 2021;71(3):209–49.
2. Sickles EA, D'Orsi CJ, Bassett LW et al. ACR BI-RADS® mammography. ACR BI-RADS® Atlas, Breast Imaging Reporting and Data System. Reston, VA, American College of Radiology, 2013:121–40.

3. Henrot P, Leroux A, Barlier C, Génin P. Breast microcalcifications: the lesions in anatomical pathology. Diagn Interv Imaging. 2014;95(2):141–52.

4. Mordang JJ, Gubern-Mérida A, Bria A, Tortorella F, Mann R, Broeders M et al. The importance of early detection of calcifications associated with breast cancer in screening. Breast Cancer Res Treat. 2018;167(2):451–8.

5. Wong DJ, Gandomkar Z, Wu WJ, Zhang G, Gao W, He X et al. Artificial intelligence and convolution neural networks assessing mammographic images: a narrative literature review. J Med Radiat Sci. 2020;67(2):134–42.

6. Chen KC, Chin CL, Chung NC, Hsu CL. Combining multi-classifier with CNN in detection and classification of breast calcification. International Conference on Biomedical and Health Informatics. Springer. 2019:304–11.

7. Rehman Ku, Li J, Pei Y, Yasin A, Ali S, Mahmood T. Computer vision-based micro-calcification detection in digital mammograms using fully connected depthwise separable convolutional neural network. Sensors. 2021;21(14):4854.

8. Mustafa WA, Kader MMMA. A review of histogram equalization techniques in image enhancement application. J Phys Conf Ser. 2018;1019:012026.

9. Shorten C, Khoshgoftaar TM. A survey on image data augmentation for deep learning. J Big Data. 2019;6(1):1–48.

10. Selvaraju RR, Cogswell M, Das A, Vedantam R, Parikh D, Batra D. Grad-cam: visual explanations from deep networks via gradient-based localization. Proc IEEE Int Conf Comput Vis. 2017:618–26.

11. Lee RS, Gimenez F, Hoogi A, Miyake KK, Gorovoy M, Rubin DL. A curated mammography data set for use in computer-aided detection and diagnosis research. Sci Data. 2017;4(1):1–9.

12. He K, Zhang X, Ren S, Sun J. Deep residual learning for image recognition. Proc IEEE Comput Soc Conf Comput Vis Pattern Recognit. 2016:770–8.

Longitudinal Analysis of Disease Progression Using Image and Laboratory Data for Covid-19 Patients

Francesca De Benetti[1], Verena Bentele[1], Egon Burian[2,3], Marcus Makowski[2],
Nassir Navab[1,4], Rickmer Braren[2], Thomas Wendler[1]

[1]Chair for Computer Aided Medical Procedures and Augmented Reality, TU Munich
[2]Department of Diagnostic and Interventional Radiology, TU Munich
[3]Department of Diagnostic and Interventional Neuroradiology, TU Munich
[4]Computer Aided Medical Procedures Lab, Laboratory for Computational Sensing+Robotics,
Johns Hopkins University
francesca.de-benetti@tum.de

Abstract. In search of prognostic markers for Covid-19 disease outcome, we propose a workflow that integrates short-term changes in longitudinal CT imaging and laboratory data with disease outcome. For longitudinal imaging data analysis, we use deformable registration and quantify the change in status (healthy, ground glas opacity and consolidation) of the lung parenchyma at a voxel level. We identify lung tissue transformed to worse (pathological) status and increasing inflammatory parameters (i.e., CRP and IL-6) to be prognostic of extended hospital stay and worsened patient outcome. We apply the methodology to compute the predictive value of these features in the first and the second Covid-19 wave.

1 Introduction

Since the Coronavirus Disease of 2019 (Covid-19) was reported in late 2019, it has developed into a pandemic. Due to high potential for critical clinical course and severe outcome, finding prognostic parameters at an early stage of hospitalization is of high interest. Analysing dynamic changes of longitudinal laboratory data and image progression profiles can provide important insights in disease progression and outcome prediction [1, 2]. To detect image changes, deformable registration of longitudinal lung CTs is required [3, 4].

In this work, we aim to fill the lack of off-the-shelf methods for disease progression analysis with voxel-level comparison, while applying them to the first two Covid-19 waves in which different treatment was administered.

The main contributions of this work are: 1) We introduce an automatic methodology to quantify disease progression in the lungs for voxel-wise comparison. 2) We propose a simple method to assess the correlation between outcome, longitudinal laboratory and image data. 3) We apply the method on intensive care unit (ICU) Covid-19 patient cohort from the first and second wave.

2 Materials and methods

2.1 Dataset

The data contains 50 patients presented at our institution that were confirmed to be Covid-19 positive by RT-PCR, showing characteristic symptoms and image findings. All patients were admitted in ICU due to an increased breathing rate, and low blood oxygen levels. The collection includes 25 patients in the first (May-April: 22 male, 3 female; 62 ± 16 years) and 25 patients in the second (June-November: 20 male, 5 female; 71 ± 12 years) wave, and was performed retrospectively in accordance with ethical approvals 245/19 S-SR and 111/20 S.

Low dose non-contrast thorax CT scans were taken with elevated arms and in full inspiration by a 256-row multidetector CT scanner (iCT, Philips Healthcare, Best, The Netherlands: 120 kVp/200 mAs/0.6 mm). On average there were 20 ± 11 days between first (at T_0; 2 ± 7 days after tested Covid-19 positive) and follow up CT (at T_1).

Each patient is represented by static (demographic and clinical) and longitudinal (laboratory and image) data. Lung CT scans and laboratory values were collected at the same time (± 1 day). Differences in longitudinal data, denoted by Δ, is always calculated subtracting the value at T_0 to the value at T_1.

Our dataset is composed by 2 demographics (sex and age), 19 clinical, 54 laboratory and 46 image-derived features, accounting for 121 values per patient.

- The clinical parameters describe the treatment (i.e., extracorporal membrane-oxygenation, hemodialysis or duration of invasive ventilation), as well as, short and long term outcome parameters: death (0: "no"; 1: "yes"), hospital stay (days), ICU stay (days) and outcome 30 days after diagnosis (7 categories - from 1: "passed away" to 7: "discharged to home").
- The laboratory data includes blood count, clinical chemistry, inflammation and coagulation parameters with their Δ. If some values could not be collected, they were replaced by the cohort's (gender- and wave-specific) mean. Parameters with >25% of values missing were treated only as static.
- The image-derived parameters include static parameters (such as the volume of each pathology) with their Δ, and the progression analysis parameters (Sec. 2.3). Both absolute (ml) and percent values are included. The pathologies considered were ground-glass-opacity (ggo), consolidation (cons) and pleural effusion (plef).

The complete list of features is available[1].

2.2 Image data preprocessing: segmentation and registration

2.2.1 Segmentation. The CT dataset was manually annotated by trained MD candidates using the software ImFusion Labels (version 0.17.2, ImFusion, Munich, Germany). For a better workflow, we first created a base label (lung incl. pleural effusion), which was used to get a mask from the CT. Within that mask, we labelled ventilated lung tissue (healthy), consolidation, ggo and pleural effusion. The lung label was created by removing pleural effusion from the base label.

---

[1]github.com/FrancescaDB/Longitudinal-Analysis-of-Covid-19-Disease-Progression

2.2.2 Registration. The deformable registration brings the two volumetric data in the same coordinate space and it ensures the match between the lung voxels, a mandatory requirement for the voxel-wise progression analysis. Compared to CT-based deformable registration, performing it on lung label maps gives better results in a shorter amount of time (Fig. 1).

After being resampled to isotropic spacing of 1 mm, the label maps are cropped to minimize the total size of the images. Then, the registration is performed using the Free Form Deformation algorithm and the BSpline transform of SimpleITK (version 1.2.4). The transformation computed on each lung label map is then applied to the corresponding pathology label map at T_1.

2.3 Progression analysis

The progression analysis aims to compute the type of transition of each voxel from its status (healthy, ggo, cons) in T_0 to its status in T_1. After encoding the presence of each status in a set of binary label maps, the number of voxels transitioning from one status to another is computed intersecting the two corresponding binary maps.

The results of the progression analysis are included in the features list as volumes (in ml) and in percentages of "common lung" (defined as the intersection of the two lung label maps after the registration).

Two additional binary features, namely "lung improving" and "lung worsening", are derived from the progression analysis and are defined as the sum of the lung progressing from every pathology to healthy and from consolidation to ggo, and the sum of the lung progressing from healthy to each pathology and from ggo to consolidation, respectively.

2.4 Correlation analysis and feature selection

Due to the high dimensionality and a limited number of samples in the dataset, the analysis is carried out with naïve correlation methods: phi coefficient, Pearson and point biserial [5], using the scikit-learn (version 0.23.2) and the scipy (version 1.4.1) packages. The significance (p-value) is computed too assuming 5% as threshold. The correlation heatmaps are computed including first wave patients only, second wave only and both waves together.

A filter method based on correlation was used for feature selection [6]. After extracting items with correlation above 0.5 [5], an additional manual analysis was performed.

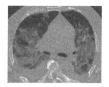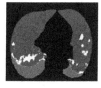   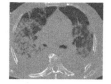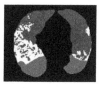

(a) CT and label map at T_0 (b) CT and label map at T_1

Fig. 1. CT (left) and pathology label map (right) at T_0 and at T_1. Nomenclature of label maps: pleural effusion: green, consolidation: yellow, ggo: blue, healthy: red.

The focus was set on laboratory and image-derived features associated with severe Covid-19 course [2]. Furthermore, similar or dependent features were sorted out and parameters that show disease progression were favoured.

3   Results

We evaluated the performance of our deformable registration in terms of dice score between the fixed lung label map (at T_0) and the moving lung label map (at T_1), achieving 0.94 ± 0.01 (n=50).

Due to their impact on disease progression in other lung diseases, three inflammatory parameters, namely CRP (mg/dl), IL-6 (pg/ml) and procalcitonin (ng/ml) were selected for further analysis. Data imputation was requested in 1, 23 and 6% of the patients for CRP, IL-6 and procalcitonin respectively.

Focusing on dynamic changes, we detected that the proportion of healthy lung affects the outcome positively. Also, lung tissue transformed to worse pathological status (Fig. 2) as well as increase of CRP and IL-6 indicated worse outcome (Fig. 3). While increases in CRP and IL-6 affect mostly the mortality and outcome after 30 days, changes in image features have also impact on the length of hospital and ICU stay.

Comparing the correlation heatmaps of the two waves, we see slight differences. An example would be the correlation between lung worsening and death: in the first wave the worsening of lung conditions is a strong predictor of patient's death, whereas in the second wave this relation is weaker. This can be, at least partially, explained with the administration of better therapeutic means due to the accumulated knowledge in the second wave.

Correlation analysis between longitudinal imaging and laboratory feature can be found in the additional material. Especially increasing CRP shows strong correlation with disease-related progression to worse lung status in CT images.

4   Discussion

In this paper, we present a metholodogy for analysing correlations between longitudinal image and laboratory data, as well as static data. Our evaluation on an in-house Covid-19 cohort is however limited by the relatively small group size and missing data which required imputation.

We applied our method to manually segmented lung CTs, to have the highest possible degree of precision. However, automated segmentation algorithms for lungs and Covid-19-related pathologies, such as [7], will be included in the future.

CNN-based image registration has been proposed previously for lung yielding dice scores of 0.95 ± 0.03 [8]. There, Hering et al. use different a pyramid approach and enforce physically plausible deformation fields by adding regularization losses. They evaluate this on a inspiration/exhalation dataset. Our approach requires a segmentation mask and is simpler, however can perform similarly to the proposed method (0.94 ± 0.01) and cope better for changes inside the lung. A comparison of our method with imaging data similar to the one used by Hering et al. is part of our future work.

We observed that the presence of pleural effusion has a negative impact on the performance of the registration, because the pleural effusion compresses the lung tissue and therefore the shape of the lung can be quite different from a lung without pleural effusion. The bigger the volume of the pleural effusion, the lower the dice score was. Using here also image data beyond the mask itself may result in better results. We plan to investigate this in follow-up studies.

As for the progression analysis, voxel-wise comparison of longitudinal image data is a standard methodology in medical imaging [4] and has also been applied to Covid-19 longitudinal CT scans to assess pneumonia progression [3]. In particular, the detection of local changes regional or voxel-wise analysis gives better results than an average analysis over the complete organ [4]. Nevertheless, we believe our approach, based on binary label map comparison, is more robust than the one proposed by Pu et al. because the comparison of the baseline and follow-up CT scans can be subject to interpolation errors in registration [3].

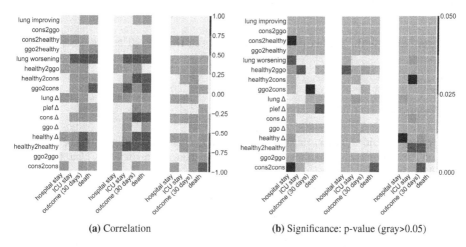

(a) Correlation   (b) Significance: p-value (gray>0.05)

Fig. 2. Correlation (and its significance) between dynamic change of image-features and outcome parameters; lung improving/worsening and state transition in percentage of common lung, lung/cons/ggo/healthy Δ in percentage of initial lung volume and plef Δ in ml (left to right: both waves, 1st wave, 2nd wave)

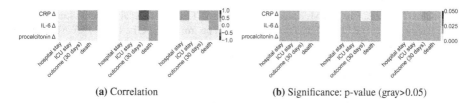

(a) Correlation   (b) Significance: p-value (gray>0.05)

Fig. 3. Correlation (and its significance) between dynamic change of inflammatory parameters and outcome parameters (left to right: both waves, 1st wave, 2nd wave).

Among the many methods available to perform feature selection [6, 9], the high dimensionality and small number of samples forced us to use a very simple approach. Indeed, more complex feature selection methods (such as *wrapper*) are more prone to overfit [9]. Moreover, we propose a methodology that can be applied to problems where the target feature is not defined a priori. This requires the use of *unsupervised* feature selection methods, such as the correlation [6].

In accordance with the literature, our results show that Covid-19 patients with high dynamic in pathological lung transformation to worse status and increasing inflammatory parameters tend to present a severe clinical course with worse prognosis [1, 2]. Furthermore, as shown in the additional material, laboratory values (in particular CRP and lung remodeling) are known to correlate [2]. Comparing the correlation maps of both waves, there is a decrease of prognostic value of features in the second Covid-19 wave. Possible explanations could be the small dataset or overall improved patient management and has to be further evaluated. All in all, our approach proved the prognostic value of longitudinal imaging and laboratory data in terms of Covid-19 disease and has the potential to discover non trivial longitudinal feature interaction.

Acknowledgement. Verena Bentele and Francesca De Benetti contributed equally to this work.

References

1. Wang YC, Luo H, Liu S, Huang S, Zhou Z, Yu Q et al. Dynamic evolution of COVID-19 on chest computed tomography: experience from Jiangsu province of China. Eur Radiol. 2020;30(11):6194–203.
2. Gao YD, Ding M, Don X, Zhang Jj, Azkur AK, Azkur D et al. Risk factors for severe and critically ill COVID-19 patients: a review. Allergy. 2021;67(2):428–55.
3. Pu J, Leader JK, Bandos A, Ke S, Wang J, Shi J et al. Automated quantification of COVID-19 severity and progression using chest CT images. Eur Radiol. 2020;31(1):436–46.
4. Battaglini M, Giorgio A, Stromillo ML, Bartolozzi ML, Guidi L, Federico A et al. Voxel-wise assessment of progression of regional brain atrophy in relapsing-remitting multiple sclerosis. J Neurol Sci. 2009;282(1-2):55–60.
5. Khamis H. Measures of association: how to choose? J Diagn Med Sonogr. 2008;24(3):155–62.
6. Kuhn M, Johnson K. Applied predictive modeling. Springer New York, 2013.
7. Kim ST, Goli L, Paschali M, Khakzar A, Keicher M, Czempiel T et al. Longitudinal quantitative assessment of COVID-19 infection progression from chest CTs. Proc MICCAI. Springer International Publishing, 2021:273–82.
8. Hering A, Häger S, Moltz J, Lessmann N, Heldmann S, Ginneken BV. CNN-based lung CT registration with multiple anatomical constraints. Med Image Anal. 2021;72:102139.
9. Soares I, Dias J, Rocha H, Carmo Lopes M do, Ferreira B. Feature selection in small databases: a medical-case study. Springer International Publishing, 2016:814–9.

Adipose and Muscular Tissue Removal for Direct Volume Rendering of the Visceral Region in Abdominal 3D CT Images

Nico Zettler, Derya Dogan, Andre Mastmeyer

Faculty of Optics and Mechatronics, Department of Digital Health Management, Aalen University
andre.mastmeyer@hs-aalen.de

Abstract. A two-stage approach for segmentation and removal of subcutaneous tissue layers to expose the visceral region is presented. Starting from the outer skin layer, the first step is to find the boundary between the subcutaneous adipose tissue and the muscle tissue. Subsequently, the boundary between muscle and the inner visceral region is determined. Thus adipose tissue, muscle and bone structures can be segmented and removed within the abdomen, providing the viewer with an unobstructed direct volume rendering. To evaluate the procedure, segmentations of the individual compartments of subcutaneous adipose tissue and muscle tissue were compared with corresponding expert ground truth. The implied simultaneous fat and muscle segmentation (DSC>90%) used for tissue removal is also of high diagnostic value.

1 Introduction

Virtual reality (VR) simulation of the organ situs in 3D CT images is of major importance for training and planning of surgical interventions in a visuo-haptic abdominal 4D VR simulator [1–3] respecting breathing motion (3D+t). In previous work, we primarily dealt with simulating needle punctures into pathological structures such as dilated bile ducts (PTC/PTCD) or lesions for biopsy or ablation simulation [4]. Hereto, fastly and accurately generated patient models are required, i.e. segmentation masks of the relevant abdominal organ group: liver, spleen, pancreas and kidneys. The fully-automatic CNN methods also used by our group and others don't deliver sufficiently correct masks currently, but only yield mask proposals. This rises the necessity to interactively correct the masks of variable quality, which currently only can take place in 2D segmentation editors. One of our project goals is to provide a 3D VR segmentation editor using specialized visuo-haptic methods. As part of this endeavor, a free sight of the organs in the abdominal cavity is needed. This work contributes to this intermediate goal and uniquely in the literature by removing tissues impeding a clear direct volume rendering (DVR) of the visceral organs in the abdomen.

Recently, several semi- and fully-automated segmentation approaches were published for subcutaneous adipose tissue (SAT) and visceral adipose tissue (VAT) [5]. Due to the negative range of Hounsfield units (HU) of adipose tissue being distinctive from other tissues in the abdomen, CT images are preferred. Using basic techniques, thresholding was the most widely used approach, followed by watershed. Semi-automated approaches then emerged such as active contour and shape models. Zhao et al. and various other groups [5–7] started from the abdominal center and working with HU intensity profiles along axial, radial lines and connected sparse points towards the skin barrier. Muscle segmentation in CT images is especially challenging as in the abdomen, muscles and neighboring organs have significant intensity range intersections. Therefore, single- and multi-atlas based methods [8, 9] were used and extended with level-sets [10]. In contrast to previous publications, we generate separate masks for SAT and muscle segmentation using one algorithm.

2   Materials and methods

For our method evaluation, 10 abdominal CT scans with different noise, field of view, number of slices (105 to 245), pathologic lesions, slice thickness (1 to 2 mm), contrast agent and obesity status were used.

First, in the top slice of the abdominal scan initial segmentation boundaries are determined to yield a slice center of mass. Second, the algorithm iterates slice-wise from top to bottom and adjusts the segmentation boundaries.

2.1   Top slice boundary detection

2.1.1   Inner SAT border segmentation. First, the boundary between the subcutaneous adipose tissue (SAT) and the muscle layer is detected. To find a suitable starting point, the outer contour of the skin layer is initially calculated similar to Hussein et al. [7] by detecting the skin outline as the longest connected contour in a binary threshold image. Differently to the proposed method, we only use the top slice of the scan to find the initial segmentation boundaries, which are then adapted in all further slices. We also calculate the slice center c_s as the center of mass of all outline pixels. To detect the inner SAT boundary, we trace 40 radial lines from the outline towards center c_s using Bresenham's line algorithm at an angle step of 9°. As a value range from -190 to -30 HU is often used to describe fat tissue in CT scans [6][1], possible candidates for the boundary between SAT and muscle region are found when, for two consecutive pixels p_1 and p_2, the intensity value changes from $I(p_1) \leq -30$ to $I(p_2) > -30$ (positive ascent). Given that some outliers may occur, a refinement step repositions candidates that are too far from the average distance of all other candidates from the original outline pixel. In addition to the candidate's position, we record the next five pixel neighborhood in- and outwards (Fig. 1a).

2.1.2   Subcutaneous muscle layer segmentation. To find the boundary between the muscle and visceral region of the body, the lines are traced further towards the slice center (Fig. 1b). Since the majority of the boundary in the top slice is adjacent to the lung region with strongly negative HU values, we find candidates for the muscle segmentation

---

[1]https://bit.ly/3DZbyL1

boundary by looking for the sharpest change from positive to negative intensities along the line. For each pixel on the Bresenham line, the 8 neighbors are categorized into four forward and four backward pixels depending on the angle to the slice center (Fig. 1c: green: forward pixels, red: backward pixels).

Let $\min_{\text{green}}(p)$ be the mask minimum intensity among forward pixels and $\max_{\text{red}}(p)$ be the mask maximum intensity among backward pixels for a pixel p. For all pixels p on a Bresenham line B, a candidate for the inner muscle boundary $p_b \in B$ is defined as (Fig. 1c)

$$p_b = \arg\max_{p \in B} \left(\max_{\text{red}}(p) - \min_{\text{green}}(p)\right) \qquad (1)$$

Also, we stop tracing the Bresenham line when an intensity value of $I(p) \leq -200$ HU is reached to avoid outliers in the lung area. Posterior, the spinal area is included in the muscle layer as it is in close proximity to the hip muscles of the lower body and can later be easily separated from the muscle tissue. As seen in Figure 2a, Bresenham lines are traced in a fan-like rotation radiating from the outline pixel in the bottom mid at 7.5° increments. On the spine specific Bresenham lines, potential candidates for the segmentation boundary p_b are calculated as before using Equation 1.

2.1.3 Boundary candidate connection.

To complete the segmentation boundaries for SAT and muscle regions, the detected boundary candidates must be connected without intersecting the visceral organs to be segmented. Other approaches propose the use of structuring elements and smoothing procedures [5, 6] leading to leakage between muscle and fat regions, as the main focus is on a correct SAT vs. VAT segmentation without considering muscle tissue. To this end, we use a modified shortest route algorithm for gray scale images, inspired by [11]. For two subsequent boundary candidates p_{b_1} and

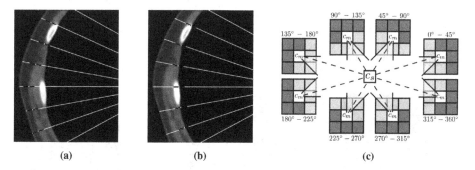

(a)   (b)   (c)

Fig. 1. The tracing for SAT and muscle borders starts at the outline leading towards the center of mass c_s. (a) Initial candidates for the boundary between SAT and muscle tissue found by tracing lines from the body outline towards the slice center. (b) Candidates for the inner muscle boundary determined by further tracing the lines and finding the strongest transition from positive to negative values. (c) Example of the eight different mask configurations used to calculate the maximum intensity change in the 3x3 neighborhood. For the mask center c_m, four forward (green) and four backward pixels (red) are considered depending on the angle to the slice center c_s.

p_{b_2}, we calculate a cost value for every potential shortest path pixel x connecting p_{b_1} and p_{b_2}. The cost value for the inner muscle boundary is computed as

$$\text{cost}_M(x) = \min_{\text{green}}(x) - \max_{\text{red}}(x) + |I(x)| + d(x, p_{b_2}) \tag{2}$$

where $d(x, p_{b_2})$ is the euclidean distance [mm] between x and p_{b_2}. For inner SAT boundary connection, the neighborhood intensity difference is reversed, as we look for the steepest ascent between (-) adipose tissue and (+) muscular pixels

$$\text{cost}_S(x) = \min_{\text{red}}(x) - \max_{\text{green}}(x) + |I(x)| + d(x, p_{b_2}) \tag{3}$$

The shortest path is found by traversing the set of pixels that result in the minimum cost sum. Figure 2b-c show the resulting segmentation boundaries.

2.2 Top-down segmentation boundary adjustment

After the initial segmentation boundaries have been calculated for the top slice, iterations are performed from top to bottom through all other slices, and the next boundaries are determined by using the result of each previous slice. Starting with the boundary candidates, the neighborhood mask from Figure 1c is used on the next five pixels of the Bresenham line in both directions to find the most significant change in intensity. If a change has been found, the boundary candidate is moved accordingly along the corresponding direction. Next, all boundary candidates are connected again by the shortest path algorithm. This process is repeated for every slice.

In most scans, boundary candidates where e.g. the liver and muscle touch are treated with outlier prevention considering the neighbors from the slice above using average distances from the slice center and a shortest path heuristic to prevent the algorithm from intersecting visceral tissues. The final step is to compose the respective SAT and muscle layer based on the segmentation boundaries to create two label masks for tissue removal in the DVR by full voxel transparency. Since all bone structures (spine, cartilage, ribs, etc.) are enclosed in our muscle layer, they can be removed via the closed muscle label mask, thus providing an unobstructed view of the visceral region. For the evaluation, we used Dice-similarity coefficient (DSC) and average Hausdorff distance (AHD) as metrics from ITK 5.3 modules.

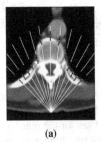 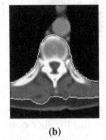 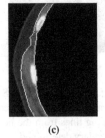

(a) (b) (c)

Fig. 2. (a) Spine approach by using a rotating sampling from the bottom-mid outline pixel found by descending from c_S. (b-c) Connected segmentation boundaries of SAT and muscle (+ spine) region according to the shortest path algorithm.

Tissue type	DSC [0, 1]	AHD [mm]
SAT	0.94±0.02	0.20±0.10
Muscle	0.90±0.03	0.88±0.39
Muscle*	0.92±0.03	0.20±0.09

Tab. 1. Overlap and surface metrics (Mean±Std.). Muscle*: Including voxels in the spine with intensities similar to muscle in the expert segmentation.

3   Results

The method's HU thresholds have been found from CT literature and considering the full-width-half-maximum (FWHM) principle of true object borders in CT imaging. The DSC or AHD results in Tabular 1 show good values of over 90% or <1 mm. Figure 3a shows the step-by-step removal of the individual segmented tissue layers as colored DVR. SAT, muscle tissue and bones are removed in the first three images. In the fourth image, the remaining visceral adipose tissue (VAT) is masked out by applying the fat threshold from section 2.1.1, which clears up the view of the visceral area. In the fourth and fifth image, a potential area for segmentation correction is obvious. The red area is indicating the true border of the liver top, where the proposed segmentation (undersegmented in green) has to be aligned with using our future 3D VR segmentation editing.

4   Discussion and conclusion

Overall, the results in this study show that multi-type subcutaneous tissue removal is feasible in one algorithm. We showed an example of an undersegmentation case in Figure 3b. For visual oversegmentation detection, there will be the option of rendering the proposed masks border transparently if needed. An open topic to be focused will also be the dedicated segmentation of intestinal structures. We conclude, using the proposed preprocessing of SAT and muscle removal to be valuable for our envisioned 3D VR visuo-haptic segmentation editor and in diagnostics [10]. This assistant will provide much more efficient manual segmentation editing by local 3D tools. Futhermore, we consider a bounding box or hull approach for localized one-organ editing in future work.

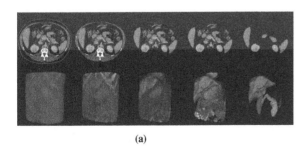 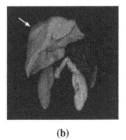

(a)   (b)

Fig. 3. (a) Steps of the proposed insight preventing tissue removal layer after layer. (b) Enlarged Figure 3a image, rightmost: Undersegmentation of liver top (green) vs. red liver border from DVR. Green: Liver. Magenta: R. kidney. Blue: Spleen. Cyan: L. kidney. Yellow: Pancreas. Intestinals removed by $r = 1$ cm dilation, inverted masking.

Potentially, this work shall also help to faster generate the needed ground truth image data to apply CNNs hereto.

Acknowledgement. DFG-Project MA 6791/1-1.

References

1. Mastmeyer A, Wilms M, Handels H. Population-based respiratory 4D motion atlas construction and its application for VR simulations of liver punctures. Proc. SPIE MI: Image Processing. Vol. 10574. 2018:1057417.
2. Mastmeyer A, Wilms M, Handels H. Interpatient respiratory motion model transfer for virtual reality simulations of liver punctures. J World Soc Comput Graph. 2017;25(1):1–10.
3. Mastmeyer A, Fortmeier D, Handels H. Random forest classification of large volume structures for visuo-haptic rendering in CT images. Proc. SPIE MI: Image Processing. 2016:97842H.
4. Kath N, Handels H, Mastmeyer A. Robust GPU-based virtual reality simulation of radio-frequency ablations for various needle geometries and locations. Int J Comp Ass Radiol and Surg. 2019;14(11):1825–35.
5. Hui SC, Zhang T, Shi L, Wang D, Ip CB, Chu WC. Automated segmentation of abdominal subcutaneous adipose tissue and visceral adipose tissue in obese adolescent in MRI. Magn Reson Imaging. 2018;45:97–104.
6. Zhao B, Colville J, et al. Automated quantification of body fat distribution on volumetric computed tomography. J Comp Assis Tomogr. 2006;30:777–83.
7. Hussein S, Green A, Watane A, Reiter D, Chen X, Papadakis GZ et al. Automatic segmentation and quantification of white and brown adipose tissues from PET/CT scans. IEEE Trans Med Imaging. 2017;36(3):734–44.
8. Yokota F, Otake Y, Takao M, al. et. Automated muscle segmentation from CT images of the hip and thigh using a hierarchical multi-atlas method. Int J Comp Ass Radiol and Surg. 2018;13:977–86.
9. Zhang W, Liu J, Yao J, Summers RM. Segmenting the thoracic, abdominal and pelvic musculature on CT scans combining atlas-based model and active contour model. SPIE Medical Imaging 2013: Computer-Aided Diagnosis. Vol. 8670. International Society for Optics and Photonics. 2013:867008.
10. Prescott JW, Best TM, al. et. Anatomically anchored template-based level set segmentation: application to quadriceps muscles in MR images from the osteoarthritis initiative. J Digit Imaging. 2011;24:28–43.
11. Ikonen L, Toivanen P, Tuominen J. Shortest route on gray-level map using distance transform on curved space. Scandinavian Conference on Image Analysis - SCIA. 2003:305–10.

Elektromagnetisches Instrumententracking für die Schlaganfallbehandlung mittels Thrombektomie

Ann-Kathrin Greiner-Perth[1], Eva Marschall[1], Tobias Kannberg[1],
Benjamin J. Mittmann[2,3], Bernd Schmitz[4], Michael Braun[4], Alfred M. Franz[2]

[1]Institut für Medizintechnik und Mechatronik, Technische Hochschule Ulm (THU)
[2]Institut für Informatik, Technische Hochschule Ulm (THU)
[3]Medizinische Fakultät, Universität Heidelberg
[4]Sektion Neuroradiologie, Bezirkskrankenhaus Günzburg
alfred.franz@thu.de

Zusammenfassung. Bei der Schlaganfallbehandlung mittels Thrombektomie werden Blutgerinnsel mithilfe von Instrumenten wie Kathetern und Führungsdrähten aus dem Gefäßsystem entfernt. Werden diese Instrumente mit kleinen elektromagnetischen (EM) Sensoren versehen, kann man sie durch einen EM Feldgenerator (FG) im Körper lokalisieren. Mithilfe dieser Trackingdaten und präoperativen Bilddaten könnten dem Arzt während des Eingriffes zusätzliche Informationen, wie z.B. der aktuelle Abstand zum Blutgerinnsel, angezeigt werden, was eine effektivere Durchführung unterstützen würde. Die Firma Polhemus Inc. bietet mit dem Liberty TX1 einen kleinen FG an, der nah am Eingriffsort platziert werden kann und potentiell wenige Störungen in der intraoperativen Bildaufnahme verursacht. Daneben gibt es das etablierte System Aurora von Northern Digital Inc. (NDI) mit dem Tabletop FG. Mithilfe eines standardisierten Messprotokolls wurden beide FGen unter klinischen Bedingungen auf ihre Genauigkeit und Robustheit geprüft. Der NDI Tabletop FG erreichte bei der Platzierung auf der Patientenliege eine Positionsgenauigkeit von 0,38 mm und einen mittleren Jitter von 0,02 mm, der Polhemus TX1 FG eine Genauigkeit von 0,24 mm und einen mittleren Jitter von 0,07 mm. Außerdem wurde mithilfe eines open-science Gefäßphantoms eine katheterbasierte Intervention nachgestellt, um den Einfluss der FGen auf die digitale Subtraktionsangiographie (DSA) zu untersuchen. Der TX1 FG erzeugte durch die geringe Baugröße im Gegensatz zum Tabletop FG kaum Artefakte. Aufgrund der Kompaktheit, den tendenziell besseren Genauigkeitsergebnissen und der hohen Robustheit stellt der TX1 FG für das Instrumententracking eine interessante Alternative dar. Derzeit hat das Polhemus System allerdings noch die Einschränkung, dass dessen kleinster Sensor mit einem Durchmesser von 1,8 mm minimal größer ist als der maximale Innendurchmesser eines bei der Thrombektomie eingesetzten Aspirationskatheters von 1,77 mm.

1 Einleitung

Beim ischämischen Schlaganfall tritt ein Gefäßverschluss der Hirngefäße oder der hirnversorgenden Gefäße im Halsbereich auf. Das primäre Ziel der Akuttherapie ist die Wiedereröffnung des verschlossenen Gefäßes [1]. Bei der mechanischen Thrombektomie wird ein Blutgerinnsel mit Hilfe eines Katheters entfernt, wobei die Navigation des Katheters eine herausfordernde Aufgabe darstellt. Die Lokalisation des Katheters während der Thrombektomie könnte die Navigation erleichtern und damit die Reperfusion der Arterien früher ermöglichen [2].

Aktuell wird die Position des Katheters sukzessiv mithilfe intraoperativer Durchleuchtung überprüft. Neben den derzeit erforschten, bildbasierten Methoden [3] ist es möglich mit elektromagnetischem (EM) Tracking Katheter und Führungsdrähte in der interventionellen Radiologie zu lokalisieren [4]. Dabei messen Sensoren, welche in den Instrumenten integriert sind, ein durch einen externen Feldgenerator (FG) emittiertes EM Feld. Dadurch kann die Position der Instrumente innerhalb des Trackingvolumens, also dem Bereich in dem lokalisiert werden kann, bestimmt werden [5]. Durch den Einsatz von größeren FGen kann eine höhere Reichweite des Trackingvolumens generiert werden. Jedoch wirkt sich die Größe des FGs auf die praktische Einsatzfähigkeit im klinischen Alltag aus, da große FGen schwieriger zu handhaben sind. Eine weitere Schwierigkeit von EM Tracking ist die geringere Robustheit gegenüber externer Störquellen in klinischer Umgebung [6]. Dies ist ein bekanntes Problem, weshalb es bereits etablierte Protokolle zur Bewertung der Genauigkeit von Trackingsystemen gibt, wie z.B. von Hummel et al. [7]. Außerdem ist von Interesse, wie sich der Einsatz von EM Trackingsystemen auf die intraoperative Bildgebung auswirkt.

Für die Durchführung einer Thrombektomie wurden EM Trackingsysteme bislang noch nicht eingesetzt. Insbesondere der Liberty TX1 FG von der Firma Polhemus Inc. (Colchester, USA) wurde noch nicht für diesen Zweck getestet, obwohl Polhemus mittlerweile auch den Micro Sensor 1.8 (Abb. 1a) mit einem Durchmesser von 1,8 mm anbietet [8]. Ziel dieses Projektes war es, zu untersuchen, ob sich der TX1 FG (Abb. 1b), ein vergleichsweise kleiner FG (23 mm x 28 mm x 15 mm), für den Einsatz bei der Thrombektomie eignet. Durch seine Kompaktheit und die damit verbundene erhöhte praktische Anwendbarkeit im klinischen Alltag könnte der Polhemus TX1 FG neue Einsatzbereiche in der Navigation durch EM Trackingsysteme eröffnen. Verglichen wurde das Polhemus System mit dem bereits etablierten Trackingsystem Aurora von der Firma NDI (Northern Digital Inc., Waterloo, Kanada) mit dem Aurora 6DOF FlexTube Sensor (Artikel 610060) (Abb. 1a). Der Aurora Tabletop FG (Abb. 1b) hat eine Größe von 507 mm x 762 mm x 34 mm und besitzt ein großes elliptisches Trackingvolumen (Hauptachse 600 mm, Nebenachse 420 mm, Höhe 600 mm).

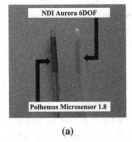
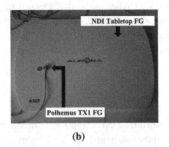
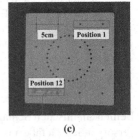

(a)   (b)   (c)

Abb. 1. a) EM Sensoren. b) EM Feldgeneratoren. c) Hummel-Messplatte mit 4x3-Gitter.

2 Material und Methoden

Zur Bewertung der Trackinggenauigkeit wurden Versuche im Bezirkskrankenhaus Günzburg durchgeführt, bei denen beide Systeme auf einer Patientenliege in der Angiographie der Neuroradiologie getestet wurden. Um eine Vergleichbarkeit der Messergebnisse zu gewährleisten, erfolgten neben den klinischen Messungen zusätzliche Referenzmessungen unter Laborbedingungen an der Technischen Hochschule Ulm (THU). Zur Untersuchung des NDI Aurora Tabletop FGs und des Polhemus Liberty TX1 FGs dienten Positionsmessungen, die nach dem standardisierten Messprotokoll von Hummel et al. durchgeführt wurden [7]. Dabei war das Ziel, die Trackinggenauigkeit der beiden Systeme in einem definierten Trackingvolumen zu ermitteln. Da es sich bei dem erforderlichen Arbeitsvolumen für das Instrumententracking während einer Thrombektomie um ein kleines Trackingvolumen im oberen Halsbereich handelt, wurde für die Messungen die in einer anderen Studie empfohlene Hummel-Messplatte mit einem reduzierten 4x3-Gitter verwendet [6], dessen Lochdistanz 50 mm beträgt. Hierfür wurde eine kleine Version der Messplatte 3D-gedruckt (Abb. 1c).

Für die Durchführung der Positionsmessung wurde der jeweilige Sensor der Trackingsysteme mithilfe einer Halterung an definierten Positionen auf der Messplatte platziert. In jeder Messposition auf der Messplatte wurden jeweils 150 Sensorwerte aufgezeichnet. Aus den Messwerten benachbarter Sensorpositionen wurde im Anschluss die betragsmäßige Differenz zwischen den berechneten mittleren euklidischen Distanzen und der realen Lochdistanz auf der Hummel-Messplatte (50 mm) ermittelt. Der Mittelwert dieser Differenzen dient zur Beurteilung der Positionsgenauigkeit der Systeme. Zur Bewertung der Präzision der Trackingsysteme wird die Präzision (engl. Jitter) der aufgenommenen Sensorwerte um eine Messposition betrachtet. Diese ist als die Wurzel der mittleren quadratischen Abweichungen (RMSE) der 150 Messwerte definiert [7].

Um den Einfluss der Positionierung der FGen zum Trackingvolumen zu untersuchen und eine geeignete Platzierung für eine hohe Genauigkeit zu identifizieren, wurden die FGen mit unterschiedlicher Orientierung zur Messplatte aufgebaut. Das Inferior-Setup, bei dem der FG unterhalb der Hummel-Messplatte platziert wurde, entspricht dem Standard-Setup für den NDI Tabletop FG (Abb. 2a). Für den zweiten Aufbau, dem Lateral-Setup, wurde der FG seitlich, neben der Hummel-Messplatte positioniert (Abb. 2b). Die Positionsmessungen des Tabletop FGs erfolgten in der Klinik und im

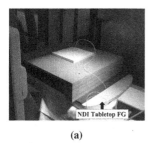 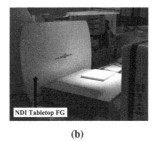 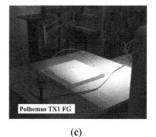

(a)   (b)   (c)

Abb. 2. Klinische Versuchsaufbauten: a) Tabletop FG (Inferior-Setup). b) Tabletop FG (Lateral-Setup). c) TX1 FG (Lateral-Setup).

Labor jeweils in beiden Setups. Für das Polhemus Liberty System mit dem deutlich kleineren TX1 FG wurden die Positionsmessungen im Labor ebenfalls in beiden Setups durchgeführt, in der Klinik nur im Lateral-Setup (Abb. 2c), da aufgrund der kompakten Baugröße des TX1 FGs keine signifikanten Abweichungen bei der unterschiedlichen Orientierung relativ zum Trackingvolumen erwartet wurden.

Zur Beurteilung des Einflusses der FGen auf die intraoperative Bildgebung wurde die Durchführung einer vaskulären Intervention in der Angiographie nachgestellt. Dafür wurde das open-science Gefäßphantom verwendet, das im Rahmen eines Forschungsprojektes an der THU entwickelt wurde [9]. Das neurovaskuläre Gefäßphantom dient zur Simulation katheterbasierter Interventionen und Evaluierung von Computerassistenzsystemen. Mithilfe des Phantoms wurde untersucht, ob die zwei FGen Störungen bei der Aufnahme von DSA-Daten hervorrufen. Dazu wurden das Phantom und die Trackingsysteme auf der Patientenliege platziert. Der Tabletop FG wurde unterhalb des Phantoms und der TX1 FG neben dem Phantom positioniert. Während der Intervention wurden DSAen des Phantoms und der FGen erstellt und anschließend qualitativ beurteilt.

3 Ergebnisse

Die Ergebnisse der Positionsmessungen nach dem Hummel-Protokoll sind in Abbildung 3 dargestellt. Der ermittelte Positionsfehler des Tabletop FGs beträgt im Labor 0,49 mm im Inferior-Setup und 0,39 mm Lateral-Setup, in der Klinik 0,38 mm im Inferior-Setup und 1,64 mm im Lateral-Setup. Der Positionsfehler des TX1 FGs beträgt im Labor 0,21 mm und in der Klinik 0,24 mm im Lateral-Setup. Der mittlere Jitter des Tabletop FGs beträgt im Labor 0,03 mm im Inferior-Setup und 0,08 mm im Lateral-Setup. In der Klinik wurde ein mittlerer Jitter von 0,02 mm im Inferior-Setup und 0,14 mm im Lateral-Setup ermittelt. Für den TX1 FG wurde im Lateral-Setup ein Jitter von 0,05 mm im Labor und 0,07 mm in der Klinik gemessen.

Zur Untersuchung des Einflusses der FGen auf die intraoperative Bildgebung wurden die erzeugten DSAen des Phantoms betrachtet. Eine DSA des einzelnen Gefäßbaums dient als Referenzaufnahme (Abb. 4a). Die Aufnahme des Phantoms mit dem Tabletop FG (Inferior-Setup) zeigt im Vergleich zur Referenz eindeutige Artefakte, die große Teile

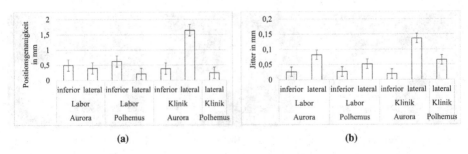

Abb. 3. Ergebnisse der Messungen nach Hummel et. al. [7]: a) Positionsgenauigkeit in mm (50 mm Distanzen). b) Jitter in mm (Präzision).

des darzustellenden Gefäßbaums überlagern und diesen dadurch unkenntlich machen (Abb. 4b). Vermieden werden kann diese Überlagerung potentiell durch die seitliche Platzierung des Tabletop FGs im Lateral-Setup, wodurch eine Durchleuchtung in AP (anterior-posterior) ohne Darstellung des Tabletop FGs möglich ist. Der TX1 FG, der in der Aufnahme neben dem Gefäßbaum platziert ist (Abb. 4c), ist im Vergleich zum Tabletop FG deutlich kleiner. Durch die kleine Baugröße und die seitliche Platzierung kann eine Überlagerung des FGs und des Gefäßbaums vermieden werden.

4 Diskussion

Mit dem Ziel EM Trackingsysteme zukünftig in der Angiographie einzusetzen, wurden in dieser Arbeit der Tabletop FG und der TX1 FG sowohl unter klinischen als auch unter Laborbedingungen auf die Trackinggenauigkeit und Präzision geprüft, um aus dem Vergleich die Robustheit bewerten zu können. Das NDI Aurora System erzielte im Labor in beiden Setups eine hohe Positionsgenauigkeit mit einem Fehler von unter 0,5 mm, wobei im Inferior-Setup ein besseres Präzisionsergebnis (Jitter) erreicht werden konnte. Auch in der klinischen Messung konnte im Inferior-Setup ein EM Trackingergebnis mit einer hohen Genauigkeit von 0,38 mm und geringem Jitter erzielt werden. Dahingegen lieferten die klinischen Messungen im Lateral-Setup sowohl höhere Positions- als auch Präzisionsfehler. Dies lässt sich potentiell mit dem größeren Einfluss von Störfeldern in der Sagittalebene begründen, da die Abschirmung der Patientenliege wegfällt. Mit dem Polhemus Liberty System wurden im Lateral-Setup in der Klinik und im Labor vielversprechende, robuste Trackingergebnisse mit einem geringen Positionsfehler von unter 0,25 mm erreicht. Auch ein hohes Präzisionsergebnis mit einer Abweichung von unter 0,1 mm konnte in beiden Umgebungen erzielt werden. Verglichen mit Literaturwerten [6], lieferten die untersuchten Systeme für den Jitter mit tendenziellen Werten unter 0,1 mm ähnliche Ergebnisse. Einzig für den Tabletop FG im Lateral-Setup weicht das Präzisionsergebnis in der Klinik von der Literatur ab. Die Werte der ermittelten Positionsfehler sind mit den Literaturwerten ebenfalls vergleichbar. Allerdings fällt auf, dass im Gegensatz zur vorherigen Studie keine deutliche Verschlechterung von den klinischen zu den Laborergebnissen besteht, außer beim Tabletop FG im Lateral-Setup. Besonders mit dem TX1 FG konnte eine gleichbleibend hohe Genauigkeit in beiden Umgebungen erzielt werden. Ein großer Vorteil des TX1 FGs ist dessen geringe Größe,

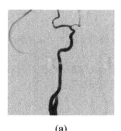 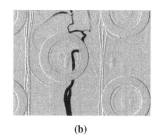 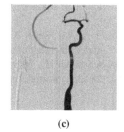

(a)   (b)   (c)

Abb. 4. DSA mit Gefäßphantom: a) Referenzaufnahme. b) Tabletop FG. c) TX1 FG.

wodurch eine einfachere Installation und Handhabung möglich ist. Außerdem konnte anhand der aufgenommenen DSAen gezeigt werden, dass der TX1 FG im Gegensatz zum Tabletop FG nur wenige Artefakte erzeugt. Daher kann eine Überlagerung der darzustellenden Gefäße durch eine geeignete Platzierung des FGs vermieden werden. Eine Herausforderung beim Einsatz des Polhemus Liberty Systems stellt allerdings die Größe des Polhemus Microsensor 1.8 dar, da dessen Durchmesser mit 1,8 mm den maximalen Innendurchmesser eines bei der Thrombektomie eingesetzten Aspirationskatheters von 1,77 mm derzeit noch überschreitet. Eine Entwicklung eines kleineren Sensors könnte diese Schwierigkeit überwinden, wobei die erreichbare Trackinggenauigkeit erneut zu ermitteln wäre. Außerdem ist zukünftig der Einfluss des laufenden C-Bogens auf das EM Tracking zu untersuchen.

Danksagung. Diese Arbeit entstand im Rahmen eines Projekts, das unter dem Förderkennzeichen ZF4640301GR8 vom Bundesministerium für Wirtschaft und Energie gefördert wird. Wir danken Thomas Szimeth für die Unterstützung beim 3D-Druck.

References

1. Lehrner J. Klinische Neuropsychologie: Grundlagen - Diagnostik - Rehabilitation. Wien: Springer, 2006.
2. Yoo AJ, Andersson T. Thrombectomy in acute ischemic stroke: challenges to procedural success. J Stroke. 2017:121–30.
3. Heimann T, Mountney P, John M, Ionasec R. Real-time ultrasound transducer localization in fluoroscopy images by transfer learning from synthetic training data. Med Image Anal. 2014:1320–8.
4. Condino S, Calabrò EM, Alberti A, Parrini S, Cioni R, Berchiolli RN et al. Simultaneous tracking of catheters and guidewires: comparison to standard fluoroscopic guidance for arterial cannulation. Eur J Vasc Endovas Surg. 2014:53–60.
5. Franz AM, Haidegger T, Birkfellner W, Cleary K, Peters TM, Maier-Hein L. Electromagnetic tracking in medicine: a review of technology, validation, and applications. IEEE Trans Med Imaging. 2014:1702–25.
6. Maier-Hein L, Franz AM, Birkfellner W, Hummel J, Gergel I, Wegner I et al. Standardized assessment of new electromagnetic field generators in an interventional radiology setting. Med Phys. 2012:3424–34.
7. Hummel JB, Bax MR, Figl ML, Kang Y, Maurer C, Birkfellner WW et al. Design and application of an assessment protocol for electromagnetic tracking systems. Med Phys. 2005:2371–9.
8. Franz AM, Seitel A, Cheray D, Maier-Hein L. Polhemus EM tracked micro sensor for CT-guided interventions. Med Phys. 2019:15–24.
9. Stevanovic L, Mittmann BJ, Pfiz F, Braun M, Schmitz B, Franz AM. Open-Science Gefäßphantom für neurovaskuläre Interventionen. Proc BVM. 2020:172–7.

Abstract: Synthesis of Annotated Pathological Retinal OCT Data with Pathology-Induced Deformations

Hristina Uzunova[1], Leonie Basso[2], Jan Ehrhardt[2], Heinz Handels[1,2]

[1]German Research Center for Artificial Intelligence, Lübeck
[2]Institut für Medizinische Informatik, Universität zu Lübeck
hristina.uzunova@dfki.de

In recent years, neural networks drastically gained on popularity in the medical image processing domain since they proved to be suitable to reliably solve many complex tasks. However, neural networks typically require a large amount of ground truth annotated training images to deliver accurate results. Yet, the annotation of medical images is a very time-consuming process and mostly requires expert knowledge. This problem gets further aggravated by the common presence of pathological structures in medical images. Since their shape and appearance is usually less homogeneous than normal anatomical structures, their variability is enormous, thus they are hard to model. Furthermore, pathological structures commonly severely displace the surrounding anatomy, e.g. pathological fluids in retinal OCTs, and thus significantly impede image processing methods like segmentation. To approach the problem of missing annotated pathological data, in this work [1], a GAN-based pipeline for the generation of realistic retinal OCTs with available pathological fluids and the simultaneous generation of ground truth anatomical and pathological annotations is established. Pathological fluids between the retinal layers can cause small local deformations, as well as large global distortions, which makes it even more challenging to simulate such deformations in a realistic manner. For this reason, the emphasis of this work lies on a new approach for the simulation of the pathology-induced deformations in retinal OCTs. Here, a cGAN-based method using cycle-consistency loss is applied to model the deformations from the pathological to the healthy image domain. Compared to naive methods for the modeling of pathological deformations, the proposed approach generates more realistic data evaluated quantitatively and qualitatively in the performed experiments. Furthermore, the generated images are used for the training of a segmentation neural network and prove their suitability for data augmentation purposes.

References

1. Uzunova H, Basso L, Ehrhardt J, Handels H. Synthesis of annotated pathological retinal OCT data with pathology-induced deformations. Accepted at SPIE Medical Imaging 2022: Image Processing, International Society for Optics and Photonics.

Comparison of Evaluation Metrics for Landmark Detection in CMR Images

Sven Koehler[1,2], Lalith Sharan[1,2], Julian Kuhm[1], Arman Ghanaat[1],
Jelizaveta Gordejeva[1], Nike K. Simon[1], Niko M. Grell[1], Florian André[1],
Sandy Engelhardt[1,2]

[1]Department of Internal Medicine III, Heidelberg University Hospital, Heidelberg
[2]DZHK (German Centre for Cardiovascular Research), partner site Heidelberg/Mannheim
sven.koehler@med.uni-heidelberg.de

Abstract. Cardiac magnetic resonance (CMR) images are widely used for cardiac diagnosis and ventricular assessment. Extracting specific landmarks like the right ventricular insertion points is of importance for spatial alignment and 3D modelling. The automatic detection of such landmarks has been tackled by multiple groups using Deep Learning, but relatively little attention has been paid to the failure cases of evaluation metrics in this field. In this work, we extended the public ACDC dataset with additional labels of the right ventricular insertion points and compare different variants of a heatmap-based landmark detection pipeline. In this comparison, we demonstrate very likely pitfalls of apparently simple detection and localisation metrics which highlights the importance of a clear detection strategy and the definition of an upper-limit for localisation based metrics. Our preliminary results indicate that a combination of different metrics are necessary, as they yield different winners for method comparison. Additionally, they highlight the need of a comprehensive metric description and evaluation standardisation, especially for the error cases where no metrics could be computed or where no lower/upper boundary of a metric exists. Code and labels: https://github.com/Cardio-AI/rvip_landmark_detection

1 Introduction

It is common to acquire cardiac magnetic resonance (CMR) image in a short-axis (SAX) orientation, which is clinically used for ventricular assessment. However, while the normal of the multi-slice stack points along the long axis of the heart, there is a remaining degree of freedom around this axis (e.g. right ventricle could be to the left or on the lower/upper side of the image slice (Fig. 2c-d)). Recent works show that deep neural network models perform better if based on standardised, in plane-rotated CMR images [1]. For rotation and to facilitate automated analysis and reporting, landmark points such as the two right ventricular insertion points (RVIP), need to be identified on the images. They define the septum, span over several z-slices and are important for 3D cardiac modelling, particularly for fitting bi-ventricular meshes or to determine the standard myocardial segments [2].

Multiple approaches have been previously adopted to tackle the task of landmark detection in this domain. [3, 4] followed a reinforcement learning approach to detect

Springer Fachmedien Wiesbaden GmbH, ein Teil von Springer Nature 2022
K. Maier-Hein et al. (Hrsg.), *Bildverarbeitung für die Medizin 2022*,
Informatik aktuell, https://doi.org/10.1007/978-3-658-36932-3_43

anatomical landmarks from CMR images. [5] presented a method for localising landmarks in CMR images using a cyclic motion mask. [6] proposed a model based on deep distance metric learning. [7] developed a CNN based solution for robust landmark detection for different CMR image contrasts. However, these works do not focus on the different metric definitions and their respective impact on assessment of model performance.

A very recent work [8] has started a timely discussion on the effects of choosing different evaluation metrics for segmentation tasks. In general, independent of the task, it is important to report how *NA* cases are treated or whether an upper/lower bound to a metric exist or need to be defined.

In this paper, we aim to show the influence of the definition of different apparently simple detection and localisation metrics in the particular use-case of RVIP landmark detection. We show that, depending on the metric, improved model variant comparison tailored to the post-processing task are possible. The results emphasise that more attention should be paid to evaluation metric definition and that authors are encouraged to provide more comprehensive descriptions.

2 Materials and methods

2.1 Data pre-processing and ground truth

To ensure good reproducibility and comparability of the presented approaches, we make use of the publicly available ACDC dataset [9]. This dataset consists of SAX CMR images from 100 patients and covers adults with normal anatomy and pathological cases. We manually labeled the anterior and inferior RVIPs as circular regions of 5 pixels, which we make openly available on our GitHub page. The images are pre-processed while training as follows: In-plane resampling to a uniform spacing of $1.2 \, \text{mm}^2$, linear interpolation for images, nearest neighbour for the masks. Centre crop/pad to network input size of 224^2 pixels. The CMR images are further clipped by the 0.999 quantile and min/max-normalised. The following augmentations are applied online with a probability of 80%: random grid distortion, 90° rotation, shifts and downsampling. In a separate experiment (Var.2), we apply random histogram matching to deal with the different pixel value distributions.

2.2 Model pipeline

To handle slices without RVIPs we formulate this problem as a slice-based segmentation task, using a combined binary cross-entropy and dice loss. The network has a U-Net architecture, consisting of four down-/up-sampling blocks [10]. All parameters are configurable, the implementation details and model definition are publicly available on GitHub. The training-subset was shuffled and split in a 4-fold cross-validation manner with respect to the pathologies as done by [11]. We present four different model variants: the baseline model (Base), the model with histogram matching performed (Var.1), and two models with Gaussian distribution applied to the masks, with values $\sigma = 2$ (Var.2), and $\sigma = 4$ (Var.3). Each model was trained for 500 epochs with early stopping.

As post-processing we apply a threshold $t = 0.5$ on the predicted heatmaps and retain only the biggest connected component per channel. Finally, we inverted all operations to compute the metrics in the original CMR image space.

2.3 Evaluation

2.3.1 Detection-based metrics. The crucial aspect in detection based metrics is *how* the True Positives (TP), False Positives (FP), and False Negatives (FN) are actually defined. This definition may be heavily dependent on the use-case. The Positive Predictive Value (PPV) PPV = TP/(TP + FP) and the True Positive Rate (TPR) TPR = TP/(TP + FN) can then be derived. We analyse three different evaluation strategies to compute the TP, FP, and FN. (1) Firstly, we adopt a line-based strategy, where we only consider the slices where both RVIPs are detected (Fig. 1a (i)). This case is relevant for rotational alignment of the images, as the axis between the anterior (Ant) and inferior (Inf) RVIP is only defined when both the landmarks are predicted. In this case, only slices that contain both points in the ground-truth (GT) and predicted (PRED) are considered as TP. When only one of the points is predicted, it is considered as a FN. The slices without GT points but two predicted points are considered as FP. (2) In the second case, we adopt a point-based detection strategy, where single predicted points are also considered in the computation, i.e. the evaluation is done for each individual landmark (TPR$_{Ant}$, TPR$_{Inf}$, similarly PPV$_{Ant}$, PPV$_{Inf}$) (Fig. 1a (ii)). (3) Figure 1a (iii) shows the third variant, a thresholded point-based strategy. Here, we define a radius of 15 mm around the GT points as done in [6]. Points inside this radius are counted as TPs, and all others are FPs.

2.3.2 Localisation-based metrics. Computing the Euclidean distance ($|d|$) between the GT and PRED point is a common localisation metric. As for this metric, no upper

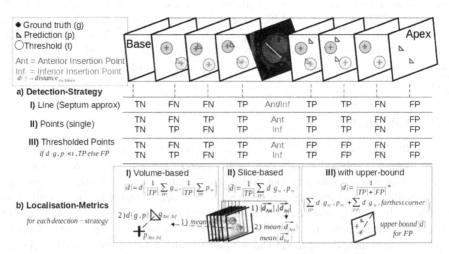

Fig. 1. Example cases for our three different detection strategies (a), they influence the total number of true positives, and could be combined with each localisation metrics (b).

Tab. 1. Comparison of localisation metrics for different experiments (Base: Baseline, Var.1: + Hist. matching, Var.2: + Gauss $\sigma = 2$, Var.3: + Gauss $\sigma = 4$).

Detection-Strategy		(i) Line			(ii) Points	
	Exp.	$\|d\|_{Ant} \downarrow$	$\|d\|_{Inf} \downarrow$	$\Delta_\alpha \downarrow$	$\|d\|_{Ant} \downarrow$	$\|d\|_{Inf} \downarrow$
(i) Volume-based	Base	5.92 ± 4.83	3.86 ± 5.32	3.80 ± 4.09	7.16 ± 6.88	5.79 ± 7.17
	Var.1	$\mathbf{5.58} \pm 6.25$	4.16 ± 5.75	4.60 ± 7.12	6.88 ± 7.71	4.86 ± 6.51
	Var.2	6.26 ± 7.08	3.54 ± 3.83	4.13 ± 5.24	6.93 ± 8.06	5.40 ± 9.08
	Var.3	5.86 ± 4.95	$\mathbf{3.33} \pm 3.47$	$\mathbf{3.67} \pm 3.41$	$\mathbf{6.67} \pm 5.72$	$\mathbf{4.17} \pm 5.57$
(ii) Slice-based	Base	4.42 ± 5.66	3.96 ± 7.07	$\mathbf{2.70} \pm 3.09$	5.08 ± 9.04	3.89 ± 6.96
	Var.1	$\mathbf{3.79} \pm 7.20$	3.02 ± 4.39	3.31 ± 5.77	$\mathbf{4.05} \pm 7.67$	3.00 ± 4.08
	Var.2	3.88 ± 4.97	3.12 ± 7.10	3.63 ± 7.51	4.08 ± 5.47	3.51 ± 8.14
	Var.3	4.42 ± 5.67	$\mathbf{2.48} \pm 2.20$	3.81 ± 9.00	4.58 ± 6.77	$\mathbf{2.71} \pm 2.89$
(iii) Slice-based, ↑-bound	Base	50.33 ± 65.01	49.68 ± 65.98	30.85 ± 39.20	35.05 ± 46.46	29.93 ± 59.14
	Var.1	$\mathbf{37.07} \pm 46.70$	$\mathbf{36.83} \pm 45.74$	$\mathbf{24.25} \pm 29.92$	$\mathbf{29.62} \pm 42.46$	$\mathbf{14.80} \pm 28.56$
	Var.2	48.53 ± 64.66	47.58 ± 63.89	30.79 ± 38.75	36.82 ± 57.30	27.39 ± 46.82
	Var.3	55.05 ± 74.88	53.76 ± 75.66	34.66 ± 44.92	39.44 ± 61.48	34.57 ± 58.76

bound exists, but slices without a detected point must be handled. We analyse different variants to compute the distance and penalise false predictions. (1) In the first method, we compute a volume-based distance, where the mean location of the GT and PRED points are computed across all TP slices. Then, the distance between the mean points is computed (Fig. 1b (i)). (2) In the second method, the distances are computed in a slice-based manner, considering also single detected points, following we take the mean of the distances per volume (Fig. 1b (ii)).

Computing the distances with a volume-based method reduces the outlier bias and yields a good approximation of the septum orientation. However, in these two methods the slices without a landmark prediction are not accounted for in the distance computation and therefore not penalised. To account for this, in our third method, (3) we apply an upper bound (↑ bound) to the cases without a prediction (FP). The upper bound distance is computed as the distance from the GT points to the farthest corner of the image (Fig. 1b (iii) and Fig. 2a). For each method we present the results ($|d|_{Ant}$ for anterior points,

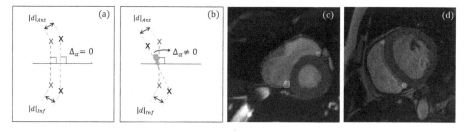

Fig. 2. (a) An example where the mean distance and the mean angle provide different comparisons. (b) Distance metrics remain the same whereas angle differs compared to (a). (c) Shows an example failure case prediction for the Ant RVIP on a rotated CMR and (d) a good prediction.

Tab. 2. Comparison of detection metrics for different experiments (Base: Baseline, Var.1: + Hist. matching, Var.2: + Gauss $\sigma = 2$, Var.3: + Gauss $\sigma = 4$).

| Detection-Strategy | (i) Line | | (ii) Points | | | |
Exp.	TPR ↑	PPV ↑	TPR_{Ant} ↑	TPR_{Inf} ↑	PPV_{Ant} ↑	PPV_{Inf} ↑
Base	0.84 ± 0.22	0.84 ± 0.22	0.89 ± 0.16	0.91 ± 0.19	0.80 ± 0.22	0.77 ± 0.24
Var.1	$\mathbf{0.88} \pm 0.16$	$\mathbf{0.85} \pm 0.19$	$\mathbf{0.91} \pm 0.15$	$\mathbf{0.96} \pm 0.10$	0.79 ± 0.21	0.79 ± 0.21
Var.2	0.85 ± 0.21	$\mathbf{0.85} \pm 0.23$	0.88 ± 0.19	0.92 ± 0.16	$\mathbf{0.81} \pm 0.23$	$\mathbf{0.80} \pm 0.22$
Var.3	0.82 ± 0.25	0.83 ± 0.26	0.88 ± 0.21	0.89 ± 0.20	0.79 ± 0.24	$\mathbf{0.80} \pm 0.24$
Base & Thresh.	(iii)		0.88 ± 0.20	0.94 ± 0.18	0.76 ± 0.25	0.73 ± 0.26
Var.1 & Thresh.	(iii)		$\mathbf{0.90} \pm 0.18$	$\mathbf{0.99} \pm 0.06$	0.77 ± 0.23	0.78 ± 0.21
Var.2 & Thresh.	(iii)		0.88 ± 0.20	0.97 ± 0.14	$\mathbf{0.78} \pm 0.24$	$\mathbf{0.79} \pm 0.23$
Var.3 & Thresh.	(iii)		0.86 ± 0.23	0.97 ± 0.15	0.77 ± 0.25	$\mathbf{0.79} \pm 0.24$

$|d|_{\text{Inf}}$ for inferior points) considering the slices where both the landmarks are detected and only single landmarks are detected, respectively (Tab. 1).

Finally, towards the motivation of rotational alignment of the CMR images based on the septal wall, we calculate the differences of the mean septum angle (Δ_α). We define this angle as the clock-wise angle between the x-axis and the septal wall (Fig. 2b). For the ↑ bound column we used an upper bound of 180°, as this reflects the maximum variation noticed in this dataset.

3   Results

Figure 2c-d shows one good/failure case of this landmark detection pipeline. Starting with the intuitive volume-based localisation metrics (i) in Table 1, it seems that Var.3 performs best in nearly all metrics. If we extend this view to the slice-based localisation metrics (ii), we see that metrics improved for all experiments (up to 3 mm for $|d|_{\text{Ant}}$, 1 mm for $|d|_{\text{Inf}}$). Simultaneously, the ranking changed. There is no clear winning method, each method performs best in one metric. One problem of the volume-(i) and slice-based (ii) methods is the lack of a fair FN case penalty. This becomes evident if we repeat the slice-based evaluation but, with an ↑ bound handling for FN cases (Fig. 1b (iii)). When a boundary is applied to the localisation metric, Var.1 with the histogram matching performs better in all metrics for both anterior and inferior points (Tab. 1 (iii)).

The detection-based results in Table 2, which by definition also reflect FN and FP cases, supports our assumption that model Var.1 with the histogram matching has a better TPR compared to the other models, whereas the precision is comparable. It can be seen that the TPR for the inferior points is higher than that of the anterior points for all experiments and evaluation methods, and the PPV is comparable. Clearly, more correct inferior points are detected. This difference gets even more clear if we apply a minimal distance threshold (2nd section of Tab. 2), here the TPR difference for Var.1 is +0.09. The threshold-based detection metrics (iii) enables a more task-dependent definition of TP cases, as we are able to include the knowledge of how accurate we need to be. There is comparable change in the PPV but an increase in the TPR, when single points are included.

4 Discussion

We investigate the performance by defining multiple, goal-dependent evaluation strategies and cross-validated the performance of this pipeline which is able to handle slices without GT points. The choice of a different strategy yields a different best-performing model. Hence, associated assumptions have to be taken into account when choosing the metric. Based on our experiments, we recommend for landmark detection the usage of at least one detection and one localisation based metric. Additionally the localisation based metric needs an upper bound in the form of a FN case handling. In this work, we have defined the upper bound on a slice-based level, meaning that the distance to the farthest corner is considered. However, this yields different values for a heterogeneous image collection of different image sizes. In future work, we will investigate these differences and compare them with a global, image-size independent, upper bound.

Acknowledgement. The research was supported by Informatics for Life project funded by the Klaus Tschira Foundation and SDS@hd service by the MWK Baden-Württemberg and the DFG through grant INST 35/1314-1 FUGG and INST 35/1503-1 FUGG.

References

1. Vigneault DM, Xie W, Ho CY, Bluemke DA, Noble JA. Net (Omega-Net): fully automatic, multi-view cardiac MR detection, orientation, and segmentation with deep neural networks. Med Image Anal. 2018;48:95–106.
2. Cerqueira MD, Weissman NJ, Dilsizian V, Jacobs AK, Kaul S, Laskey WK et al. Standardized myocardial segmentation and nomenclature for tomographic imaging of the heart. Circulation. 2002;105(4):539–42.
3. Ghesu FC, Georgescu B, Mansi T, Neumann D, Hornegger J, Comaniciu D. An artificial agent for anatomical landmark detection in medical images. Med Image Comput Comput Assist Interv. Springer. 2016:229–37.
4. Alansary A, Oktay O, Li Y, Le Folgoc L, Hou B, Vaillant G et al. Evaluating reinforcement learning agents for anatomical landmark detection. Med Image Anal. 2019;53:156–64.
5. Buján JN, Merrifield R, Wang L, Yang GZ. Automatic localisation of landmark points in CMR images using a cyclic motion mask. J Cardiovasc Magn Reson. 2012;14(1):T9.
6. Wang X, Zhai S, Niu Y. Left ventricle landmark localization and identification in cardiac mri by deep metric learning-assisted CNN regression. Neurocomputing. 2020;399:153–70.
7. Xue H, Artico J, Fontana M, Moon JC, Davies RH, Kellman P. Landmark detection in cardiac mri by using a cnn. Radiol Artif Intell. 2021;3(5):e200197.
8. Reinke A, Eisenmann M, Tizabi MD, Sudre CH, Rädsch T, Antonelli M et al. Common limitations of image processing metrics: a picture story. arXiv:2104.05642v2. 2021.
9. Bernard O, Lalande A, Zotti C, Cervenansky F, Yang X, Heng P et al. Deep learning techniques for automatic mri cardiac multi-structures segmentation and diagnosis: is the Problem Solved? IEEE Trans Med Imaging. 2018;37(11):2514–25.
10. Ronneberger O, Fischer P, Brox T. U-Net: Convolutional networks for biomedical image segmentation. Med Image Comput Comput Assist Interv. Springer. 2015:234–41.
11. Koehler S, Tandon A, Hussain T, Latus H, Pickardt T, Sarikouch S et al. How well do U-Net-based segmentation trained on adult cmr imaging data generalise...? Medical Imaging. Ed. by Fei B, Linte CA. SPIE, 2020:55.

Deep Learning Models for 3D MRI Brain Classification
A Multi-sequence Comparison

Marius Pullig[1], Benjamin Bergner[2], Amish Doshi[3], Anja Hennemuth[1],
Zahi A. Fayad[3], Christoph Lippert[2]

[1]Institute of Computer Science and Electrical Engineering, Technical University of Berlin
[2]Institute of Digital Health, Hasso-Plattner-Institute
[3]BioMedical Engineering and Imaging Institute, Icahn School of Medicine at Mount Sinai
pullig.marius@gmail.com

Abstract. This study evaluates the diagnostic performance for binary abnormality classification of deep learning models on various types of sequences from a multi-disease clinical brain MRI dataset. Additionally, it determines the influence of the sample size and the type of disease. The sequences are DWI, FLAIR, T1-weighted, T1-weighted FLAIR, T2-weighted and T2-weighted FLAIR. On the full-sized multi-disease, the best performance is achieved on the T2-weighted FLAIR sequence using a VGG-16 dataset resulting in an AUC value of 0.89. The work highlights the importance of carefully selecting MRI sequences for deep learning and identifies discrepancies to screening protocols for physicians.

1 Introduction

Neurological disorders are the world's leading cause of disability and the second largest contributor to the overall number of deaths [1]. The detection of neurological abnormalities using imaging procedures plays an important role in minimizing this burden, but the MRI analysis by radiologists is highly complex and time-consuming. Computer-aided diagnostic (CAD) supports radiologists in the detection and diagnostic of medical images. Through the application of deep neural networks, the performance of CAD systems has improved substantially in recent years. However, the deployment in clinical practice is rare. The practical workflow in the clinical context demands a CAD system to detect a multitude of diseases on the available MRI sequences. In contrast, most publications focus on single disease and single sequence datasets [2–4], leading to excellent results for a specific task but failing to generalize to more heterogeneous datasets found in the clinical context. This reflects in little knowledge on the influence of the individual MRI sequences on the diagnostic performance of deep learning models. Another barrier is the use of relatively small datasets often below 300 patients [2, 3]. Korolev et al. [2] achieve an AUC value of 0.88 with a VGG-16 on a dataset of 231 T1-weighted MR images of four states of Alzheimer's disease and Khan et al. [3] use a novel CNN model for brain tumor classification demonstrating an AUC value of 1.00 on a brain tumor dataset with 253 samples. Talo et al. [4] obtain F1-scores of up to 0.98, utilizing a multi-disease MR brain dataset containing exclusively of T2-weighted images. This results in a gap between promising research outcomes and their performance on clinical datasets. Thus,

© Der/die Autor(en), exklusiv lizenziert durch
Springer Fachmedien Wiesbaden GmbH, ein Teil von Springer Nature 2022
K. Maier-Hein et al. (Hrsg.), *Bildverarbeitung für die Medizin 2022*,
Informatik aktuell, https://doi.org/10.1007/978-3-658-36932-3_44

Tab. 1. Descriptive statistics of the individual sequence subsets. Image dimensions are given by width, length and depth.

	DWI	FLAIR	T1	T1 FLAIR	T2	T2 FLAIR
Samples	7069	4500	6344	609	10108	5069
Class 0/1	1456/5613	1063/3437	1158/5186	135/474	1892/8216	806/4263
Male/Female	1226/2005	1530/2416	1712/2501	225/316	3259/5010	1752/2352
Age	54.2±17.5	57.0±18.4	54.5 ±18.1	49.5±23.9	55.8±18.8	57.2±19.7
Width	170.3± 64.1	406.5± 98.4	448.9± 93.6	609.2± 291.6	449.8± 91.6	504.5± 41.2
Length	170.0± 63.9	406.3± 98.3	433.3± 116.1	598.1± 304.2	448.2± 91.9	503.0± 46.7
Depth	31.6± 4.9	31.9± 4.6	25.7± 4.9	26.0± 5.1	32.0± 4.5	29.3± 4.4

additional studies on multi-disease abnormality classification are needed. This work is based on a large clinical brain MRI dataset consisting of 152,107 MR images from 9,910 patients. It provides the foundation to address the research objectives of this research. First, this work determines the diagnostic performance of deep learning models on various types of 3D MRI sequences from a clinical multi-disease brain dataset for binary abnormality classification. Second, it investigates the influence of the dataset size of a clinical multi-disease brain MRI and of the type of disease on the diagnostic performance.

2 Materials and methods

2.1 Dataset

The IRW Brain MRI dataset [5] comprises 152,107 MR images from 9,910 patients. The data are collected in the daily clinical work, resulting in a high variation of MRI sequences, scanner types, magnetic field strengths, and number of slices per MRI scan. The scanners models are Optima MR450w, Signa HDxt, Signa Excite and Discovery MR750 from GE Medical Systems and Aera, Skyra, Amira and Avanto from Siemens Healthineers. The magnetic field strength is 1.5 Tesla or 3.0 Tesla. Studies with an abnormality are labelled as "0", without an abnormality as "1". For this research the most frequent axial sequences are used: diffusion weighted imaging (DWI), fluid attenuated inversion recovery (FLAIR), T1-weighted, T1-weighted FLAIR, T2-weighted and T2-weighted FLAIR. The statistical details are listed in Tabular 1 and MR image examples without an abnormality are shown in Figure 1. In addition to the anamnestic patient data, a medical report is linked to each individual brain study. These reports are processed to map one or multiple disease to each study. The most prevalent diseases are clustered into the following non-exhaustive groups to create additional labels: glioblastoma, hemorrhage, infarct, and other benign tumor.

2.2 Methodology

The preprocessing of the data includes data cleansing, augmentation, resizing, and feature scaling. Data cleansing consists of the removal of outliers in regards to spatial depth and inconsistency within an image series. Data augmentation methods are rotation, flipping, Gaussian noise and contrast. The image is resized by a 10 % crop and rescaled to 30x128x128 voxels. Feature rescaling comprises clipping of pixel values to the 0.99-quartile and z-score normalization.

The two convolutional neural networks (CNN) are derived from the VGG-16 [6] and the ResNet-50 [7] as they are widely used in state-of-the art research [2–4]. The networks are modified to transform the asymmetric input size of 30x128x128 into symmetric feature maps in deeper layers, inspired by Du et al. [8]. The settings of the hyperparameters and results are presented for the VGG-16 model as it demonstrates a higher diagnostic performance. The settings are based on state-of-the-art studies [2–4] and evaluated with a reduced grid search. An adam optimizer is established with a mini-batch size of 12, an initial learning rate of 10^{-4} and a decay on plateau of 0.4 every 4th epoch without improvement on the validation loss. For regularization, a dropout layer with a dropout rate of 0.4 is implemented. Additionally, the augmentation factor is set to 0.7 for the VGG-16. The class imbalanced is addressed with a weighted binary cross-entropy loss. The training is terminated after 15 epochs without a decline on the validation loss. The main evaluation metrics are the area under the ROC curve (AUC) and the F1-score in order to consider the class imbalance.

The experiments are conducted on four Tesla V100 16GB supported by two Intel Xeon CPU E5-2690 v4 2.60GHz with a total of 24 cores. For the experiments, the six subsets DWI, FLAIR, T1, T1 FLAIR, T2 and T2 FLAIR are each split into a 65 % training, 15 % validation and 20 % test set. These splits are conducted on patient level and are stratified. First, all samples are used to train, validate and test the models to demonstrate the diagnostic performance for binary abnormality classification on large heterogeneous datasets. Second, the subsets are under-sampled in order to compare the performance on the individual MRI sequences on uniform-sized datasets. The number of samples used per subset is 609, determined by the sequence with the smallest sample size: T1-weighted FLAIR. Third, the performance on single-disease groups is evaluated.

3 Results

The metrices for the VGG-16 model on the multi-disease full-sized dataset are shown in Tabular 2 and Figure 2. The best results are achieved on the T2-weighted FLAIR sequence with an AUC value of 0.89. On the uniform-sized datasets, the model demon-

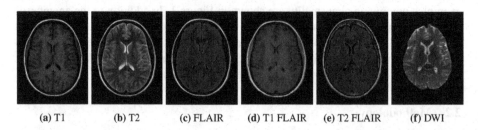

(a) T1   (b) T2   (c) FLAIR   (d) T1 FLAIR   (e) T2 FLAIR   (f) DWI

Fig. 1. Axial views of MRI sequences from patients without a diagnosed abnormality.

Tab. 2. Metrices for binary classification on full-sized (1) and uniform-sized (2) multi-disease datasets.

	DWI		FLAIR		T1		T1 FLAIR	T2		T2 FLAIR	
Dataset size	1	2	1	2	1	2	1/2	1	2	1	2
AUC	0.75	0.6	0.81	0.59	0.75	0.54	0.84	0.84	0.71	0.89	0.79
F1-score	0.77	0.33	0.77	0.68	0.77	0.90	0.67	0.72	0.72	0.86	0.78
Precision	0.88	0.83	0.93	0.83	0.92	0.81	0.96	0.98	0.92	0.97	0.97
Sensitivity	0.68	0.2	0.66	0.58	0.66	1.00	0.51	0.57	0.59	0.78	0.65
Specificity	0.69	0.86	0.83	0.54	0.73	0.00	0.90	0.95	0.76	0.84	0.88

Tab. 3. AUC values for VGG-16 on full-sized subsets for a single-disease binary classification.

	DWI	FLAIR	T1	T1 FLAIR	T2	T2 FLAIR
Glioblastoma	0.80	-	0.96	-	0.99	1.00
Hemorrhage	0.76	0.87	0.81	0.85	0.91	0.97
Infarct	0.83	0.90	0.85	0.95	0.94	0.94
Other benign tumor	0.73	0.72	0.71	-	0.77	0.82

strates a lower performance than on the full-sized dataset, shown in Tabular 2 and in Figure 2. The highest AUC value is achieved on the T1-weighted FLAIR sequence with 0.84. The sequences DWI, FLAIR, T1-weighted have the largest decline in their AUC values compared to the results on the full-sized datset. The model is not able to distinguish between the classes in the sequences DWI and T1-weighted. DWI yields a F1-score of 0.33 and T1-weighted a sensitivity of 1.00 and a specificity of 0.00.

The results of the single-disease classification for the VGG-16 are listed in Tabular. 3. Empty cells indicate a test set with less than five abnormal samples which are rejected as the sample size is not representative. On the single-disease dataset, the AUC values are generally higher than the corresponding values of the full-sized dataset. The T2-weighted FLAIR sequence yields superior results on the groups glioblastoma and hemorrhage with AUC values of 1.00 and 0.97, respectively.

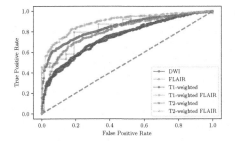 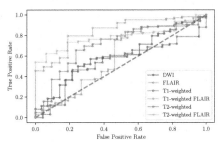

Fig. 2. ROC curves for binary classification on full-sized (left) and uniform-sized (right) multi-disease datasets.

4 Discussion

The main objective of this research is to assess the diagnostic performance for binary abnormality classification of deep learning models on the MRI sequences for brain images:
diffusion weighted imaging (DWI), fluid attenuated inversion recovery (FLAIR), T1-
weighted, T1-weighted FLAIR, T2-weighted and T2-weighted FLAIR. All sequences
are suitable to produce useful predictions despite the heterogeneous nature of the dataset.
The AUC values of studies based on more homogenous datasets [2–4] are higher, however the single-disease evaluation of the IRW Brain MRI dataset yields comparable result
in most of the selected disease groups with AUC values up to 1.00. Consequently, the
first conclusion of this research is that highly homogeneous datasets are not necessary.
However, the implementation of CAD systems in clinical routine requires improvements
of the diagnostic performance, especially in regards to the sensitivity rate. Thus, further
studies on improving the diagnostic performance are required and should be conducted
on heterogeneous datasets to narrow the gap between research and clinical practice.

The T2-weighted FLAIR sequence is the basis for superior diagnostic performance
with an AUC value of 0.89 for the VGG-16 model on the full-sized dataset. The T2-
weighted FLAIR, the T1-weighted FLAIR and the T2-weighted sequence demonstrate
high AUC values in both models. The relative low AUC values on the DWI and the
FLAIR sequence may be influenced by a higher variance of scanners and pixel values.
The results yield indications for screening protocols for patients with a non-specific con-
dition as the data contains multiple diseases from the clinical routine. Non-specific brain
MRI screening protocols for physicians typically include T1-weighted, T2-weighted and
FLAIR sequences [9]. The second conclusion of this work is to incorporate T1-weighted
FLAIR and T2-weighted FLAIR images in screening protocols, as they exhibit superior
AUC values compared to T1-weighted, FLAIR and DWI in both models. In addition,
a general screening protocol for deep learning algorithm to determine to most relevant
sequences for specific and non-specific conditions would be of great value. Advanc-
ing these findings on other datasets and comparing them to screening protocols for
physicians is suggested.

The superior diagnostic performance for the uniform-sized subsets is achieved on
the T1-weighted FLAIR sequence with the VGG-16. Apart from this sequence, the
ranking of the AUC values is similar to the ones of the full-sized subsets. The diagnostic
performance results clearly show the positive effect of larger datasets as the AUC
values are lower compared to the full-sized datasets. There are two main reasons behind
the limited usage of large heterogeneous datasets for MRI brain imaging. First, the
widespread availability of such datasets is not yet given. While other deep learning fields
have seen massive increases in data collection such as social media [10], large medical
image databases are still scarce. Second, available medical image datasets as well as
the data collection methods show minor harmonization. Thus, the third conclusion is
to implement more exhaustive and standardized data collection processes in order to
drastically increase the data quality and reduce time-consuming pre-processing steps.
In particular, standardized source data from patient anamnestic are required and would
help to overcome potential biases of the algorithms. This could be accompanied by
additional data from healthy subjects.

References

1. Feigin VL, Nichols E, Alam T, Bannick MS, Beghi E, Blake N et al. Global, regional, and national burden of neurological disorders, 1990–2016: a systematic analysis for the Global Burden of Disease Study 2016. Lancet Neurol. 2016.
2. Korolev S, Safiullin A, Belyaev M, Dodonova Y. Residual and plain convolutional neural networks for 3D brain MRI classification. IEEE ISBI. 2017.
3. Khan HA, Jue W, Mushtaq M, Mushtaq MU. Brain tumor classification in MRI image using convolutional neural network. Mathematical biosciences and engineering: MBE. 2020.
4. Talo M, Yildirim O, Baloglu UB, Aydin G, Acharya UR. Convolutional neural networks for multi-class brain disease detection using MRI images. Comput Med Imaging Graph. 2019.
5. BioMedical Engineering and Imaging Institute. Imaging research warehouse. http://researchroadmap.mssm.edu/reference/systems/irw.
6. Simonyan K, Zisserman A. Very deep convolutional networks for large-scale image recognition. ICLR. 2015.
7. He K, Zhang X, Ren S, Sun J. Deep residual learning for image recognition. IEEE CVPR. 2016.
8. Du Tran, Bourdev L, Fergus R, Torresani L, Paluri M. Learning spatiotemporal features with 3D convolutional etworks. IEEE ICCV. 2015.
9. Mikulis DJ, Roberts TPL. Neuro MR: protocols. Journal of magnetic resonance imaging: JMRI. 2007.
10. Taigman Y, Yang M, Ranzato M, Wolf L. DeepFace: closing the gap to human-level performance in face verification. 2014.

Towards Super-resolution CEST MRI for Visualization of Small Structures

Lukas Folle[1], Katharian Tkotz[2], Fasil Gadjimuradov[1], Lorenz A. Kapsner[2,6],
Moritz Fabian[3], Sebastian Bickelhaupt[2], David Simon[4], Arnd Kleyer[4],
Gerhard Krönke[4], Moritz Zaiß[3], Armin Nagel[2,5], Andreas Maier[1]

[1]Pattern Recognition Lab, Friedrich-Alexander-Universität Erlangen-Nürnberg (FAU), Erlangen, Germany
[2]Institute of Radiology, University Hospital Erlangen,
Friedrich-Alexander-Universität Erlangen-Nürnberg (FAU), Erlangen, Germany
[3]Institute of Neuroradiology, University Hospital Erlangen,
Friedrich-Alexander-Universität Erlangen-Nürnberg (FAU), Erlangen, Germany
[4]Department of Internal Medicine 3, University Hospital Erlangen,
Friedrich-Alexander-Universität Erlangen-Nürnberg (FAU), Erlangen, Germany
[5]Division of Medical Physics in Radiology, German Cancer Research Center (DKFZ),
Heidelberg, Germany
[6]Medizinisches Zentrum für Informations- und Kommunikationstechnik, Universitätsklinikum
Erlangen, Erlangen, Deutschland
lukas.folle@fau.de

Abstract. The onset of rheumatic diseases such as rheumatoid arthritis is typically subclinical, which results in challenging early detection of the disease. However, characteristic changes in the anatomy can be detected using imaging techniques such as MRI or CT. Modern imaging techniques such as chemical exchange saturation transfer (CEST) MRI drive the hope to improve early detection even further through the imaging of metabolites in the body. To image small structures in the joints of patients, typically one of the first regions where changes due to the disease occur, a high resolution for the CEST MR imaging is necessary. Currently, however, CEST MR suffers from an inherently low resolution due to the underlying physical constraints of the acquisition. In this work we compared established up-sampling techniques to neural network-based super-resolution approaches. We could show, that neural networks are able to learn the mapping from low-resolution to high-resolution unsaturated CEST images considerably better than present methods. On the test set a PSNR of 32.29 dB (+10%), a NRMSE of 0.14 (+28%), and a SSIM of 0.85 (+15%) could be achieved using a ResNet neural network, improving the baseline considerably. This work paves the way for the prospective investigation of neural networks for super-resolution CEST MRI and, followingly, might lead to a earlier detection of the onset of rheumatic diseases.

1 Introduction

Patients affected by rheumatic diseases such as psoriatic arthritis (PsA) or rheumatoid arthritis (RA) suffer from synovial inflammation, which can lead to cartilage and bone destruction if no treatment is initiated [1]. But, if detected at an early stage, rheumatic

© Der/die Autor(en), exklusiv lizenziert durch
Springer Fachmedien Wiesbaden GmbH, ein Teil von Springer Nature 2022
K. Maier-Hein et al. (Hrsg.), *Bildverarbeitung für die Medizin 2022*,
Informatik aktuell, https://doi.org/10.1007/978-3-658-36932-3_45

diseases can be controlled well through the prescription of disease modifying anti-rheumatic drugs (DMARD) [2]. The early detection, however, still remains a challenging task, even with the use of neural networks [3]. Chemical exchange saturation transfer (CEST) magnetic resonances imaging (MRI) of joints allows for the visualization of biochemical alterations of tissue and, thus, is a promising tool for the detection of disease onset. One major obstacle of CEST MRI is the inherently low resolution [4]. This is due to the fact that a high signal to noise ratio (SNR) is needed for a reproducible CEST contrast, which restricts image resolution. For the application in a rheumatic setting, imaging of thin structures such as the joint tissue of the knee is thus very challenging. Super-resolution focuses on the task of computing high-resolution (HR) images from low-resolution (LR) images by exploiting prior information [5]. One very prominent method for extracting and exploiting this information are neural networks [6]. Previously, neural network-based super-resolution mostly focused on increasing the resolution of common MR sequences such as fast-spin-echo and double echo in steady-state [7, 8]. So far, no evaluation of super-resolution techniques for CEST MRI has been performed. One established method along different MRI sequences is k-space zero-filling and thus will serve as the baseline for our comparison [9]. In this work, we will investigate the feasibility of applying super-resolution neural networks for CEST MRI scans by comparing different neural network architectures and loss functions for 7T unsaturated knee CEST MR images.

2   Theory and methods

In the following, the acquisition of the CEST MR scans will be described, followed by an overview of the deep learning methods and current interpolation techniques. The main motivation of CEST MRI is the imaging of other metabolites than free water, which mainly contributes to normal 1H images - described in [10, 11]. This contrast utilizes the chemical exchange of bound hydrogen atoms with free water. To add metabolic information, the magnetization at the resonance frequency of the bound hydrogen proton is saturated. Due to the chemical exchange the saturation is transferred to the free water signal and results in a signal decrease in the subsequent acquired MR image. Typically, images with saturation at different resonance frequencies are acquired, resulting in voxel-wise spectral information showing the abundance of the metabolic groups. However, due to the repeated flipping and relaxation of the magnetization during the image acquisition the magnetization converges to a steady state, that is independent of the previous saturation. Thus, a higher resolution, which corresponds to a longer acquisition phase, will reduce the metabolic weighting in the resulting image. The only possibility to avoid this is a segmented k-space acquisition, which, however, prolongs the acquisition process significantly. For the training of super-resolution networks, however, HR data is necessary. For our experiments, the training and test data consisted only of unsaturated images. All scans were acquired using a 7 T MR Siemens Magnetom Terra (Siemens Healthcare, Erlangen, Germany) with a 1Tx/28Rx knee coil (Quality Electrodynamics LLC, Mayfield Village, Ohio, USA). The high-resolution CEST images were acquired with a 3D GRE sequence [12] and had a slice thickness of 2.5 mm and a pixel spacing of 0.802 mm resulting in volume dimensions of $192 \times 192 \times 40$.

A repetition time of 13 ms was chosen, including three echos at 1.81 ms, 6.43 ms, and 11.05 ms to achieve a higher variety of the image contrast. In total, 39 HR volumes were available from 13 healthy volunteers with three different echo times that were split in to 23 training volumes, 8 validation, and 8 testing volumes. No data was shared across the three sets. All participants gave written informed consent before the measurement and were recruited under the approval of the local ethics committee (Ethik-Kommission, Friedrich-Alexander-Universität, Erlangen-Nürnberg). For the training and quantitative comparison, LR images were generated by down-sampling of the HR images by a factor of two. Trilinear interpolation as a further established method was dropped due to the inferior performance to the k-space zero-filling. Pre-processing steps included z-score normalization and, for the training phase, random 3D crops of size ($64 \times 64 \times 16$), random flipping along all three axes, and random rotations (15 degree in-plane, 5 degree through-plane). To estimate how close a predicted image is to the HR image, structural similarity (SSIM), peak signal to noise ratio (PSNR), and normalized root mean square error (NRMSE) were evaluated. Two different network architectures were compared throughout this work, namely a ResNet-based network [13] and a DenseNet-based net-

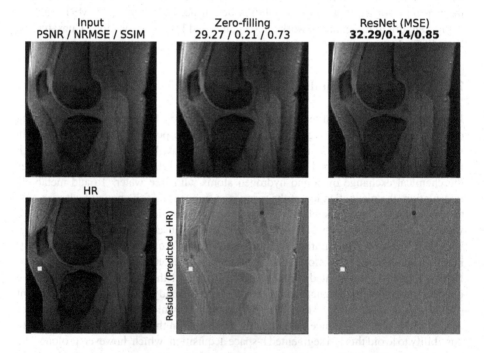

Fig. 1. Comparison of traditional k-space zero-filling and the best performing neural network prediction. Input to both methods is the low-resolution image LR (top left) and target is the ground-truth high-resolution image HR (bottom left). Residuals between prediction and HR are depicted below the predictions (pixel values in [-0.23, 0.38] for all residuals). Yellow square and blue dot mark regions with high difficulty for both methods due to high-frequency image components or blood flow.

Tab. 1. Comparison of k-space zero-filling and the neural network for the test cases of the dataset. PSNR: peak signal to noise ratio (dB); (NR) MSE: (normalized root) mean square error; SSIM: structural similarity; SD: standard deviation; ↑: higher is better; ↓: lower is better. Best performance marked in bold.

Method	Loss function	PSNR (SD) ↑	NRMSE (SD) ↓	SSIM (SD) ↑
K-space zero-filling	n/a	29.27 (0.77)	0.21 (0.04)	0.73 (0.03)
	MSE	**32.29** (1.19)	**0.14** (0.03)	**0.85** (0.01)
ResNet	SSIM	31.08 (0.98)	0.16 (0.03)	0.84 (0.01)
	Perceptual	31.65 (0.99)	0.18 (0.04)	0.77 (0.03)
	MSE	31.07 (0.87)	0.16 (0.03)	0.83 (0.01)
DenseNet	SSIM	30.70 (1.02)	0.17 (0.03)	0.83 (0.01)
	Perceptual	31.93 (1.10)	0.17 (0.04)	0.80 (0.02)

work [14], both adapted to 3D images. A Wasserstein generative adversarial network (GAN) [15] during initial experiments could not be trained to convergence and thus was removed from the comparison. The DenseNet-like model consisted of four Dense-Blocks with a growth rate in each block of 16 and 32 initial channels resulting in a total of 411k parameters. The ResNet-like model consisted of 16 residual blocks each with 32 channels leading to 528k parameters. For the ResNet and the DenseNet, different loss functions were compared: mean-squared error loss (MSE), SSIM loss, and a perceptual loss. The perceptual loss was calculated based on the distance of feature vectors extracted from a VGG network trained in ImageNet [16, 17]. Training was stopped when no improvement on the validation set SSIM was perceived for 100 epochs. Adam with a constant learning rate of $1e^{-4}$ was used for all models. The complete dataset was split into 60% training samples, 20% validation samples, and 20% test samples. For comparison to the predictions of the neural networks, k-space zero-filling was used. K-space zero filling is applied to the raw k-space MR data. Thereby the outer regions of the k-space, which contain the high frequency information, are padded with zeros in all three directions up to the desired resolution. Typically, filters are applied to smooth the hard edges in k-space, but were removed in our comparison to achieve higher SSIM and PSNR.

3 Results

Table 1 shows the quantitative comparison of the different neural network configurations together with the baseline, k-space zero-filling on the test set. Overall, the ResNet models outperformed the DenseNet models consistently across all metrics and loss functions except for the perceptual loss. Further, mean-squared error loss leads to better results for both models. Finally, k-space zero-filling could be considerably outperformed using the best neural network configuration by an increase of the performance using the ResNet trained with MSE loss of PSNR +3.02 dB, NRMSE +0.07, and SSIM +0.12. Figure 1 provides a qualitative comparison of the neural-network-based method (ResNet MSE loss) over the currently used method (k-space zero-filling) together with the LR input and the HR ground-truth (GT). It can be seen that the residual between the prediction and the GT is substantially improved by the network over the zero-filling approach. Regions the network is not able to recover typically have either very high frequencies such as subcutaneous fat anterior to the patella (yellow square) or strong blood flow such as the popliteal artery (blue dot). The regions of high interest for arthritis research, the tibiofemoral joint and patellofemoral joint, are resolved with high accuracy by the network.

4 Discussion

In this work, we demonstrated the application of neural network for super-resolution on CEST MR imaging and compared different network architectures and loss functions. We believe, that the results of this work have the potential to further advance the application of the CEST contrast in arthritis research, as our findings enable imaging of smaller structures in the knee joint which play a vital role in the early detection of rheumatic diseases. The presented work considerably outperformed the baseline method. Overall, ResNet inspired models as well as the mean-squared error loss function performed best in our experiments. Our approach has some limitations. We did not test the combination of loss functions and the implication of the loss function on the image appearance. In future work, we want to focus on those points specifically. Additionally, the general reasoning behind the predictions of neural networks is inherently hard to understand and errors in the prediction might be hard to spot. Thus, in future work, we want to focus on the data consistency of the predictions and provide an easy to use software tool to compare LR image and HR prediction at the click of a button. Further, we want to make use of all the information from the k-space by incorporating the reconstruction step into our method. Currently, parts of this information are lost due to the lossy reconstruction. Finally, we aim to perform a qualitative evaluation of the best performing configuration on prospectively acquired low-resolution CEST MRI at different frequencies and compare the resulting CEST contrast with currently used methods.

Acknowledgement. This work was supported by the emerging field initiative (project 4 Med 05 "MIRACLE") of the University Erlangen-Nürnberg and MASCARA - Molecular Assessment of Signatures Characterizing the Remission of Arthritis Grant 01EC1903A. We would like to thank the d.hip data center for computational support. Katharina Tkotz and Lukas Folle contributed equally to this work.

References

1. McInnes IB, Schett G. The pathogenesis of rheumatoid arthritis. N Engl J Med. 2011;365(23). PMID: 22150039:2205–19.
2. Schett G, Emery P, Tanaka Y, Burmester G, Pisetsky DS, Naredo E et al. Tapering biologic and conventional DMARD therapy in rheumatoid arthritis: current evidence and future directions. Ann Rheum Dis. 2016;75(8):1428–37.
3. Folle L, Liu C, Simon D, Meinderink T, Liphardt AM, Krönke G et al. Differential diagnosis of RA and PsA using neural networks on three-dimensional bone shape of finger joints. Ann Rheum Dis. 2021;80(Suppl 1):86.

4. Wu B, Warnock G, Zaiss M, Lin C, Chen M, Zhou Z et al. An overview of CEST MRI for non-MR physicists. eng. EJNMMI Phys. 2016;3(1). 27562024[pmid]:19–9.

5. Köhler T, Huang X, Schebesch F, Aichert A, Maier A, Hornegger J. Robust multiframe super-resolution employing iteratively re-weighted minimization. IEEE Trans Comput Imaging. 2016;2(1):42–58.

6. Köhler T, Bätz M, Naderi F, Kaup A, Maier A, Riess C. Toward bridging the simulated-to-real gap: benchmarking super-resolution on real data. IEEE Trans Pattern Anal Mach Intell. 2019;42(11):2944–59.

7. Greenspan H, Oz G, Kiryati N, Peled S. MRI inter-slice reconstruction using super-resolution. Magn Reson Imaging. 2002;20(5):437–46.

8. Chaudhari AS, Fang Z, Kogan F, Wood J, Stevens KJ, Gibbons EK et al. Super-resolution musculoskeletal MRI using deep learning. Magn Reson Med. 2018;80(5):2139–54.

9. Luo J, Mou Z, Qin B, Li W, Yang F, Robini M et al. Fast single image super-resolution using estimated low-frequency K-space data in MRI. Magn Reson Imaging. 2017;40:1–11.

10. Zijl PCM van, Yadav NN. Chemical exchange saturation transfer (CEST): what is in a name and what isn't? Magn Reson Med. 2011;65(4):927–48.

11. Guivel-Scharen V, Sinnwell T, Wolff S, Balaban R. Detection of proton chemical exchange between metabolites and water in biological tissues. J Magn Reson Imaging. 1998;133(1):36–45.

12. Zaiss M, Ehses P, Scheffler K. Snapshot-CEST: optimizing spiral-centric-reordered gradient echo acquisition for fast and robust 3D CEST MRI at 9.4 T. NMR Biomed. 2018;31(4). e3879 NBM-17-0188.R2:e3879.

13. He K, Zhang X, Ren S, Sun J. Deep residual learning for image recognition. 2016 IEEE conference on computer vision and pattern recognition (CVPR). 2016:770–8.

14. Huang G, Liu Z, Maaten LVD, Weinberger KQ. Densely connected convolutional networks. Proc IEEE Comput Soc Conf Comput Vis Pattern Recognit. Los Alamitos, CA, USA: IEEE Computer Society, 2017:2261–9.

15. Arjovsky M, Chintala S, Bottou L. Wasserstein generative adversarial networks. Proc Int Conf Mach Learn. (ICML'17). Sydney, NSW, Australia: JMLR.org, 2017:214–23.

16. Zhang R, Isola P, Efros AA, Shechtman E, Wang O. The unreasonable effectiveness of deep features as a perceptual metric. Proc IEEE Comput Soc Conf Comput Vis Pattern Recognit. 2018:586–95.

17. Deng J, Dong W, Socher R, Li LJ, Li K, Fei-Fei L. ImageNet: a large-scale hierarchical image database. Proc IEEE Comput Soc Conf Comput Vis Pattern Recognit. 2009:248–55.

Multi-organ Segmentation with Partially Annotated Datasets

Haobo Song, Chang Liu, Lukas Folle, Andreas Maier

Pattern Recognition Lab, Department of Computer Science, Friedrich-Alexander-Universität Erlangen-Nürnberg
haobo.song@fau.de

Abstract. Efficient and fully automatic multi-organ segmentation is of great research and clinical prospect. Deep learning (DL) based methods have recently emerged and proven its effectiveness in various biomedical segmentation tasks. The performance of DL based segmentation models strongly depends on the training dataset and a large, correctly annotated dataset is always crucial. However, gathering annotation for multi-organ segmentation task is difficult and making use of public datasets with existing annotations then becomes one possible solution. In this work we propose a pipeline for training multi-organ segmentation model from partially annotated datasets. The proposed method is evaluated using left, right lungs and liver segmentation task of throat-abdomen CT scans. From average dice score, we found the proposed method can obtain very close performance using only partially annotated datasets (0.93), compared with models using fully annotated datasets (0.96).

1 Introduction

Multi-organ segmentation has long been a heated topic both for research and in clinics. In the clinical process of radiation therapy, for example, delineation of organs at risk (OARs) is required for the treatment planning. However, manually delineating OARs by clinicians is time-consuming and thus, an automated segmentation tool is widely expected. Recently, deep learning (DL) based models are heavily researched for diverse biomedical tasks, including also multi-organ segmentation [1]. Since DL based segmentation methods are commonly supervised learning methods, a large quantity of paired images and annotations are required for the successful model training. However, the size of all segmentation dataset are restricted by the difficulty of getting manual organ segmentation. To this end, making use of public dataset with verified annotation is one possible solution.

In this paper, a organ segmentation dataset where all required organs are annotated is defined as fully annotated dataset and is the optimal for training a multi-organ segmentation model. In contrast, a dataset where only one or several required organs are annotated is a partially annotated dataset. The annotations from public datasets are verified by clinicians but they can hardly serve the development of a multi-organ segmentation tool,

Springer Fachmedien Wiesbaden GmbH, ein Teil von Springer Nature 2022
K. Maier-Hein et al. (Hrsg.), *Bildverarbeitung für die Medizin 2022*,
Informatik aktuell, https://doi.org/10.1007/978-3-658-36932-3_46

Tab. 1. Fusion mode details. The fusion datasets are used only in the training phase. The number in the range represents the patient ID in the fully annotated dataset.

	FULL	PARTIAL w/o lung	PARTIAL w/o liver	Adopted training scheme
Mode 1	0-23	-	-	No
Mode 2	0-7	-	-	No
Mode 3	0-7	8-15	16-23	No
Mode 4	0-7	8-15	16-23	Yes
Mode 5	-	8-15	16-23	No
Mode 6	-	8-15	16-23	Yes

as most of these are partially annotated datasets. For segmentation models based on supervised learning, a partially annotated dataset induces incorrect annotation and can impair the performance as a result.

We offer a generic approach for fusing partially annotated datasets for training a multi-organ segmentation model. The training pipeline is adapted so that partially annotated data will be treated differently according to the annotation itself. To the best of our knowledge, not many related works have been proposed aiming to better fuse multiple partially annotated datasets. Only in [2] a special loss function has been proposed for heterogeneous annotations. For a proof of principle, we evaluate different situations of fusing partially annotated datasets by simulation of partial annotations from a fully annotated throat-abdomen CT dataset.

2 Material and methods

Since the proposed method is only related to the training process, in the experiments all trained networks share the same model and training configurations. 2D vanilla U-Net [3] is selected as the segmentation model. Adam is used as optimizer with learning rate 5e-4 and cross-entropy loss as loss function. The experiments are designed to validate the modified training pipeline by simulating different fusion modes of partially and fully annotated datasets.

2.1 Dataset

The dataset used for training contains 30 clinical torso CT images scanned by the department of radiology, university hospital Erlangen. Three abdominal organs have been manually annotated as ground truth: liver, right lung and left lung. the partially annotated dataset is generated from the fully annotated dataset to simulate different fusion modes. In this work 6 fusion modes are simulated and used for the following experiments, according to the permutation in Table 1.

Figure 1 is an example of the partial annotation simulation. When the partial annotation is generated, the "taken-away" organ is also recorded as the annotation fact with the data, so that it will be treated accordingly during the training phase.

2.2 Modified training pipeline

Our proposed training pipeline is illustrated in Figure 2a, compared with a regular training pipeline in Figure 2b. Our pipeline enables the model to treat partially annotated dataset accordingly. As mentioned previously, within one training step the model is fed with image and annotation together with the annotation fact. We have added an extra channel to each image to identify whether it is partially annotated data. When the input annotation fact indicates partially annotated data, the model will generate prediction from the current model output and add the predicted region of the missing organs to the annotation. One example is illustrated in Figure 3, the annotation fact indicates missing liver annotation. The model then generate a liver segmentation mask using the current network output and the annotation is modified. The annotation modification exists only in the running training step.

We observed that, if the partially annotated datasets are randomly mixed without annotation facts, the model training is biased because any background region can be either un-annotated organ or real background. However when we combine datasets, the annotation fact of the dataset is clearly known and such annotation fact is used in our proposed method to reduce the bias in training. Instead of eliminating loss completely from the missing annotation, our proposed method makes a prediction during training and will guide the model to keep strong activations. In this way, the model can automatically perserve in steps without valid annotation and only proceed in steps with valid annotation.

2.3 Experiments setting

As listed in Table 1, 6 fusion modes were established and experimented in this work to verify the proposed training pipeline. Mode 1 contains all fully annotated data and is designed to be the best benchmark. Mode 2, 3 and 4 contain same fully annotated data but mode 3 and 4 contain additional partially annotated data. Mode 5 and Mode 6 comprise only of partially annotated data. The proposed training pipeline is applied to model training of mode 4 and 6. For all experiments, the segmentation model is

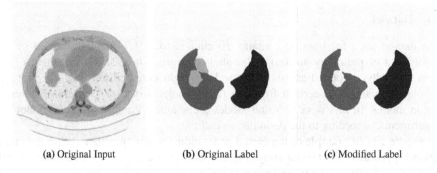

(a) Original Input   (b) Original Label   (c) Modified Label

Fig. 1. Simulation of partially-labelled missing data sets by masking.

trained to segment left, right lungs and liver. Adam is used as network optimizer and cross-entropy loss as loss function. After successful training, all modes are tested using scans from 4 extra patients with full annotation.

3   Result

From the metrics in Table 2, mode 1 shows the best performance. On average, mode 4 has 4.0 % higher dice score and 7.8 % higher IoU compared with mode 3. Mode 6 has 6.3 % higher dice score and 10.9 % higher IoU compared with mode 5. While mode 5 has lowest average dice score and IoU. Mode 4 has 3.2 % of dice score and 6.5 % of IoU superior to mode 6 (Fig. 4).

4   Discussion

From the results, we can conclude that the proposed training pipeline can effectively improve the multi-organ segmentation training using partially annotated datasets. The results of fusion mode 3 and 5 show downgraded performance using partially annotated dataset, but the proposed training pipeline can remove the downgrade, as in mode 4

Algorithm 1 Modified train step	**Algorithm 2** Regular train step
Require: *image*, *target* and *net*.	**Require:** *image*, *target* and *net*.
1: *output* ← *net*(*image*)	1: *output* ← *net*(*input*)
2: **if** *image* is partially annotated **then**	2: loss(*output*, *target*)
3: *pred* ← *output.argmax*()	3: backpropagation
4: Add missing annotation from *pred* to *target*	
5: **end if**	
6: loss(*output*, *target*)	
7: backpropagation	

(a) Modified train step   (b) Regular train step

Fig. 2. Comparison of different training steps.

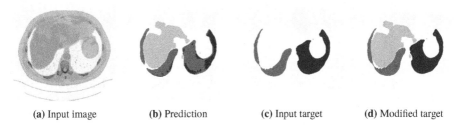

(a) Input image   (b) Prediction   (c) Input target   (d) Modified target

Fig. 3. Simulation of modifying input annotation based on current prediction.

Tab. 2. All mode results. Segmentation performance is measured by dice coefficient and IoU.

	Dice				IoU			
	Liver	L. lung	R. lung	Avg	Liver	L.lung	R.lung	Avg
Mode 1	0.953	0.981	0.978	0.970	0.911	0.963	0.957	0.943
Mode 2	0.945	0.968	0.963	0.960	0.896	0.938	0.929	0.920
Mode 3	0.938	0.939	0.901	0.926	0.883	0.885	0.819	0.863
Mode 4	0.948	0.974	0.970	0.963	0.901	0.949	0.941	0.930
Mode 5	0.920	0.888	0.826	0.877	0.852	0.799	0.704	0.787
Mode 6	0.936	0.961	0.901	0.933	0.880	0.925	0.819	0.873

and 6. From fusion mode 2 and mode 6, the proposed method can even achieve close performance compared with models using fully annotated dataset. However, the current experiments are now only based on dataset with few organs segmented and our future work will extend to the fusion of more datasets. In addition, the proposed method has only been experimented using simulation data and in future this will be used to fuse real partially annotated datasets.

4.1 Hints for using partially annotated datasets

Based on our experiments, we can provide some hints for the use of public partially annotated datasets. First of all, simply mixing partially annotated datasets is not a solution, our experiments indicate that introducing partially annotated dataset into even fully annotated dataset will on the contrary impair the performance. Secondly, fully annotated dataset is a good start point even if the size of dataset is small, our experiments also assert the importance of fully annotated dataset. Last but not least, partially annotated datasets are indeed able to assist fully annotated dataset for the development of multi-organ segmentation tool, but much further research is needed.

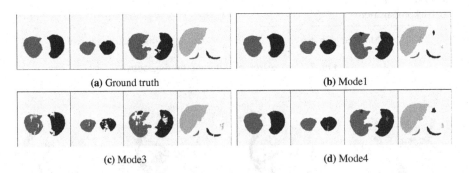

(a) Ground truth   (b) Mode1

(c) Mode3   (d) Mode4

Fig. 4. Example segmentation using models from fusion Mode 1, 3 and 4.

References

1. Maier A, Syben C, Lasser T, Riess C. A gentle introduction to deep learning in medical image processing. Z Med Phys. 2019;29(2):86–101.
2. Kemnitz J, Baumgartner CF, Wirth W, Eckstein F, Eder SK, Konukoglu E. Combining heterogeneously labeled datasets for training segmentation networks. International Workshop on Machine Learning in Medical Imaging. Springer. 2018:276–84.
3. Ronneberger O, Fischer P, Brox T. U-Net: convolutional networks for biomedical image segmentation. 2015.

Abstract: C-MORE: A High-content Single-cell Morphology Recognition Methodology for Liquid Biopsies
Toward Personalized Cardiovascular Medicine

Jennifer Furkel[1,2,3,4,5], Maximilian Knoll[3,4,5], Shabana Din[1,2], Nicolai V. Bogert[1,2], Timon Seeger[1,2], Norbert Frey[1,2], Amir Abdollahi[3,4,5], Hugo A. Katus[1,2], Mathias H. Konstandin[1,2]

[1]Department of Cardiology, Angiology and Pneumology, Heidelberg University Hospital, 69120 Heidelberg, Germany
[2]DZHK (German Center for Cardiovascular Research), Site Heidelberg/Mannheim, 69120 Heidelberg, Germany
[3]German Cancer Consortium (DKTK) Core Center Heidelberg, German Cancer Research Center (DKFZ), 69120 Heidelberg, Germany
[4]Clinical Cooperation Unit Translational Radiation Oncology, National Center for Tumor Diseases (NCT), Heidelberg University Hospital (UKHD) and DKFZ, 69120 Heidelberg, Germany
[5]Division of Molecular and Translational Radiation Oncology, Department of Radiation Oncology, Heidelberg Faculty of Medicine (MFHD) and Heidelberg University Hospital (UKHD), Heidelberg Ion-Beam Therapy Center (HIT), Heidelberg, Germany
mathias.konstandin@med.uni-heidelberg.de

Cellular morphology has the capacity to serve as a surrogate for cellular state and functionality. However, primary cardiomyocytes, the standard model in cardiovascular research, are highly heterogeneous cells and thus impose methodological challenges to analysis. Hence, we aimed to devise a robust methodology to deconvolute cardiomyocyte morphology on a single-cell level: C-MORE (cellular morphology recognition) is a workflow from bench to data analysis tailored for heterogeneous primary cells using our R package cmoRe. We demonstrate its utility in proof-of-principle applications such as modulation of canonical hypertrophy pathways and linkage of genotype-phenotype in human induced pluripotent stem cell-derived cardiomyocytes (hiPSC-CMs). Exposure of cardiomyocytes to blood plasma prior to versus after aortic valve replacement allows identification of a disease fingerprint and reflects partial reversibility following therapeutic intervention. C-MORE is a valuable tool for cardiovascular research with possible fields of application in basic research and personalized medicine [1].

References

1. Furkel et al. C-MORE: A high-content single-cell morphology recognition methodology for liquid biopsies toward personalized cardiovascular medicine. Cell Reports Medicine. 2021.

First Steps on Gamification of Lung Fluid Cells Annotations in the Flower Domain

Sonja Kunzmann[1], Christian Marzahl[1], Felix Denzinger[1], Christof Bertram[3], Robert Klopfleisch[4], Katharina Breininger[2], Vincent Christlein[1], Andreas Maier[1]

[1]Pattern Recognition Lab, FAU Erlangen-Nürnberg, Erlangen, Germany
[2]Department Artificial Intelligence in Biomedical Engineering, FAU Erlangen-Nürnberg, Erlangen, Germany
[3]Institute of Pathology, University of Verterinary Medicine, Vienna, Austria
[4]Institute of Veterinary Pathology, Freie Universität Berlin, Germany
sonja.kunzmann@fau.de

Abstract. Annotating data, especially in the medical domain, requires expert knowledge and a lot of effort. This limits the amount and/or usefulness of available medical data sets for experimentation. Therefore, developing strategies to increase the number of annotations while lowering the needed domain knowledge is of interest. A possible strategy is the use of gamification, i.e. transforming the annotation task into a game. We propose an approach to gamify the task of annotating lung fluid cells from pathological whole slide images (WSIs). As the domain is unknown to non-expert annotators, we transform images of cells to the domain of flower images using a CycleGAN architecture. In this more assessable domain, non-expert annotators can be (t)asked to annotate different kinds of flowers in a playful setting. In order to provide a proof of concept, this work shows that the domain transfer is possible by evaluating an image classification network trained on real cell images and tested on the cell images generated by the CycleGAN network (reconstructed cell images) as well as real cell images. The classification network reaches an average accuracy of 94.73 % on the original lung fluid cells and 95.25 % on the transformed lung fluid cells, respectively. Our study lays the foundation for future research on gamification using CycleGANs.

1 Introduction

On a number of tasks, computer vision algorithms have demonstrated human-level performance, especially in the areas of object detection and classification [1]. One major reason for this is the growing amount of labeled data sets which synergizes well with the advent of increasingly powerful deep learning (DL) algorithms. However, these data sets usually need to be enriched with information about their content. Most commonly performed by human annotators, this is a very time consuming, subjective and tedious task, which is also expensive and often needs prior training. Especially in the medical domain, i.e. for annotating cells in pathological whole slide images (WSIs), expert annotators usually have to get several years of practical experience. In other areas, where this constraint is not as severe, crowdsourcing is a popular approach to obtain label information. Usually crowdsourcing annotations is performed by hosting data on an interactive platform like the EXACT online annotation tool [2], where multiple

© Der/die Autor(en), exklusiv lizenziert durch
Springer Fachmedien Wiesbaden GmbH, ein Teil von Springer Nature 2022
K. Maier-Hein et al. (Hrsg.), *Bildverarbeitung für die Medizin 2022*,
Informatik aktuell, https://doi.org/10.1007/978-3-658-36932-3_48

annotators can assess the data simultaneously. EXACT hosts a partially annotated WSI data set [3] for the cyto-pathological diagnosis of equine asthma. However, large regions on multiple WSIs are still unlabeled. In order to overcome the issue, we propose the use of gamification approaches where game elements are applied in a non-gaming context [4]. Gamification aims to provide users with an exciting and rewarding annotation experience. An exemplary collection of successfully applied gamification in the medical domain is part of the Medical Data Donors project [5].

In order to decrease the necessary domain knowledge for untrained annotators, we propose to transform cells into flower images. The task of differentiating between various types of flowers should be possible for many human annotators. In the center of flower images the blossom is usually displayed, with a more or less homogeneous background and possibly more flowers in the background. This corresponds very well to the image perception in the cell domain where a cell is also usually located in the center of the image and other incomplete cells may be present at the edges. Figure 2 demonstrates our analogy. As a gamification strategy for the task of annotating cells, we propose the following approach (Fig. 1): in order to perform the domain transfer from cell to flower domain, we leverage the CycleGAN architecture [6]. Successful applications are e.g. style transfer, object transfiguration and season transfer as presented in Zhu at el. [6] and Bousmalis at el. [7]. As a proof of concept, we apply one CycleGAN model to each single cell type to create flower images. In the annotation game setting, the user would only see the flower image, which originates from a cell, and gets the task to annotate it in a playful way. Embodiments of the game are open for creativity but may include different tasks for different flowers (cut all sunflowers, water all daisies, etc.). In order to evaluate the performance of the CycleGAN – and therefore show that this domain transfer is possible – we evaluate cycle consistency by checking the performance of a cell type classification network using the transformed data created by transforming flowers back to the cell domain.

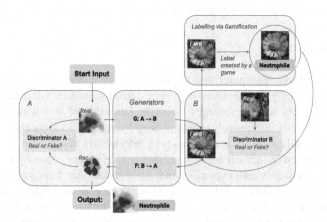

Fig. 1. Applying gamification for the task of annotating lung fluid cells: a CycleGAN architecture allows transformation of real cell images to reconstructed flower images and vice versa.

2   Materials and methods

Before going into details about the architecture and experiment design, we will present the characteristics of the two data sets used in this study, one containing lung fluid cell data and the other one flower images.

2.1   Lung fluid cells data set

The lung fluid cell data set consists of six cytological samples of equine bronchoalveolar lavage fluid (BALF), which were cytocentrifugated and stained using May Grunwald Giemsa. This data set was provided by Marzahl et al. [3]. Afterwards, the glass slides were digitized using a linear scanner (Aperio ScanScope CS2, Leica Biosystems, Germany) at a magnification of 400x with a resolution of 0.25 μm/px [3]. Two of the six WSIs are fully annotated and four partially annotated by a trained pathologist. The 87,738 bounding box annotated cells include neutrophils (12,556), multinuclear cells (310), mast cells (1,553), macrophages (24,498), lymphocytes (46,397), erythrocytes (339) and eosinophiles (105) [3]. Example images for the individual cell types can be seen in the top row of Figure 2. For subsequent processing, the single cells were cropped from the WSIs.

2.2   Flowers data set

The F17 Category Flower Data set [8] contains images of 17 different kinds of flowers with 80 images for each class. For our method, we took seven random flower types to match with a corresponding lung fluid cell type. The seven classes are coltsfoot, buttercup, daisy, windflower, daffodil, crocus, and sunflowers, as displayed in the bottom row of Figure 2. The images have large scale, pose and light variations, and there are also classes with significant variations of images within the class and close similarity to other classes [8].

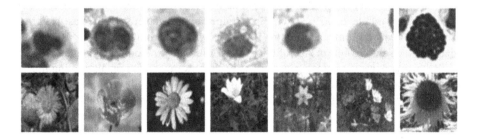

Fig. 2. Pairs of lung fluid cells (top) and flowers (bottom) from left to right: neutrophils and coltsfoot, multinuclear and buttercup, mast cells and daisy, macrophages and windflower, lymphocytes and daffodil, erythrocyte and crocus, eosinophile and sunflowers.

2.3   Image transformation

In order to transform the images to the respective other domain, we decided to use a Generative Adversarial Network (GAN), which includes a generator and a discriminator and use an adversarial loss to learn the mapping such that the translated images are interchangeable with the images in the target domain. One approach is the CycleGAN architecture [6] which is an extension of the GAN architecture and involves simultaneous training of two generator and two discriminator. It captures unique characteristics of one image collection and learns how these characteristics could be transformed into another domain without paired input-output examples. Also, the CycleGAN makes further use of cycle consistency. So, that the output of the first generator propagated through the second generator should create a fake image that matches the original image. The discriminators try to classify whether the image is real or fake. Few disadvantages are information loss and incorrect conversion.

Since we first want to test whether the lung fluid cells can be converted, we trained CycleGANs with cell and flower pairs as shown in Figure 2. The architecture design and implementation for the CycleGAN is based on a publicly available Github repository (available at `https://github.com/junyanz/pytorch-CycleGAN-and-pix2pix`) which used an L1 loss function and Adam optimizer with a learning rate of 0.0002 for both generators and discriminators.

2.4   Experimental design

The first step is to find out if our approach is able to transform images from cells to flowers by using the CycleGAN architecture [6]. For that, we train each model for 200 epochs, with an input resolution of 64×64, and a batch size of 32. Both data sets with seven lung fluid cell types and seven flower types were divided into training (80 %), testing (10 %) and validation (10 %). In order to validate the capability of a successful domain transfer, we used the testing data of the original cell type images and reconstructed cell images to evaluate with a image classification network. The network should recognize the individual cells and should not notice any difference between real and reconstructed cells if the cycle consistency holds true. The image classification network is based on the ResNet18 architecture [9] which is pre-trained on ImageNet from the FastAi library. The model reached convergence after 10 epochs with a learning rate of 3×10^{-3}, batch size of 64, and a resolution size of 64×64. Additionally, random augmentations such as flip, rotation, random erasing and intensity shifts were applied on all training images of the data set. In order to tackle the severe class imbalance, cell types with a frequency below 2,000 were randomly oversampled to include 2,000 samples in the training set.

3   Results

Exemplary qualitative results for the CycleGAN approach are displayed in Figure 3. In the first row, the original domain is displayed, in the second row the reconstructed domain is shown, and in the last row the reconstructed cells are visualised. The individual cells were transformed to the corresponding domain as shown: neutrophils to coltsfoot, multinuclear to buttercup, mast cells to daisy, macrophages to windflower, lymphocytes to daffodil, erythrocyte to crocus, as well as eosinophils to sunflowers. While we see several convincing results for the converted flowers, e.g., for neutrophils (coltsfoot), the visual quality for others, e.g. daisy and crocus, may not be optimal yet (Fig. 3). A possible explanation for this can be a suboptimal ratio of available cell to flower data.

Our classification network – which should differentiate between different cell types – was trained on real cells and tested on a real cell test set and a reconstructed cell test set. The corresponding confusion matrices (CMs) are depicted in Figure 4. When the network is trained and tested on the original cell images it is able to achieve an average accuracy of 94.73 %. While it reaches accuracies of up to 100.0 % for individual classes, the multinuclear cells are often misclassified as macrophages. These cell types are challenging to differentiate for the model, since the only difference really is the number of nuclei. Macrophages have one nuclei and multinucleated cells have multiple. When testing on reconstructed data, the performance stays within the same range indicating that the domain transfer did not lead to a loss of information.

4 Discussion

Our method provides a proof of concept that domain conversion from lung fluid cells to flowers is possible (Fig. 3). This conversion may lower the hurdles of necessary expertise, time, and cost for crowdsourcing annotations. Additionally, a classification network did not find large differences between real or reconstructed images, which is confirmed by the average accuracy of 94.73 % on the real cell test set and an average accuracy of 95.25 % on the reconstructed cell test set. Currently, information about the labels of each cell type is necessary in order to exchange them to flowers. In future work, we would like to address this in an unsupervised or semi-supervised manner. Instead of using the cell type information as input, we could add another discriminator and loss function that takes the cell type as an additional target. Additionally, a better choice of

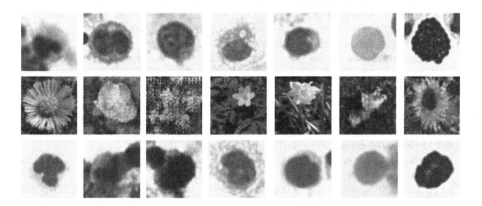

Fig. 3. Results of the domain transformation from real lung fluid cells (first row) to fake flowers (second row) and reconstructed lung fluid cells (third row).

Fig. 4. Confusion matrices for the image classification network trained on the original cell type images and tested on the real cell images (left) and tested on the reconstructed cell images (right).

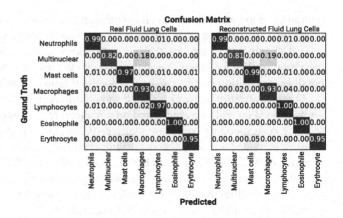

flowers is also essential and we will analyze the gamification potential of other datasets. Specifically, we are interested in finding a suitable target data set that is optimized to allow users the differentiation of the source classes. As the current study focused on the technical feasibility, the development and evaluation of a suitable annotation game is an important next step towards translation.

References

1. Marzahl C, Aubreville M, Bertram C, Gerlach S, Maier J, Voigt J et al. Is crowd-algorithm collaboration an advanced alternative to crowd-sourcing on cytology slides? Bildverarbeitung für die Medizin 2020. 2020:26–31.
2. Marzahl C, Aubreville M, Bertram CA, Maier J, Bergler C, Kröger C et al. EXACT: a collaboration toolset for algorithm-aided annotation of images with annotation version control. Sci Rep. 2021;11(1):1–11.
3. Marzahl C, Bertram CA, Wilm F, voigt J, Bartom AK, Klopfleisch R et al. Learning to be EXACT, cell detection for asthma on partially annotated whole slide images. 2021.
4. Khakpour A, Colomo-Palacios R. Convergence of gamification and machine learning: a systematic literature review. Technology, Knowledge and Learning. 2021;26.
5. Servadei L, Schmidt R, Eidelloth C, Maier A. Medical monkeys: a crowdsourcing approach to medical big data. On the Move to Meaningful Internet Systems. OTM 2017 Workshops. Springer. 2017:87–97.
6. Zhu JY, Park T, Isola P, Efros AA. Unpaired image-to-image translation using cycle-consistent adversarial networks. arXiv. 2020.
7. Bousmalis K, Silberman N, Dohan D, Erhan D, Krishnan D. Unsupervised pixel-level domain adaptation with generative adversarial networks. Proceedings of the IEEE Conference on Computer Vision and Pattern Recognition (CVPR). 2017.
8. Nilsback ME, Zissermann A. 17 category flower dataset. URL: https://www.robots.ox.ac.uk/~vgg/data/flowers/17/. (accessed: 26.10.2021).
9. He K, Zhang X, Ren S, Sun J. Deep residual learning for image recognition. 2016 IEEE Conference on Computer Vision and Pattern Recognition (CVPR). 2016:770–8.

Computation of Traveled Distance of Pigs in an Open Field with Fully Convolutional Neural Networks

Marcin Kopaczka[1], Lisa Ernst[2], Mareike Schulz[2], René Tolba[2], Dorit Merhof[1]

[1]Institute of Imaging and Computer Vision, RWTH Aachen University
[2]Institute of Laboratory Animal Science, University Clinic Aachen
marcin.kopaczka@lfb.rwth-aachen.de

Abstract. The proceedings of the workshops *Bildverarbeitung für die Medizin* are published in a unified form electronically and as bound proceedings. LATEX serves as the base for both types of publication. The template of this PDF can be used as a template, all files can be obtained from the pages of the workshop. In order to be able to guarantee a unified appearance and a smooth process, we ask you to comply with the specifications described here. If necessary, submission in MS Word format is possible, however, and extra fee is charged for this.

1   Introduction and previous work

The open field test is a common part of laboratory animal experiments. Since its introduction in the 1930s [1], it has gained wildespread use in psychological and pharmacological studies [2, 3] for representative overviews. Due to the relevance of the test and the usually controlled experimental conditions which allow highly consistent image data, numerous commercial and academic solutions for automated analysis of animal movement patterns in the open field have been proposed. Notable examples include [4, 5] as non-commercial academic approaches and [6] as a widely adapted commercial solution. While the test has been originally proposed for rodents and most OF tests are performed with rats or mice, it has been successfully adapted to large-animal studies as well. However, most of the automated analysis methods are specialized at analyzing the behavior of rodents and therefore the image processing algorithms are not always applicable to other animals. This can be attributed to several factors: First, mice and rats are the most commonly used species in animal experiments with 65.3% of all experimental animals used in Germany in 2019 being mice and 8.92% being rats, while pigs which are in focus of this work account only for 0.87% of experiments [7], therefore explaining the demand for automation methods in rodent experiments. Furthermore, an open field experiment for large animals is demanding in terms of personnel, time and space and is therefore less common than in rodent studies. Finally, the experimental conditions and open field parameters are more difficult to standardize when working on a large animal experiment, therefore imposing a further challenge for automated analysis systems.

In this paper, we address the automated tracking of pigs in an open field experiment. The open field for pigs is not as commonly used as for rodents and far less standardized, with both field dimensions as well as analyzed parameters varying strongly between individual publications [8]. So far, only a limited number of publications have therefore addressed tracking of pigs. In [9], the authors applied threshold-based animal segmentation and static background subtraction to enable localization of a pig in an open field. While computationally inexpensive and methodologically well-established, background subtraction methods like the one presented in the paper are known to suffer from performance loss in recordings with poor contrast or non-static backgrounds. In the more recent work presented in [10], data of a pen with multiple pigs was acquired using a 3D depth camera and subsequently fed into a pipeline that applied the hungarian algorithm to perform frame-to-frame tracking of individually detected point clouds corresponding to each animal. While the method was capable of multi-animal tracking, it relied on depth cameras instead of regular 2D RGB or grayscale hardware. Next to the technical challenges imposed by 3D imaging, these sensors usually lack the versatility of cameras with interchangeable lenses and offer only a fixed field of view which does not always fit to the layout of the open field setup. Therefore, we aim at developing a method which utilizes current advances in deep learning to allow detection and tracking of an animal using widely available 2D cameras which are commonly used to acquire open field recordings of rodents and therefore are part of standard laboratory equipment in many facilities. In detail, we apply a fully convolutional deep neural network with a multi-task loss to perform learning-based detection and tracking of the animal by regressing keypoint coordinates.

2 Materials and methods

This section will describe both data acquisition and preparation as well as the methods for keypoint detection and tracking.

2.1 Image data and annotations

The training data consisted of a set of videos of a single pig filmed from above in an open field and acquired at a resolution of 1280 x 1024 pixels. For training and validation, a total of 1650 individual frames from 55 videos was selected with 30 frames acquired from

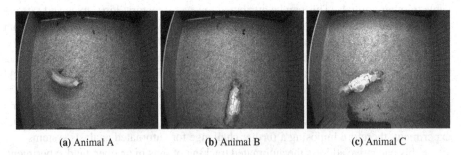

(a) Animal A   (b) Animal B   (c) Animal C

Fig. 1. Sample images with automatically detected keypoints for the three animals in the test set (Sec. 2.1 for the dataset definition).

each video. The individual frames were selected systematically for maximal variance using the k-means frame clustering algorithm provided by [5]. For testing, consecutive frames from 3 full 10-minute videos were extracted at a rate of 1 frame per second, resulting in 1800 test frames. Subsequently, keypoints for the tail base and neck were annotated manually in every selected frame.

2.2 Fully convolutional keypoint detection network

For keypoint detection, we propose a fully convolutional neural network consisting of a feature extraction stage which is implemented using the EfficientNet-B0 architecture [11]. The final fully connected layers were removed to expose the results of the convolutional layers for further processing. To increase the size of the final output, the strided convolutions in the two network were replaced by convolutional layers with a stride of 1. As a result, the output of the feature extraction stage is a 1280-channel 2D signal which is downsampled by a factor of 8 resulting in a 80 x 60 x 1280 volume. This volume is forwarded into a transposed convolution with two output channels to obtain the heatmaps for the keypoints, with one keypoint heatmap predicted per channel.

For keypoint detection, we apply a weighted combination of two loss functions. The heatmap images themselves are created by computing the binary cross entropy between the predictions and ground truth heatmaps which are created by placing two-dimensional Gaussian lobes at the manually annotated keypoint coordinates. Additionally, the keypoint coordinates are directly computed by utilizing a softargmax layer on the heatmaps and subsequently computing the L1-distances between actual and predicted keypoint locations. This additional loss has been shown to improve localization precision in [12]. The final loss is a linear combination of both individual losses where the cross entropy loss is weighted with a factor of 0.01.

2.3 Keypoint processing and tracking

Initial experiments had shown that the detection is robust for most of the cases, however the detections in single individual frames may be inaccurate. As this issue usually affects only individual frames while neighbouring frames have well-placed keypoints, the outliers can be filtered out. Therefore, after obtaining the keypoint coordinates, detection outliers are removed by first picking the median of the predictions from 30 consecutive frames, resulting in a 1 fps localization which is consistent with the annotations made for the test videos. Subsequently, the center point of the animals is obtained by computing the mean between tail and neck coordinates. In a final step, the center coordinates are filtered again with a moving median filter with a window size of 3 to obtain animal centerpoint predictions for every second of the recording. As the most relevant metric for behavioral assessment is given by the total traveled distance over the entire recording, the cumulative distance between all detections in a video is measured and subsequently divided by the length of a meter in pixels to obtain the traveled distance in meters.

Tab. 1. Total traveled distance of the individual animals in the test videos when measured manually and with our method.

	Animal A	Animal B	Animal C
Manual Distance [m]	85.68	56.29	45.57
Our Method [m]	86.53	57.77	45.95
Difference [m]	+0.85 (1.0%)	+1.48 (2.6%)	+0.38 (0.8%)

3   Experiments and results

The training data of 1650 images was split into 1530 images from 51 randomly selected videos for training and 120 frames from the remainiang 4 videos for validation to ensure that the algorithms are trained and validated on different sets of recordings. Training was performed for 100 epochs using the Adam optimizer at a learning rate of 10^{-4}. For image augmentation during training, the images were resized to half size for faster inference, randomly flipped in both directions and subsequently randomly rotated by up to 15°. Additionally, region dropout was applied to further enhance the robustness of the predictor. The validation and test videos were not augmented, only the resize operator was applied to maintain consistent image sizes.

After training, the three manually annotated test videos showing three different animals A, B and C were analyzed with the network and the traveled distance by tracking the detected keypoints was computed as described in Section 2.3 for both manual and predicted coordinates. Sample images are shown in Figure 1. The plots in Figure 2 show the cumulative distance over the video duration for both methods, the total distances are displayed in Table 1. Results show that the distance is measured with a total difference of < 1.5 metres or 2.6%. Additionally, the distance plots acquired using both methods allow analysis of movement patterns such as phases of exploration and rest. Additionally, we display the occupancy heatmaps that show the preferred positions in the open field in Figure 3. It can be seen that both manual and automated analysis return almost identical heatmaps, therefore making both methods equally suitable for occupancy analysis.

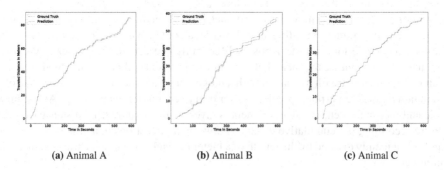

(a) Animal A   (b) Animal B   (c) Animal C

Fig. 2. Manual vs. predicted distances for animals A, B and C.

Fig. 3. Manual vs. predicted coordinates of the three test animals as heatmap to display preferred occupancy in the open field arena.

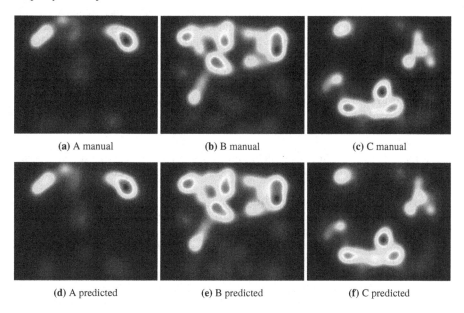

(a) A manual	**(b)** B manual	**(c)** C manual
(d) A predicted	**(e)** B predicted	**(f)** C predicted

4   Discussion

Results indicate that the presented approach allows precise keypoint localization and tracking of pigs in an open field. An analysis of the cumulative traveled distance and occupation heatmaps shows a strong correlation with the human annotator while removing the need for manual annotations in further similar videos. Quantitative analysis shows that the distance computed from the automatically detected keypoints is systematically slightly larger than the manually measured distance. This can be explained by the fact that the automatically detected keypoints may still expose slight jitter even after filtering which in sum leads to a higher total distance.

5   Conclusion and outlook

We present and validate a deep learning-based approach for keypoint tracking of pigs in an open field. Results show strong consistency with human annotations, making the approach feasible for large-scale analysis. In the future, we aim at analyzing additional videos to evaluate its applicability for fast and reliable automated open field tracking in large studies.

Acknowledgement. This research was funded by the German Research Foundation, reference number ME 3737/18-1, TO 542/5-1 and TO 542/5-2.

References

1. Hall C, Ballachey EL. A study of the rat's behavior in a field. A contribution to method in comparative psychology. University of California Publications in Psychology. 1932.
2. Walsh RN, Cummins RA. The open-field test: a critical review. Psychol Bull. 1976;83(3):482.
3. Seibenhener ML, Wooten MC. Use of the open field maze to measure locomotor and anxiety-like behavior in mice. J Vis Exp. 2015;(96):e52434.
4. De Chaumont F, Coura RDS, Serreau P, Cressant A, Chabout J, Granon S et al. Computerized video analysis of social interactions in mice. Nat Methods. 2012;9(4):410–7.
5. Mathis A, Mamidanna P, Cury KM, Abe T, Murthy VN, Mathis MW et al. DeepLabCut: markerless pose estimation of user-defined body parts with deep learning. Nat Neurosci. 2018;21(9):1281–9.
6. Noldus LP, Spink AJ, Tegelenbosch RA. EthoVision: a versatile video tracking system for automation of behavioral experiments. Behav Res Methods Instrum Comput. 2001;33(3):398–414.
7. Verwendung von Versuchstieren. 2019.
8. Schulz M, Kopaczka M, Zieglowski L, Tolba R. The open field test as a tool for behavior analysis in pigs: is a standardization of setup necessary? A systematic review. bioRxiv. 2021.
9. Lind NM, Vinther M, Hemmingsen RP, Hansen AK. Validation of a digital video tracking system for recording pig locomotor behaviour. J Neurosci Methods. 2005;143(2):123–32.
10. Matthews SG, Miller AL, Plötz T, Kyriazakis I. Automated tracking to measure behavioural changes in pigs for health and welfare monitoring. Sci Rep. 2017;7(1):1–12.
11. Tan M, Le Q. Efficientnet: rethinking model scaling for convolutional neural networks. International Conference on Machine Learning. PMLR. 2019:6105–14.
12. Kopaczka M, Jacob T, Ernst L, Schulz M, Tolba R, Merhof D. Robust open field rodent tracking using a fully convolutional network and a Softargmax distance loss. Bildverarbeitung für die Medizin 2020. Springer, 2020:242–7.

Spatiotemporal Attention for Realtime Segmentation of Corrupted Sequential Ultrasound Data
Improving Usability of AI-based Image Guidance

Laura Graf[1], Sven Mischkewitz[2], Lasse Hansen[1], Mattias P. Heinrich[1]

[1]Institut für Medizinische Informatik, Universität zu Lübeck
[2]ThinkSono GmbH, Potsdam
l.graf@uni-luebeck.de

Abstract. Image-guided diagnostics with AI assistance, e.g. compression-ultrasound for detecting deep vein thrombosis, requires stable, robust and real-time capable analysis algorithms that best support the user. When using anatomical segmentations for user guidance the spatiotemporal consistency is of great importance, but point-of-care modalities deliver signal which in many frames is hard to interpret. Since 2D+t models with 3D CNNs are not applicable for many mobile end devices, we propose a new spatiotemporal attention approach that re-uses deep backbone features from previous frames to learn and optimally fuse all available image information. Proof-of-concept experiments demonstrate an improvement of over 8% for the segmentation compared to simpler 2D+t models (using several frames as multi-channel input).

1 Introduction

Many clinical diagnostic pathways involve an ultrasound examination performed by expert medical staff, such as the duplex compression ultrasound for assessing deep-vein thrombosis. Machine learning (ML) based image processing promises to assist users without the years of training necessary for dealing with the anatomic structures in the noisy data with shadows and artifacts obfuscating the view. Ultrasound devices are affordable and available outside of hospitals and in remote areas. The modality is fast to apply, non-invasive and does not bear risks of radiation and can together with ML yield improvements for everyone in the health care system. However, regardless of the promise, major hurdles remain for the wide spread use of automated analysis. When considering the assistance in ultrasound diagnosis, the partly bad image quality in a scan has to be handled. It is an open question how to apply deep learning models which are developed for direct use on expensive, large GPUs and return results with seconds delay to real time ultra sound devices with 40-60 frames per second (fps). At the point of care powerful GPUs are not necessarily available, so there is a demand for models which work for mobile computing devices. Furthermore, 3D image processing methods temporally lag behind the models applicable for 2D data. Ultrasound is a modality where due to varying image quality processing of temporal context from neighboring frames is important. At the current time mobile end-devices usually do not support 3D convolutions natively, so there is a need for alternatives not relying on these.

For practical application enhancing the scanned image data with semantic guidance or providing localization to find standard views is very helpful. This poses the challenge for the algorithm to run in real time and to not be reliant on frames subsequent to the current time frame in order to guide the user. Segmentation of anatomical structures can provide an intuitive understanding of the view and beside the quantitative information about the relevant structures utilizable in many clinical scenarios also delivers the input for further processing steps. The segmentation of the different vessels in the tissue in ultrasound sequences is complex, due to dynamic and anatomic variation of the structures. The need for a fast and memory efficient segmentation for 3D data is not met by current models, where often the input gets downsized [1], resulting in information loss, especially in the case of medical application where fine structures are often more important compared to common vision video processing. On the other hand, the fast single frame, 2D models do not consider the temporal context and thus fail to address the variations in image quality, such as shadows introduced by bone structures, lack of gel or movement of the probe. In previous works, different hybrids of 2D/3D processing have been proposed, such as in one paper [2] where the authors segment organs in CT scans applying bidirectional Convolutional Long Short-Term Memory in an architecture varying the popular U-Net to include spatial inter-slice correlations instead of a merging of final 2D net outputs. Different from our concept, they assume the availability of data from after the current time point. In very recent computer vision work, Sparse Spatiotemporal Transformers [3] use sparse attention over spatiotemporal features for video object segmentation, reporting improved robustness and scalability to high resolution media input. Transformers do not incorporate the innate structure of the videos and have to learn arrangements from tokens, often needing more training data.

Our main contribution is to perform segmentation of ultrasound sequences in a resource efficient way that leverages context of the current and previous frames but also does not decrease resolution and thereby spatial information. An attention module is applied to learn to estimate the reliability and importance of image frames that may not clearly show the anatomic structures. We compute the attention vectors from deep features of a 2D network and apply them on the 2D network features of higher spatial resolution. Afterwards the feature maps are fused and passed to the classification head. The method improves the baseline by over 8% by applying temporal features in the latent space instead of directly using multiple frames as input channels, it enables an application in the ultrasound guidance scenario. The developed modules run with 10.65GMACs, which is suitable for the real time segmentation for the frame rate of an ultrasound device.

2 Materials and methods

2.1 Data

We evaluated the performance on ultrasound data acquired by performing a compression ultrasound exam to assess deep vein-thrombosis. The probe head was moved along the patient's leg following the vein while applying pressure to check for a blood clot. This is an actual case of where the guidance and automatic segmentation can support especially non-expert users at a point-of-care facility, due to the difficulty of making out the right vessels in the noisy ultrasound video. It can guide the user to know which way to move the device. Here it is of utmost importance for the user interaction to be mindful of how good support can actually be provided for a person interacting with the software. Non-cohesive segmentation of structures, as it is output by a network not taking into account the temporal context, could mean a hindrance more than an improvement for the procedure.

Predating work has shown promising results for automatic interpretation and guidance for free-hand ultrasound of the veins for deep vein thrombosis diagnosis for scanning patients without specialist attendance [4].

Reference labels are given by expert annotations for all the frames. We complicate the task by flipping every third frame (altering flips in x and/or y dimension), so it does not contain the right information compared to the reference, to show the effect of the attention module.

2.2   Method

Our network builds upon a small MobileNetV3 [5], which is optimized for the use with memory and runtime restrictions of backbone for mobile device inference and comprises a lite reduced atrous spatial pyramid pooling (LR-ASPP) for performing very efficient semantic segmentation with state-of-the-art results [5]. The full configuration is shown in Figure 1. The 2D backbone network's feature maps only have to be calculated for the current input frame and we can re-use the maps from the $n - 1$ preceding frames. The features of these n frames are then fed into the spatio-temporal Attention/Fusion module. The attention part uses deep features (with low spatial resolution and strong semantic information) as input and consists of 2D (spatial) and 1D (temporal) convolutions to leverage temporal context without requiring 3D CNNs. It outputs a weighting map, similar to Attention-gated U-Nets [6], for each frame and is concatenated to both lower and higher level features as input for the fusion module. Here, the combined spatio-temporal information and estimated weights, that represent the confidence in each frame, are fused. The outputs are 2D feature-maps of equal size as the original MobileNetV3 backbone, which are then directly fed into the LR-ASPP classifier for the final segmentation prediction. The computational complexity of the Attention/Fusion module is nearly ten times lower than that of the backbone leading to negligible overhead at inference time. By restricting ourselves to 2D and 1D convolutions we can directly enable an implementation that runs on mobile end-devices, which usually do not support 3D convolutions natively.

By applying the attention module on the features extracted from a 2D network only, the whole process is efficient for full resolution image frames and does not rely on the availability of all frames at the time of processing. It also requires much less memory space than alternative 2D+t approaches.

We compare our method to the naive approach of segmenting the frames with a 2D network as well as a 2D network trained on the frames of n time points like our network but treating the frames as multi-channel input of the MobileNet and not explicitly calculating attention.

For the training of the 2D model we did not flip any frames. We train the networks using a cross entropy loss. For better efficiency we used mixed precision for all parameters. We did not include gradients for the backbone feature calculations of the previous frames and only backpropagate to the features of the current frame.

3   Results

We analysed 175 compression ultrasound sequences with lengths between 50 and 128 frames for a baseline 2D network, a standard 2D+t network and our proposed spatio-temporal attention method. Dice's coefficients for the 2D network are very small for the frames of the input sequence which are flipped and largest for our network with Attention/Fusion Module with an advantage of four percentage points over the 2D+t network that convolves over the n, here reported for $n = 5$ frames directly. For the whole image with every third frame flipped, the Dice's coefficients result to 64.9% and 59.1% for the vein and artery labels respectively for the 2d+t network, 52.9% and 54.6% for the simple 2D approach and outperforming both other approaches, 68.1% and 64.0% for our network (Tab. 1). When incorporating only three other frames in the decision of a frame, the results worsen by 3% while those of the multichannel network worsen by 10%, performing very badly on corrupted frames.

We also reviewed qualitative results, and found that the baseline networks – without a deeper spatio-temporal processing – frequently confused labels of vein and artery across frames. One representative example can be seen in Figure 2.

As for efficiency, the attention/fusion part and classifier run in under 1ms. The network has a total parameter count of 6,489,222. The attention/fusion addition to the MobileNet needs 10.65GMACs, resulting in a segmentation speed topping that of modern ultrasound device frame rates.

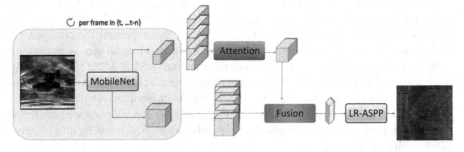

Fig. 1. Overview of our network -First, the small MobileNet backbone extracts features on the single frame. The deeper features of the n frames get passed through an attention module to obtain attention features for the sequence. These are used on the backbone features of higher spatial resolution calculated for each of the n frames to then pass the fused vector into a lightweight classification head.

Tab. 1. Our method performs better, on corrupted as well as not corrupted frames, than MobileNet on the single frames and a network that takes multiple frames as image channels as input. The table reports a mean of Dice's coefficients for corrupted frames as well as those for all frames-for vein labels and the harder to trace artery labels respectively, as well as the standard deviation among different whole videos. Our approach shows consistent advantage across all labels.

Method	Dice on corrupted frames	Vein	Artery	Std.
2D Network	15.2%	51.9%	49.6%	14.3%
2D+t (multichannel input)	61.4%	64.9%	59.1%	15.5%
Ours	64.5%	68.1%	64.0%	14.2%

4   Discussion

The results show that a 2D segmentation network alone performs insufficiently well on highly dynamic compression ultrasound sequences (in particular when considering distortions), due to the noise that makes many of the single frames hard to define. By including multiple frames as multi-channel input this can be substantially improved but it is not an optimal solution for sequences of varying image quality. Our method which incorporates an additional attention/fusion module improves the result by 8%, since attention helps the network to recognize the context and reliability of each of the n frames. Visual inspection of the results confirmed that label switch-ups can be avoided by considering temporal relations and more accurate label predictions are possible when fusing (pre-computed) features of the other frames if the frame is distorted. Precision for the label of a non flipped frame also exceeds that of a sole 2D model, which might be

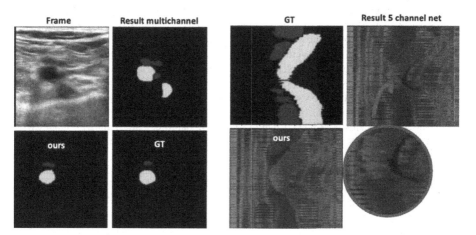

Fig. 2. Visual results of the obtained segmentations shown for a selected B-mode scan and (right grid) as spatial+temporal slice through all time points. Our result shows substantially better agreement with the reference labels ("GT") and in particular avoids mix-up among the labels (vein and artery) along the sequence and therefore improves usability.

partially due to a regularizing effect of the fusion in the heavily reduced feature space, because the (temporal) shape space is additionally regulated.

Our contribution that combines a 2D feature extractor and attention weighting for the fusion of features from multiple frames can pave new ways of making ultrasound examination guidance applicable on resource limited devices; a use case that requires real time processing of the most recent frame. Our method can handle the potentially varying image quality in the recording without resource intensive 3D convolutions. The inference speed allows processing at the high frame rate required for ultrasound exams.

We plan to extend the proof-of-concept experiments to gain insight into where precisely the fusion in the feature space helps, how much temporal context is useful for certain data and how multi-scale models compare.

In the future we will explore further design optimisations and evaluation metrics to enhance the spatio-temporal segmentation of ultrasound used in cooperative human-AI systems with demanding realtime requirements. We will also assess which type of ML output can best aid the user for the exam in terms of trustworthiness and simple-to-use technology.

Acknowledgement. I want to thank the people working for ThinkSono for supplying the ultrasound footage used for these experiments and for the insights into their project for support of diagnosis of deep vein thrombosis.

References

1. Wang W, Zhou T, Porikli F, Crandall D, Van Gool L. A survey on deep learning technique for video segmentation. preprint arXiv:2107.01153. 2021.
2. Novikov AA, Major D, Wimmer M, Lenis D, Bühler K. Deep sequential segmentation of organs in volumetric medical scans. IEEE T-MI. 2018;38(5):1207–15.
3. Duke B, Ahmed A, Wolf C, Aarabi P, Taylor GW. Sstvos: sparse spatiotemporal transformers for video object segmentation. IEEE/CVF CVPR. 2021:5912–21.
4. Kainz B, Heinrich MP, Makropoulos A, Oppenheimer J, Mandegaran R, Sankar S et al. Non-invasive diagnosis of deep vein thrombosis from ultrasound imaging with machine learning. NPJ Digit Med. 2021;4(1):1–18.
5. Howard A, Sandler M, Chu G, Chen LC, Chen B, Tan M et al. Searching for mobilenetv3. ICCV. 2019:1314–24.
6. Schlemper J, Oktay O, Schaap M, Heinrich M, Kainz B, Glocker B et al. Attention gated networks: learning to leverage salient regions in medical images. Med Image Anal. 2019;53.

Virtual DSA Visualization of Simulated Blood Flow Data in Cerebral Aneurysms

Rebecca Preßler[1], Kai Lawonn[1], Bernhard Preim[2], Monique Meuschke[2]

[1]Institute of Computer Science, University of Jena, Germany
[2]Department of Simulation and Graphics, University of Magdeburg, Germany
rebecca.debora.pressler@uni-jena.de

Abstract. Cerebral aneurysms represent an essential problem in neuroradiology. In clinical practice, they are frequently diagnosed and treated based on digital subtraction angiography (DSA) which provides an impression of the blood flow dynamics. In contrast, computational hemodynamics enables precise quantification of flow-related properties based on a patient-specific 3D anatomy extracted from CT or MRI. To support the qualitative interpretation of simulated flow data, we imitate the appearance of DSA data from simulated flow data. This research is motivated by shortcomings of previous visualization techniques which may overwhelm physicians and are not familiar to them. The virtual DSA representations can be generated without manual parameter adaption by the user. We applied our method to different cerebral aneurysm data sets and performed a qualitative evaluation compared to real DSA images together with two radiologists.

1 Introduction

Cerebral Aneurysms are local dilatations of the arteries in the brain. The rupture of the vessel wall has fatal consequences for the patient. Therefore, it is important to investigate the aneurysm and to decide about appropriate treatment. The location, size and morphology as well as the blood flow provide information about the risk of rupture and treatment success. In clinical routine, digital subtraction angiography (DSA) images are frequently used to assess aneurysm rupture risk and to plan treatment. Since a catheter with a contrast agent must be inserted and moved in the target anatomy, DSA is an invasive procedure which carries risks for the patient. The color intensity of DSA images is caused by the attenuation of x-rays, depending on the amount of contrast agent in a vessel, which ultimately represents the strength of the volume flow. Since computing power has significantly improved in the last decades, blood flow can be simulated with increasing spatial and temporal resolution and thus increasing accuracy. Several works aims at performing patient-specific blood flow simulations often by means of computational fluid dynamics (CFD) [1]. Ford et al. [2] showed that patient-specific CFD blood flow simulations are well validated and coincide strongly with measured in vivo hemodynamics. There are numerous possibilities to visualize simulated blood flow where many works used cerebral aneurysms as use case. Different techniques were

© Der/die Autor(en), exklusiv lizenziert durch
Springer Fachmedien Wiesbaden GmbH, ein Teil von Springer Nature 2022
K. Maier-Hein et al. (Hrsg.), *Bildverarbeitung für die Medizin 2022*,
Informatik aktuell, https://doi.org/10.1007/978-3-658-36932-3_51

developed to visualize the 3D extracted vessel representation as context information, where other techniques are used to visually analyze simulated vector fields, representing the internal blood flow. Usually integral lines are used in the form of streamlines or path lines to represent the qualitative blood flow behavior. A path line describes the trajectory of a flow particle over time, starting from a seed point. Additionally to the spatial and temporal information of a line, another attribute such as velocity can be color-coded [3]. More advanced techniques aim to extract qualitative flow patterns, such as vortices or inflow jets, that appear to be related to aneurysm progression and rupture [4]. For this purpose, usually partition-based methods are employed that decompose the vector field into areas of similar flow according to a predefined degree of similarity. To visualize the extracted flow patterns in relation to morphological features, interactive focus-context approaches [5–7] are often used. They provide the user with numerous options to visually explore the data. A comprehensive overview about the visual exploration of medical flow data can be found in [4]. However, physicians are not very familiar with such complex scientific visualizations. The use of existing methods for exploration of simulated data require a high training time, which is not available in clinical routine. Therefore, we propose a method to generate virtual DSA representations from simulated blood flow data. Thus, familiar blood flow visualizations can be created without the invasive nature of real DSA. As input, integral lines are used. Different areas of darkness are created by blurring and blending these lines. We present how the virtual DSA representation is generated and which parameters influence the visualization, as well as the clinical application possibilities.

2   Materials and methods

In this section, we describe the generation of the virtual DSA representation. Therefore, we provide an overview about the general concept first and explain details about the implementation and rendering afterwards.

2.1   Data acquisition

For blood flow simulation, we first extract a 3D vessel surface from clinical CTA images. For this purpose, we follow the suggested pipeline by Mönch et al. [8]. The aneurysm and its parent vessel are separated from the surrounding tissue using a threshold-based segmentation. The 3D vessel surface is extracted via Marching Cubes, applied to the segmented image data. To prepare a geometric model as input for the flow simulation, it is necessary to manually correct artifacts and to optimize the mesh quality. Then, the 3D vessel surface is transformed to an unstructured volumetric grid as input for the simulation. Patient-specific hemodynamics are calculated numerically using CFD, solving the Navier-Stokes equation [9]. Details of the CFD simulation are presented in [10]. As a result, we receive data with a high temporal resolution comprising 93 time steps ($\Delta t = 0.01$ s). Finally, path lines have been seeded on the centers of the ostium triangles (the surface that separates the aneurysm from the healthy vessel) resulting in a homogeneously distributed number of vertices.

2.2 General concept of virtual DSA

The virtual DSA representation is generated based on blood flow-representing path lines. Each path line point, in addition to its 3D position, has a temporal component representing the integration time during the cardiac cycle. The generation of the DSA representation is performed in two render passes. In the first pass, the path lines are drawn as dotted lines and the rendering result is saved in a texture. In the second pass, this texture is blurred by a convolution kernel to create the typical coloring of DSA images. We experiment with three different kernel sizes: 3×3, 5×5 and 7×7 as well as two blurring methods: the Gaussian and the average filter. The idea is to change the line-based appearance of the blood flow into a more fluid-like shape. To reach this, the size of the path line dots are increased to get thicker lines with small gaps between the single dots. The filtering then creates a more soften look.

2.3 Implementation

Our virtual DSA representation is developed in JavaScript and WebGL and embedded in HTML. We choose these languages to provide an easy access to the tool over the internet. Furthermore, we use the dat.gui to create a simple user interface, and glMatrix libraries to extend the default functionality of JavaScript. After the vessel surface and the path lines have been loaded, their 3D vertex positions as well as further attributes such as the corresponding vertex normals and time values of the path lines are uploaded to the GPU. For this purpose, vertex buffer objects (VBOs) linked to a vertex array object (VAO), are used, where the data can be accessed by the attached shaders. These attributes are accepted by corresponding shader programs and processed further in separate rendering methods, one for rendering the vessel surface and one for rendering the path lines. Together they produced the virtual DSA visualization. In the following paragraphs, we explain details regarding the two rendering methods starting with the vessel surface rendering, followed by the path line rendering.

2.3.1 Vessel surface rendering. Similar to a real DSA rendering, the vessel wall is rendered as a light gray surface on a dark gray background to act as contextual information. In addition, the contour of the vessel is highlighted a bit darker. Since the path lines are animated based on their temporal information, there is no flow at the beginning of the animation. At this point, the user sees a light gray vessel, which serves as orientation during the path line animation. For rendering the vessel surface, a vertex and a fragment shader is needed. The vertex shader reads in the vertex positions as an attribute and calculates the positions of the coordinates. Besides that, it calculates the normal of every face and passes the result to the fragment shader. With this information the fragment shader decides if the fragment belongs to the contour or not. The calculation works with the dot product of the normal and the view direction vector. If the dot product of both is zero the fragment is a part of the contour and should be colored in darker gray otherwise it should be light gray.

2.3.2 Path line rendering. The rendering of the path lines for the virtual DSA is more complex. To create the two render passes we first need a framebuffer and a texture.

In the first render pass, we call a different draw-path-lines function. In comparison to the otherwise called draw function for path lines, the uniforms and attribute buffers were given to another pair of shaders and the rendering context of drawElements is called with gl.POINTS instead of gl.LINE_STRIP. Because of that it is now possible to change the size of the points and thus the thickness of the lines. Moreover, each path line point is assigned an alpha value of 0.01. During the first render pass, we activate additive blending. This blends the black semi-transparent path line points additively for each frame of the animation. Since areas with strong blood flow should appear dark in the final image, the result of the blending is inverted at the end. After the point-based drawing of the path lines, the blending result is saved to the texture, which will be attached to the framebuffer. Now another shader program is loaded and the positions of a screen-filling quad are passed to the vertex shader. On this quad the texture will be displayed. Before the rendered image is shown to the user, the texture image will be blurred in the fragment shader. Regarding the size of the path line points, we used a value of 10. Larger or smaller values, either resulted in large holes in the image or allowed blood flow to leak out of the vessel. Moreover, a 5×5 Gaussian filter works best to imitate the coloring of real DSA images. With smaller or larger kernel sizes, the resulting visualizations look either very blocky or too washed out.

3 Results

We generated virtual DSA images for five data sets, where the results were evaluated with two radiologists (16 and 18 years of work experience) by conducting informal interviews. The radiologists are familiar with the diagnosis of cerebral aneurysms based on real DSA images. They should assess if the virtual DSA images support the risk assessment and treatment planning of cerebral aneurysms. Figure 1 shows five virtual DSA images (a-e) of an aneurysm data set, generated for five time steps within the cardiac cycle compared to a real DSA image (f). The radiologists emphasized that the virtual DSA images looked very similar to real DSA images, so the physicians felt immediately familiar with the virtual images and did not need extensive explanations to interpret the visualizations. A key advantage of virtual DSA images over real images, they say, is that the virtual images allow analysis of blood flow through the cardiac cycle without exposing the patient to further radiation, as would be necessary in real images. Occurring flow patterns, such as vortices and inflow jets can be analyzed which helps to assess the rupture risk and to decide about an optimal treatment. Moreover, the context visualization of the vessel wall in the virtual images supports the assessment of morphological aspects such as the aneurysm shape, which is also an important point regarding risk analysis and treatment planning.

4 Discussion

Both radiologists concluded that the virtual DSA images where the blood flow is animated during the cardiac cycle, are easy to interpret regarding morphological and hemodynamic aspects and, therefore, support aneurysm analysis. Moreover the virtual DSA images are very suited to document patient data as well as to educate students regarding DSA examinations. To further improve treatment planning, they would like to have a virtual integration of different treatment options such as stents, clips or coils in the future. The treatment options would have to be considered in the simulation and could then be explored comparatively in the form of the virtual DSA representation. For medical research related to a better understanding of rupture causes, such as forces acting on the vessel wall, e.g., wall shear stress or pressure, more complex visualizations are better suited. However, physicians dealing with aneurysms in clinical routine need familiar and easy to understand visualizations, such as virtual DSA images, to improve diagnosis and treatment.

4.1 Limitations

Due to necessary assumptions regarding the flow and boundary conditions for the CFD simulations, it cannot be guaranteed that the simulation results accurately reflect patient-specific conditions. Therefore, visual differences between real and virtual DSA images are possible. In addition, the virtual DSA is influenced by the seeding strategy of the path lines. More seeding points and other integration methods can lead to changes in the DSA representation. Finally, real-time imaging during interventions is not possible with the virtual DSA visualization, but instead it can be used for planning interventions.

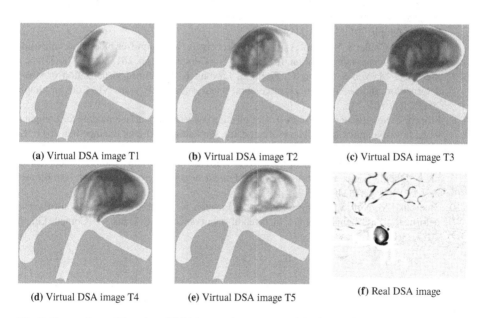

(a) Virtual DSA image T1 (b) Virtual DSA image T2 (c) Virtual DSA image T3

(d) Virtual DSA image T4 (e) Virtual DSA image T5 (f) Real DSA image

Fig. 1. Comparison of five virtual DSA images (a-e) generated for five cardiac time steps (T1-T5) to a real DSA image (f). While the real DSA image just shows a strong contrast agent accumulation in the aneurysm, the virtual images show occurring flow patterns, such as vortices, in the aneurysm.

4.2 Future work

In the future, it would be conceivable to allow the user to manipulate the blurring parameters like point size or blurring method. Another important point for future research is an extensive evaluation of our method with physicians to assess the suitability in clinical routine based on a large number of aneurysm data sets.

References

1. Berg P, Stucht D, Janiga G, Beuing O, Speck O, Thévenin D. Cerebral blood flow in a healthy circle of willis and two intracranial aneurysms: computational fluid dynamics versus four-dimensional phase-contrast magnetic resonance imaging. J Biomech Eng. 2014;136(4).
2. Ford M, Stuhne G, Nikolov H, Habets D, Lownie S, Holdsworth D et al. Virtual angiography for visualization and validation of computational models of aneurysm hemodynamics. IEEE Trans Med Imaging. 2005;24(12):1586–92.
3. Preim B, Botha C. Visual computing for medicine: theory, algorithms, and applications. The Morgan Kaufmann Series in Computer Graphics, 2013:666–74.
4. Oeltze-Jafra S, Meuschke M, Neugebauer M, Saalfeld S, Lawonn K, Janiga G et al. Generation and visual exploration of medical flow data: survey, research trends and future challenges. Comput Graph Forum. 2019;38 (1):87–125.
5. Gasteiger R, Neugebauer M, Beuing O, Preim B. The FLOWLENS: a focus-and-context visualization approach for exploration of blood flow in cerebral aneurysms. IEEE Trans Vis Comput Graph. 2011;17(12):2183–92.
6. Lawonn K, Glaßer S, Vilanova A, Preim B, Isenberg T. Occlusion-free blood flow animation with wall thickness visualization. IEEE Trans Vis Comput Graph. 2015;22(1):728–37.
7. Meuschke M, Voß S, Beuing O, Preim B, Lawonn K. Combined visualization of vessel deformation and hemodynamics in cerebral aneurysms. IEEE Trans Vis Comput Graph. 2017;23(1):761–70.
8. Mönch T, Neugebauer M, Preim B. Optimization of vascular surface models for computational fluid dynamics and rapid prototyping. Int. Workshop on Digital Engineering. 2011:16–23.
9. Sanchez M, Ambard D, Costalat V, Mendez S, Jourdan F, Nicoud F. Biomechanical assessment of the individual risk of rupture of cerebral aneurysms: a proof of concept. Ann Biomed Eng. 2013;41(1):28–40.
10. Meuschke M, Voß S, Beuing O, Preim B, Lawonn K. Combined visualization of vessel deformation and hemodynamics in cerebral aneurysms. IEEE Trans Vis Comput Graph. 2017;23(1):761–70.

Reconstruction of 1D Images with a Neural Network for Magnetic Particle Imaging

Anselm von Gladiss[1], Raphael Memmesheimer[1], Nick Theisen[1],
Anna C. Bakenecker[2], Thorsten M. Buzug[2,3], Dietrich Paulus[1]

[1]Institute for Computational Visualistics, University of Koblenz-Landau
[2]Fraunhofer Research Institution for Individualized and Cell-Based Medical Engineering IMTE,
Lübeck
[3]Institute of Medical Engineering, University of Lübeck
vongladiss@uni-koblenz.de

Abstract. Image reconstruction in Magnetic Particle Imaging is mainly performed by using a system matrix or by mapping the time signal into spatial domain and deconvolving the tracer properties. In this work, a neural network is designed and trained for reconstructing 1D images. Test data are reconstructed using both the neural network and a conventional approach. Background artefacts that appear during conventional reconstruction are not visible when reconstructing with the neural network. The images that have been reconstructed using the neural network are superior in terms of quantifiability and spatial resolution in comparison to conventionally reconstructed images.

1 Introduction

Magnetic particle imaging (MPI) visualises the spatial and temporal distribution of superparamagnetic iron oxid nanoparticles, which serve as tracer material [1]. MPI has been developed as a medical imaging modality and is established pre-clinically. Potential clinical applications are being investigated.

An oscillating magnetic field excites the tracer material whose non-linear change in magnetisation can be measured with a receive coil as a voltage signal. Superposing a magnetic gradient field generates a dynamic low-field-area and enables spatial encoding.

The measured voltage signal can be reconstructed into an image showing the spatial distribution of tracer material using a system-matrix-based approach or using x-space reconstruction. For the system-matrix-based approach the field of view (FOV) is discretised into voxels. A sample of the tracer material is shifted to each voxel sequentially and a full measurement is carried out. These calibration measurements are stored in a coefficient matrix (system matrix) for solving a linear system of equations. The spatial distribution of tracer material is then given as the solution vector. Usually, the voltage signals are translated into Fourier domain before reconstruction. As the system matrix is ill-conditioned, the solution has to be regularised [2], which reduces the dynamic range in the reconstructed images. Then, areas featuring a high concentration of tracer material may overframe image areas featuring a low concentration [3].

Using x-space-reconstruction, the parameters of both the magnetic gradient field and excitation field have to be known precisely, as the time-dependent voltage signal is mapped into image domain with respect to the magnetic low-field area. Hence, assumptions regarding inhomogeneities of the magnetic fields and the parameters of the tracer material have to be made. Especially for multi-dimensional excitation, modelling the change in magnetisation of the tracer material is insufficient [4]. Therefore, x-space-reconstruction is limited to the reconstruction of one-dimensional images.

Another approach to image reconstruction in MPI uses neural networks. Simulated 2D data have been reconstructed using a neural network and three frequency components [5] and using a convolutional neural network [6, 7]. A deep image prior has been used to reconstruct measured 3D data [8]. In this case the architecture of an untrained neural network is used for regularising the reconstruction step.

In this work, a convolutional neural network is designed for reconstructing hybrid 1D data measured in a magnetic particle spectrometer (MPS). A measured system matrix is augmented and used for training and validating the neural network. Then, the neural network is tested using the single measurements out of a second measured system matrix.

2   Materials and methods

First, the used dataset is presented. Then, both the architecture and training of the neural network are described. For comparison, the data are reconstructed using both the neural network and a conventional approach.

2.1   Dataset

Hybrid data have been measured in an MPS featuring multi-dimensional excitation [9]. However, only a one-dimensional excitation field has been used. Formerly, the data have been used in [10] for investigating the spatial resolution in MPI.

First, a system matrix of 97 emulated positions has been acquired using an excitation field amplitude of 12 mT and a magnetic offset field in the range of $[-12\,\text{mT}, 12\,\text{mT}]$. Then, a second system matrix has been acquired featuring a finer grid of 241 emulated positions within the same offset field range. A band-pass filter has been applied in Fourier domain between the 3rd and 19th harmonic.

As the system matrices consist of single measurements, they can be used directly for training and validating a neural network. The first system matrix is used for training and validating the neural network, whereas the second is used for testing it.

2.2   Neural network

The neural network consists of two dense layers and three convolutional layers (Fig. 1) and has been created with the Keras-API of TensorFlow 2. Exponential linear units (elu) have been used in the network except for the last convolutional layer where a rectified linear unit (relu) has been chosen for preventing negative intensity values in the reconstructed images.

The network has been trained in time domain using the hybrid system matrix featuring 97 emulated positions. The ground truth for the single measurements within the system matrix is given by a 1D image of 97 pixels containing zero-value-entries except for the measurement position, where the value 1 is stored. The system matrix has been augmented by scaling the single emulated positions and by providing linear combinations of the positions resulting in 7,857 positions. 20 % of the data have been chosen randomly for validating the training. As loss function the mean squared error was chosen.

2.3   Conventional reconstruction

In order to compare the reconstruction results achieved with the neural network, the data have been reconstructed using a conventional approach as well. The second system matrix has been used as 241 single-point measurements and has been reconstructed using the first system matrix in frequency domain. Frequency components between the 3rd and 19th harmonic have been selected for reconstruction. A regularised Kaczmarz-algorithm with 50 iterations and a regularisation factor of 10^{-4} have been used.

3   Results

The results of training the neural network are presented. Using the trained neural network, the test data set has been reconstructed. The results of the reconstruction step are compared to the results achieved using a conventional approach and to the ground truth data.

3.1   Neural network training

The neural network featuring the architecture shown in Figure 1 has been trained using an Adam-optimiser with a learning rate of 10^{-3} for 250 epochs. The random seeds have been initialised with a fixed value for a deterministic training. The model generalised well to the validation data. This is shown by the accuracies of 91 % and 90 % that have been achieved for the training and validation data, respectively (Fig. 2). The loss function showed values of 0.02 and 0.03.

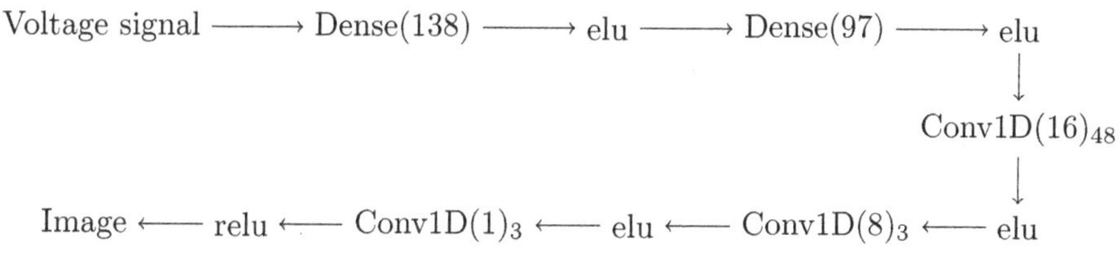

Voltage signal $\longrightarrow$ Dense(138) $\longrightarrow$ elu $\longrightarrow$ Dense(97) $\longrightarrow$ elu
$$\downarrow$$
$$\text{Conv1D}(16)_{48}$$
$$\downarrow$$
Image $\longleftarrow$ relu $\longleftarrow$ Conv1D$(1)_3$ $\longleftarrow$ elu $\longleftarrow$ Conv1D$(8)_3$ $\longleftarrow$ elu

Fig. 1. Architecture of the neural network. The voltage signal is fed to two dense layers and three convolutional layers. The parameters of the convolutional layers indicate the number of filters and the kernel size (subscripted).

3.2 Reconstruction results

The reconstruction results using the trained neural network and the conventional approach are visualised in Figure 3. The 2D images show the single reconstructed 1D images, which have been stacked row-wise.

Background artefacts cannot be seen in the neural network reconstruction results (Fig. 3 centre column). The positions of the single points are reconstructed distinctly. In comparison, the reconstruction results using the system-matrix-based approach (right column) show strong background artefacts and the positions of the single points are blurred.

However, the position of the single points reconstructed with the neural network does not match precisely the ground truth position. The deviation from the expected position increases for positions near to the centre and near to the borders of the 1D images. The system-matrix-based reconstruction results show artefacts near the central and outer positions as well in terms of increased blurriness.

Using a common scaling of the displayed grey values (Fig. 3 bottom row), the differences in reconstructed intensity values become visible. While the images reconstructed with the neural network approximately fit the intensity value range of the ground truth data, the reconstructed intensity values are smaller using the system-matrix-based approach.

4 Discussion

Hybrid 1D measurement data consisting of single point measurements at different positions have been reconstructed successfully using a neural network. The reconstructed images show no background artefacts and the single points are sharply delineated. The range of reconstructed intensity values is similar to the one given by the ground truth data, which indicates a high quantifiability of the reconstruction results achieved

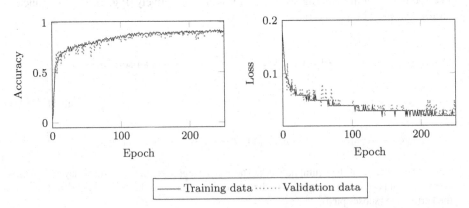

Fig. 2. Accuracy (left) and loss (right) of the neural network after each epoch of training. After 250 epochs, accuracies of more than 90 % have been reached for both the training and validation data.

with the neural network. Hence, the reconstruction results obtained with the neural network are superior to the conventional system-matrix-based approach when applying the reconstruction parameters chosen in this work.

However, the positions of the reconstructed single points do not match the positions given by the ground truth data. It has to be noted though, the ground truth data is idealised and may not match the actual truth. The positions have been set by adjusting a magnetic offset field generated with a coil by direct current sources. Because the sources are highly stable, the current has not been monitored and therefore, the actual magnetic offset field values are not known. Due to small offset currents there may be an uncertainty at low currents and therefore, fields corresponding to central positions. An unstableness of the current at central positions is indicated as well by the artefacts of the system-matrix-based reconstruction results. However, the programmed current and field values have been used for generating the ground truth data.

Artefacts near the borders of the images, which is the FOV, may appear due to the sampling trajectory. The sinusoidal trajectory features turning points here which results

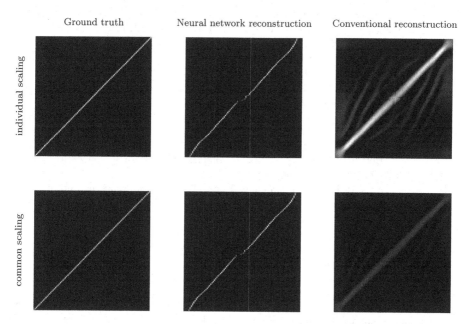

Fig. 3. Ground truth (left column) and reconstruction results of the test data using the neural-network approach (centre column) and the system-matrix-based approach (right column). In the upper row, each image has been scaled to its own grey value range, whereas the images have been scaled to a common grey value range in the bottom row. The images show the 241 reconstructed 1D images, that have been stacked row-wise. The reconstructed images using the neural network show a superior spatial resolution than using the conventional reconstruction. In the latter, the reconstructed points are blurred. Background artefacts cannot be identified visually when reconstructing with the neural network. The grey value ranges of the ground truth and neural-network-reconstruction are similar, whereas the range differs for the reconstructed images using the conventional approach.

in both no magnetic field change and no induction and in turn, a low signal-to-noise ratio.

The current work lacks a metric for comparing ground truth and test data which enables a quantitative measure of the reconstruction results. This metric needs to compare the similarity of reconstructed structures and intensity values, but should not compare the data pixel-wise, as then imprecise ground truth data or blurry reconstruction results would generate a low accuracy.

The current work will be extended by generating and reconstructing hybrid multipoint phantoms. Then, image reconstruction of multi-dimensional data using a neural network will be researched. The data will be measured in an MPS first and second in an MPI scanning device.

References

1. Gleich B, Weizenecker J. Tomographic imaging using the nonlinear response of magnetic particles. Nature. 2005;435(7046):1214–7.
2. Knopp T, Rahmer J, Sattel TF, Biederer S, Weizenecker J, Gleich B et al. Weighted iterative reconstruction for magnetic particle imaging. Phys Med Biol. 2010;55(6):1577–89.
3. Boberg M, Gdaniec N, Szwargulski P, Werner F, Möddel M, Knopp T. Simultaneous imaging of widely differing particle concentrations in MPI: problem statement and algorithmic proposal for improvement. Phys Med Biol. 2021;66(9):095004.
4. Goodwill PW, Conolly SM. Multidimensional X-Space magnetic particle imaging. IEEE Trans Med Imaging. 2011;30(9):1581–90.
5. Hatsuda T, Takagi T, Matsuhisa A, Arayama M, Tsuchiya H, Takahashi S et al. Basic study of image reconstruction method using neural networks with additional learning for magnetic particle imaging. Int J Magn Part Imaging. 2016;2(2).
6. Lecun Y, Bottou L, Bengio Y, Haffner P. Gradient-based learning applied to document recognition. Proc IEEE. 1998;86(11):2278–324.
7. Koch P, Maass M, Bruhns M, Droigk C, Parbs TJ, Mertins A. Neural network for reconstruction of MPI images. International Workshop on Magnetic Particle Imaging. 2019:39–40.
8. Dittmer S, Kluth T, Henriksen MTR, Maass P. Deep image prior for 3D magnetic particle imaging: a quantitative comparison of regularization techniques on Open MPI dataset. Int J Magn Part Imaging. 2021;7(1).
9. Chen X, Graeser M, Behrends A, von Gladiss A, Buzug TM. First measurement results of a 3D magnetic particle spectrometer. Int J Magn Part Imaging. 2018;4(1).
10. von Gladiss A, Graeser M, Cordes A, Bakenecker AC, Behrends A, Chen X et al. Investigating spatial resolution, field sequences and image reconstruction strategies using hybrid phantoms in MPI. Int J Magn Part Imaging. 2020;6(1).

Abstract: 3D Stent Graft Guidance Based on Tracking Systems

Sonja Jäckle[1], Tim Eixmann[2], Florian Matysiak[3], Malte M. Sieren[4], Marco Horn[3], Hinnerk Schulz-Hildebrandt[2,5,6], Gereon Hüttmann[2,5,6], Torben Pätz[7]

[1]Fraunhofer Institute for Digital Medicine MEVIS, Lübeck, Germany
[2]Institute of Biomedical Optics, Universität zu Lübeck, Germany
[3]Department of Surgery, UKSH, Lübeck, Germany
[4]Department for Radiology and Nuclear Medicine, UKSH, Lübeck, Germany
[5]Medical Laser Center Lübeck GmbH, Lübeck, Germany
[6]German Center for Lung Research (DZL), Großhansdorf, Germany
[7]Fraunhofer Institute for Digital Medicine MEVIS, Bremen, Germany
sonja.jaeckle@mevis.fraunhofer.de

In endovascular aneurysm repair (EVAR) procedures, the stent graft navigation and implantation is currently performed under a two-dimensional (2D) imaging-based guidance requiring X-rays and contrast agent. In [1], a novel three-dimensional (3D) stent graft guidance approach based on tracking systems is introduced. The method is based on a 3D guidance method which combines fiber optical shape sensing with electromagnetic tracking to obtain the 3D shape [2] of the tracked instrument, e.g., a stent graft system. In this work, the approach is extended to provide also the 3D stent graft shape. A calibration method for determining the start and end position of the integrated stent graft is introduced. Furthermore, an adapted and improved visualization for the stent graft guidance is described. The tracking based stent graft guidance is evaluated by conducting an EVAR procedure on a torso phantom using a stent graft system equipped with an optical fiber and three EM sensors. The physicians used the tracking-based guidance to navigate the stent graft to the landing zone, and to place and implant it. The fluoroscopy image acquired after implantation showed that the stent graft was successfully implanted. Thus, the application of the stent graft guidance is feasible in a clinical environment and promising for the reduction of radiation and contrast agent during EVAR procedures.

References

1. Jäckle S, Eixmann T, Matysiak F, Sieren MM, Horn M, Schulz-Hildebrandt H et al. 3D stent graft guidance based on tracking systems for endovascular aneurysm repair. Cur Dir Biomed Eng. 2021;7(1):17–20.
2. Jäckle S, García-Vázquez V, Eixmann T, Matysiak F, Haxthausen F von, Sieren MM et al. Three-dimensional guidance including shape sensing of a stentgraft system for endovascular aneurysm repair. Int J Comput Assist Radiol Surg. 2020;15(6):1033–42.

Superpixel Pre-segmentation of HER2 Slides for Efficient Annotation

Mathias Öttl[1], Jana Mönius[2], Christian Marzahl[1], Matthias Rübner[4],
Carol I. Geppert[2], Arndt Hartmann[2], Matthias W. Beckmann[4], Peter Fasching[4],
Andreas Maier[1], Ramona Erber[2], Katharina Breininger[3]

[1]Pattern Recognition Lab, Friedrich-Alexander-Universität Erlangen-Nürnberg (FAU)
[2]Institute of Pathology, University Hospital Erlangen, Friedrich-Alexander-Universität
Erlangen-Nürnberg (FAU), Comprehensive Cancer Center Erlangen-EMN (CCC ER-EMN)
[3]Department Artificial Intelligence in Biomedical Engineering, Friedrich-Alexander-Universität
Erlangen-Nürnberg (FAU)
[4]Department of Gynecology and Obstetrics, University Hospital Erlangen,
Friedrich-Alexander-Universität Erlangen-Nürnberg (FAU)
mathias.oettl@fau.de

Abstract. Supervised deep learning has shown state-of-the-art performance for medical image segmentation across different applications, including histopathology and cancer research; however, the manual annotation of such data is extremely laborious. In this work, we explore the use of superpixel approaches to compute a pre-segmentation of HER2 stained images for breast cancer diagnosis that facilitates faster manual annotation and correction in a second step. Four methods are compared: standard simple linear iterative clustering (SLIC) as a baseline, a domain adapted SLIC, and superpixels based on feature embeddings of a pretrained ResNet-50 and a denoising autoencoder. To tackle oversegmentation, we propose to hierarchically merge superpixels, based on their content in the respective feature space. When evaluating the approaches on fully manually annotated images, we observe that the autoencoder-based superpixels achieve a 23% increase in boundary F1 score compared to the baseline SLIC superpixels. Furthermore, the boundary F1 score increases by 73% when hierarchical clustering is applied on the adapted SLIC and the autoencoder-based superpixels. These evaluations show encouraging first results for a pre-segmentation for efficient manual refinement without the need for an initial set of annotated training data.

1 Introduction

Breast cancer, a common type of cancer that mainly affects women, can be classified into different subtypes that show differences in their aggressiveness, treatment response and prognosis [1]. Human epidermal growth factor receptor 2 (HER2) positive breast cancer is associated with a poor prognosis but targeted therapies exist that can reduce the mortality of patients suffering from this subtype [1]. To determine whether a specific treatment may benefit a patient, HER2 expression is visualized using a specific staining and scored by pathologists [1] into four classes (0, 1+, 2+, or 3+): Tumors with a score of 0 or 1+ are considered HER2-negative, and cases with a score of 3+ are regarded as HER2 positive. In routine diagnostics, breast cancer samples with a 2+

K. Maier-Hein et al. (Hrsg.), *Bildverarbeitung für die Medizin 2022*,
Informatik aktuell, https://doi.org/10.1007/978-3-658-36932-3_54

staining are further analyzed to determine positive or negative HER2 status. Recently, machine learning has been incorporated into HER2 research to better understand growth and proliferation and support the analysis of this data. For example, deep learning methods were used to segment the cell membranes [2]. These intermediate results were then utilized to determine the HER2 score. Label generation for these methods is tedious and time-consuming since fine-grained annotations are required. In this work, we evaluate superpixel methods under the premise of reducing HER2 annotation effort and to ease future work on comprehensible deep learning methods [3]. Single tumor cells per slide may present with different HER2 staining intensities and HER2 expression patterns, however, local clusters of cells often share the same HER2 score [4]. The size of areas with homogeneous HER2 score can vary greatly, and these areas show complex staining textures which motivates the use of superpixels in this context. As a baseline, we use SLIC superpixels, which are reasonably robust when the data has a non-uniform texture and achieve good results compared to other superpixel methods like the Felzenszwalb algorithm, quick shift or the normalized cuts algorithm [5]. Furthermore, we investigate different variants for this specific application, namely SLIC adapted to the color properties of HER2 stained images, as well as superpixels based on the latent representation of pretrained networks and denoising autoencoders [6]. Due to the varying size of areas with homogeneous HER2 expression, the constant size of SLIC-based superpixels would result in strong over- or undersegmentation depending on the selected superpixel size. To counteract this effect, we incorporate an additional hierarchical clustering stage to merge superpixels with similar content and evaluate the effect on the resulting pre-segmentation as a further contribution of this work.

2 Materials and methods

In this section, we first describe the four methods used to calculate superpixels, followed by the hierarchical clustering approach applied to all four superpixel methods. Furthermore, we present the data used for training and evaluation as well as the evaluation metrics.

2.1 Superpixel methods

As baseline, we use the standard SLIC algorithm described by Achanta et al. [5]. Furthermore, we adapt the representation of the HER2 images as follows.

2.1.1 Adjusted SLIC. As a preprocessing step, images are converted from RBG to haematoxylin eosin DAB (HED) color space [7] to utilize prior knowledge about the color distribution of HER2 stained images. Originally developed for hematoxylin and eosin (H&E) stained images, we use it to obtain a more uniform distribution of the hematoxylin color channel by filtering the respective image channel with a large Gaussian kernel. This channel mainly depicts cell nuclei which are not of interest for this application. Accordingly, the values of this channel are reduced to force the subsequently applied SLIC algorithm to focus on the color channels of the HER2 stain and less on the cell nuclei.

2.1.2 Pre-trained ResNet-50. A ResNet-50, pretrained as feature extractor for a mask R-CNN on the COCO segmentation dataset, is utilized to compute lower resolution features vectors from the fourth stage of the network. These feature vectors, called embeddings, are upsampled to the original image resolution and serve as input for the SLIC algorithm.

2.1.3 HER2 autoencoder. To obtain embeddings that are targeted to HER2 data, we train a denoising autoencoder to reconstuct augmented input images with the goal to determine a robust internal data representation. Our autoencoder has three levels, each with one convolutional layer in the encoder and one transposed convolutional layer in the decoder. ReLU is used as activation function. The network is trained using stochastic gradient descent (SDG) with momentum (learning rate 0.01, momentum 0.9), batchsize of 32 and mean squared error loss function, until convergence of loss on the validation set. At lowest level, 64-dimensional embeddings are calculated, which are also upsampled to the original image resolution and serve as input for the SLIC algorithm.

2.2 Hierarchical clustering

To address the problem of over- or undersegmentation that occurs when SLIC is used to segment areas of vastly different sizes, hierarchical clustering is applied. The benefits of clustering superpixels into larger regions were shown in [8]. In this work, superpixels are described by the mean value of their pixels, which can either be a color or a feature vector. Based on this mean value, the superpixels are combined using agglomerative clustering. As clustering criterion ward [9] is used, which enforces the variance within clusters to be low. In addition, only neighboring superpixels are allowed to be merged.

2.3 Dataset

The dataset used in this work consists of image regions from 20 tissue sections (five for each HER2 score), originating from 20 different patients. These sections were immuno-histochemically stained for HER2 and scanned using a PANNORAMIC 1000 scanner from 3DHistech, using a 20x objective, and are available as digital images. A total of 84 images patches of size 1.5 mm×1.5 mm were extracted to serve as the dataset. The patches were randomly split 60/20/4 on slide level into a training, validation and test set for autoencoder training and evaluation, with equal distribution of HER2 score across all subsets. The four test patches for evaluation were manually annotated into HER2 scored tumor areas, non-tumor areas and staining artefacts. These areas were segmented using polygons in the EXACT tool [10]. Annotations were performed by a medical student and reviewed by a board-certified pathologist.

2.4 Evaluation metrics

The evaluation metrics used in this work are described in detail in [6]. Achievable segmentation accuracy (ASA) describes the segmentation coverage of the superpixels and indicates whether superpixels overlap multiple ground truth segments. Boundary

F1 score is a measure for the quality of the boundary segmentation. The score is a equal weighted combination of boundary recall and boundary precision. Since the exact position of a boundary is often fuzzy, a tolerance is used in boundary measures. HER2 data has high resolution and tissue areas are hard to precisely delineate from each other, therefore a tolerance of 15 pixels (3.75 μm) is used for the evaluation of the different approaches.

3 Results

Figure 1 shows the metrics for the superpixel methods with and without hierarchical clustering. As expected, the ASA score for all versions is close to one for the initially selected superpixel size and decreases with higher superpixel diameter. A stronger decrease is visible for the baseline method, which indicates that the baseline method computes superpixels that wrongly cross tissue boundaries. For all methods the ASA score is slightly lower when hierarchical clustering is utilized, showing that some incorrect superpixel merges occur. With respect to the boundary F1 score, the baseline (peak value: 0.26) is already outperformed by adjusted SLIC (peak value: 0.32) and the autoencoder (peak value: 0.33) when no hierarchical clustering is applied. These values represent an improvement of 23% and 27% respectively. With hierarchical clustering, adjusted SLIC and the autoencoder both achieve a peak value of 0.45, representing an improvement of 73% compared to the baseline without hierarchical clustering. The pretrained ResNet-50 underperforms the baseline in all cases, except for small initial superpixel diameters. Figure 2 shows example regions of the ground truth and the output of the superpixel methods with (blue) and without hierarchical clustering (black). For all approaches the visual results are in line with the reported metrics.

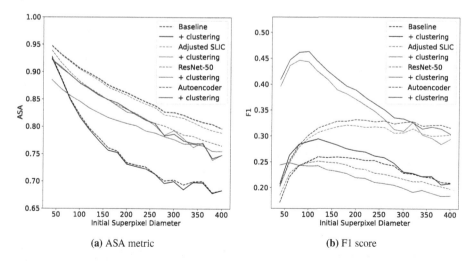

(a) ASA metric   (b) F1 score

Fig. 1. Plots of achievable segmentation accuracy (ASA) (a) and boundary F1 score (b) for the different methods for different superpixel sizes.

4   Discussion

In this work, several superpixel methods and an additional hierarchical clustering step were evaluated. We showed that superpixels from a domain adjusted SLIC and from a HER2 autoencoder outperformed a baseline SLIC in terms of boundary F1 score and achievable segmentation accuracy. These results highlight that the HER2 representations used in this methods are superior for calculating SLIC superpixels and should be considered in future segmentation task on HER2 data. Additionally, we showed that hierarchical clustering of superpixels achieves significantly higher boundary F1 scores, while decreasing the ASA score slightly. This technique reduces the annotation effort of HER2 data even further and will help to speed up the creation of ground truth annotations. Although these results are promising, the following limitations should be noted. The test dataset consists of one labelled image for each of the four HER2 scores, which restricted the use of cross validation. Additionally, all whole slide images (WSI) were scanned with the same device and only one person annotated the images. The practical annotation effort depends on a combination of boundary accuracy and the number of superpixels, but the importance of each metric can not be quantified yet. These aspects will be further explored in future work to evaluate the downstream utility for reducing annotation time with the proposed methods.

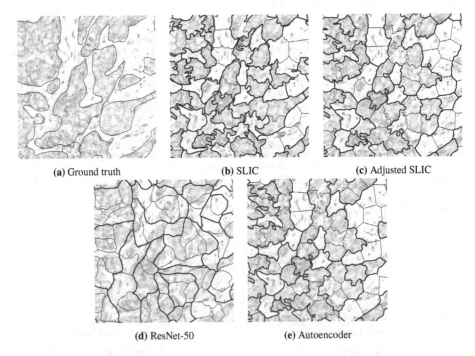

(a) Ground truth   **(b)** SLIC   **(c)** Adjusted SLIC

(d) ResNet-50   **(e)** Autoencoder

Fig. 2. Results for the superpixel methods at a inital superpixel diameter of 120 pixels. The initial superpixels are drawn with black outlining, while the clustered superpixels are visualized in blue.

Acknowledgement. This project is supported by the Bavarian State Ministry of Health and Care, project grants No. PBN-MGP-2010-0004-DigiOnko and PBN-MGP-2008-0003-DigiOnko. We also gratefully acknowledge the support from the Interdisciplinary Center for Clinical Research (IZKF, Clinician Scientist Program) of the Medical Faculty FAU Erlangen-Nürnberg.

References

1. Loibl S, Gianni L. HER2-positive breast cancer. Lancet. 2017;389(10087):2415–29.
2. Khameneh FD, Razavi S, Kamasak M. Automated segmentation of cell membranes to evaluate HER2 status in whole slide images using a modified deep learning network. Comput Biol Med. 2019;110:164–74.
3. Albayrak A, Bilgin G. Automatic cell segmentation in histopathological images via two-staged superpixel-based algorithms. Med Biol Eng Comput. 2019;57(3):653–65.
4. Marchiò C, Annaratone L, Marques A, Casorzo L, Berrino E, Sapino A. Evolving concepts in HER2 evaluation in breast cancer: Heterogeneity, HER2-low carcinomas and beyond. Seminars in Cancer Biology. Vol. 72. 2021:123–35.
5. Achanta R, Shaji A, Smith K, Lucchi A, Fua P, Süsstrunk S. SLIC superpixels compared to state-of-the-art superpixel methods. IEEE Trans Pattern Anal Mach Intell. 2012;34(11):2274–82.
6. Gaur U, Manjunath B. Superpixel embedding network. IEEE Trans Image Process. 2019;29:3199–3212.
7. Ruifrok AC, Johnston DA et al. Quantification of histochemical staining by color deconvolution. Anal Quant Cytol Histol. 2001;23(4):291–9.
8. Chaibou MS, Conze PH, Kalti K, Solaiman B, Mahjoub MA. Adaptive strategy for superpixel-based region-growing image segmentation. J Electron Imaging. 2017;26(6):061605.
9. Murtagh F, Legendre P. Ward's hierarchical agglomerative clustering method: which algorithms implement Ward's criterion? J Classif. 2014;31(3):274–95.
10. Marzahl C, Aubreville M, Bertram CA, Maier J, Bergler C, Kröger C et al. EXACT: a collaboration toolset for algorithm-aided annotation of images with annotation version control. Sci Reps. 2021;11(1):4343.

Abstract: Task Fingerprinting for Meta Learning in Biomedical Image Analysis

Patrick Godau[1,2,3], Lena Maier-Hein[1,2,4]

[1]Div. Computer Assisted Medical Interventions, German Cancer Research Center
[2]Faculty of Mathematics and Computer Science, Heidelberg University
[3]Helmholtz Information and Data Science School for Health, Karlsruhe/Heidelberg
[4]Medical Faculty, Heidelberg University
patrick.scholz@dkfz-heidelberg.de

Shortage of annotated data is one of the greatest bottlenecks related to biomedical image analysis in general, and surgical data science (SDS) in particular. Meta learning studies how learning systems can increase in efficiency through experience and could thus evolve as an important concept to overcome data sparsity. A core capability of meta learning-based approaches is the identification of similar previous tasks given a new task. We recently addressed this problem and presented the concept of task fingerprinting [1], which involves representing a task (comprising images and labels), by a vector of fixed length irrespective of data set size, types of labels or specific resolutions (Fig. 1). For the task embedding, we investigate several complementary approaches, not limiting ourselves to directly comparing the distributions of the images but also leveraging the labels for the embedding. Our initial feasibility study with 26 classification tasks from various medical and non-medical domains suggests that task fingerprinting could be leveraged for both (1) selecting appropriate datasets for pretraining and (2) selecting appropriate architectures for a new task.

Fig. 1. Concept of Task Fingerprinting. Task images and labels are embedded to fixed length feature vectors. Fingerprint similarity is used for optimizing knowledge transfer between tasks. Adapted from [1].

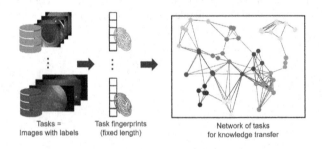

Tasks =
Images with labels

Task fingerprints
(fixed length)

Network of tasks
for knowledge transfer

References

1. Godau P, Maier-Hein L. Task fingerprinting for meta learning in biomedical image analysis. Med Image Comput Comput Assist Interv. 2021:436–46.

© Der/die Autor(en), exklusiv lizenziert durch
Springer Fachmedien Wiesbaden GmbH, ein Teil von Springer Nature 2022
K. Maier-Hein et al. (Hrsg.), *Bildverarbeitung für die Medizin 2022*,
Informatik aktuell, https://doi.org/10.1007/978-3-658-36932-3_55

Initial Investigations Towards Non-invasive Monitoring of Chronic Wound Healing Using Deep Learning and Ultrasound Imaging

Maja Schlereth[1,2], Daniel Stromer[2], Yash Mantri[3], Jason Tsujimoto[3], Katharina Breininger[1], Andreas Maier[2], Caesar Anderson[4], Pranav S. Garimella[5], Jesse V. Jokerst[6]

[1]Department Artificial Intelligence in Biomedical Engineering, FAU Erlangen-Nürnberg, Erlangen
[2]Pattern Recognition Lab, FAU Erlangen-Nürnberg, Erlangen
[3]Department of Bioengineering, University of California, San Diego
[4]Department of Emergency Medicine, San Diego
[5]Division of Nephrology and Hypertension, Department of Medicine, San Diego
[6]Department of Nanoengineering, University of California, San Diego
maja.schlereth@fau.de

Abstract. Chronic wounds including diabetic and arterial/venous insufficiency injuries have become a major burden for healthcare systems worldwide. Demographic changes suggest that wound care will play an even bigger role in the coming decades. Predicting and monitoring response to therapy in wound care is currently largely based on visual inspection with little information on the underlying tissue. Thus, there is an urgent unmet need for innovative approaches that facilitate personalized diagnostics and treatments at the point-of-care. It has been recently shown that ultrasound imaging can monitor response to therapy in wound care, but this work required onerous manual image annotations. In this study we present initial results of a deep learning-based automatic segmentation of cross-sectional wound size in ultrasound images and identify requirements and challenges for future research on this application. Evaluation of the segmentation results underscores the potential of the proposed deep learning approach to complement non-invasive imaging with Dice scores of 0.34 (U-Net, FCN) and 0.27 (ResNet-U-Net) but also highlights the need for improving robustness further. We conclude that deep learning-supported analysis of non-invasive ultrasound images is a promising area of research to automatically extract cross-sectional wound size and depth information with potential value in monitoring response to therapy.

1 Introduction

Chronic wounds affect around 6.6 million United States citizens per year (prevalence of ~2 %) [1]. These wounds often lead to patient immobility, increased risk of sepsis and amputation, pain, decreased quality of life, and a shorter life expectancy. The five-year survival rate of patients with chronic wounds is significantly lower than for age- and sex-matched controls [2]. Regular assessment of chronic wounds includes physical and visual examination or manual probing for tunneling wounds [3]. Thus, these examinations mostly evaluate the skin surface. Tracking the kinetics of wound healing

- especially below the skin surface - is still largely based on clinical experience. Using only surface information misses key information about the interface between healthy and diseased tissue and vasculature below the skin surface [4]. Assessment of cross-sectional wound size development can help to detect stagnant healing earlier. Thus, extracellular matrices or skin grafts can be applied earlier to improve the curative effects. Mantri et al. showed that non-invasive imaging such as ultrasound (US) imaging can reveal further insights into the healing processes by generating temporal and spatial information [5]. US imaging is particularly well suited for wound care because it is affordable and already broadly used in various areas of medicine. However, it can also suffer from low contrast and imaging artifacts. Image interpretation can be strongly user-dependent; thus, there is a clear need for automatic assessment of wound size to increase the clinical value of US. Wang et al. worked on a fully automatic segmentation of wound areas in photographic images [6]. With this method, they are able to monitor superficial wounds but could not image the three-dimensional wound architecture below the skin surface. Huang et al. recently reviewed machine learning approaches applied on different modalities to objectively assess burn wound severity compared to subjective methods [7]. In this study, initial results for automatic segmentation of US images are presented. We evaluated three different deep learning segmentation networks in the context of US-based wound sizing: a fully convolutional network (FCN) with a DenseNet-like encoder, a ResNet-U-Net, and a U-Net architecture [8, 9]. We also investigated the behavior of US intensities in different sections of the wound. Based on our evaluations, we identify challenges and define requirements for further research in this field to help physicians make objective wound assessments, support treatment decisions, and ultimately improve patient quality of life.

2   Material and methods

2.1   Dataset

All human subjects research was done with approval from the Internal Review Board at the University of California, San Diego. We used a commercially available LED-based photoacoustic/US imaging system (AcousticX from Cyberdyne Inc., Tsukuba, Japan). In this study, we used only the ultrasound mode and all US images were acquired at 30 frames/s. Details about the inclusion and exclusion criteria, the imaging equipment used, and manual image processing can be found in our prior work [5]. We imaged 62 patients, affected by different types of chronic leg wounds. Subjects were scanned over a four-month period for a total of 161 scans containing 15,000 images. All scans included wound and healthy adjacent tissue. Ground truth (GT) annotations were done manually in ImageJ by outlining the border between wound and healthy tissue. Each image in a sweep scan was processed individually. Ultrasound imaging and annotations of the scans were performed by two experts in this field. Each scan was annotated by one expert due to the large annotation effort. For development of the networks, the dataset was divided into training, validation and test set with the data split shown in Table 1.

	Training Set	Validation Set	Test Set
Number of Patients	37	15	10
Number of Scans	78	32	51
Number of Images	7148	3061	5052

Tab. 1. Distribution of US data for training, validating and testing.

2.2 Deep learning networks and training strategy

The three deep learning networks used for this work are FCN with a DenseNet encoder, ResNet-U-Net with a ResNet18 encoder and an adapted four-level U-Net with LeakyReLUs instead of standard ReLU activation functions. For DenseNet-FCN and the ResNet-U-Net, weights pre-trained on the ImageNet data set were used. For all networks, image input sizes of 320×320 px, Adam-Optimizer, batch size 3 and decaying learning rate (start: $1e^{-3}$, γ for weight decay: 0.1, step size: 10 epochs) were used. All networks were implemented in Python using PyTorch and trained until convergence on an Nvidia GeForce GTX 1080. Hyperparameters were selected based on the validation set.

To improve distribution of different wound type images in the training, validation, and test datasets, manifold learning-based data selection proposed by Chen was applied [10]. As many images for training are heavily correlated, random augmentation techniques were introduced to make the training more robust (i. e.: random brightness, noise, saturation, rotation, left-right flipping) [11], and the images were normalized to match ImageNet statistics.

2.3 Evaluation metrics

For quantitative evaluation of the network, we calculated precision, recall and the Dice score, also known as F1 score, of the network prediction compared to the GT annotation. Results are also visualized to compare GT with the network prediction. True positive (TP) pixels are colored green, false positives (FP) are colored yellow, false negatives (FN) are colored red and true negative (TN) areas are transparent.

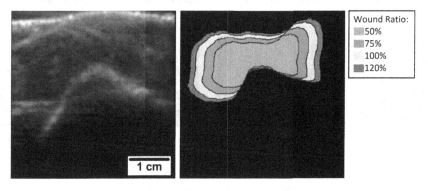

Fig. 1. Different wound regions for comparison of US intensities $\overline{m}_r$ within the wound.

Tab. 2. Dice score, precision and recall value (mean ± standard deviation over all frames) of all trained networks.

Network	FCN	ResNet-U-Net	U-Net
Dice score	0.34 ± 0.31	0.27 ± 0.32	0.34 ± 0.31
Precision	0.27 ± 0.27	0.33 ± 0.40	0.33 ± 0.33
Recall	0.71 ± 0.41	0.35 ± 0.37	0.55 ± 0.39

2.4 Wound intensity evaluation

To better understand the wound morphology and how its composition relates to measured US intensities, we analyze the average US intensity in different sections of the wound for all scans of the test set. The wound area is given by the GT segmentation mask for each scan. We introduce an evaluation scheme that adapts the segmented wound area by a dilation and erosion process. We calculated the ratio of the mean US intensity $\overline{m}_r$ of different wound regions compared to $\overline{m}_w$ over the whole wound. We used the regions 0–50 % (blue), 50–75 % (orange), 75–100 % (green) and 100–120 % (red) of the actual wound area. Figure 1 shows the different wound regions.

3 Results

Table 2 shows the quantitative evaluation of the algorithms. U-Net and FCN both achieve a Dice score of 0.34 compared to pre-trained ResNet-U-Net which has a Dice score of

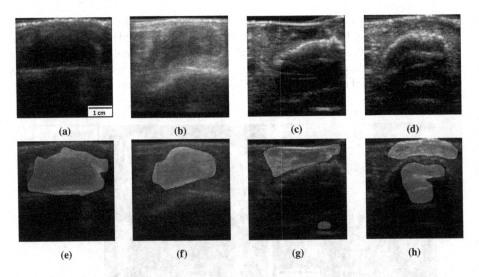

Fig. 2. (a-d) Four representative US wound images. (e-h) Visualization of corresponding segmentation predictions for FCN. Green indicates correct matches, red and yellow indicate missed (false negative) and oversegmented (false positive) areas, respectively.

Tab. 3. Comparison between US intensities measured in different ratios of wound size compared to 100 % of actual wound size.

Wound Region	0–50 %	50–75 %	75–100 %	100–120 %
US Intensity Ratio	0.89 ± 0.11	1.06 ± 0.08	1.24 ± 0.21	1.47 ± 0.37

0.27. Visualizations of the segmentation results for FCN are shown in Figure 2, where (a-d) are the original inputs, and (e-h) the corresponding color-coded outcomes. In general, the performance is promising for a number of cases, although we see a high FP rate (d,h) for others. Table 3 shows the ratio of $\overline{m}_r$ for different wound regions compared to $\overline{m}_w$ of the whole wound area. In the wound center, the US values are lower (ratio: 0.89 ± 0.11), compared to the wound borders (ratio: 1.47 ± 0.37).

4 Discussion

In this work, we showed a proof-of-concept for a non-invasive imaging technique paired with machine learning. We performed initial experiments for automatic segmentation of US wound images with deep learning which show an Dice score of 0.34 for both U-Net and FCN and 0.27 for ResNet-U-Net. The segmentation results strongly depend on the quality of the scan and the specific wound type. Quantitative results can still be improved but the visual examination of the results indicates applicability of the proposed setup. For images illustrated in Figure 2(e-g), the segmentation is very good. However, the network misclassifies the region beneath the hyperechoic bone surface (image h) as this region therefore appears dark and similar in intensity to the wound region.

The evaluation of the mean US intensity ratio in different wound regions show higher ratios for wound borders and lower intensities for the wound center compared to the whole wound area. Low echoic region can indicate the absence of healing tissue. Higher US intensity ratios at the wound edges could imply hyperdense or scar tissue. Generally, an increase in echogenicity indicates tissue regeneration and wound contraction [12]. This information about wound characteristics can help with automatic wound assessment in future work.

Based on our results, we identify the following challenges: US images are notoriously difficult to interpret because they can have low contrast as well as imaging artifacts. Given the signal variability of wound tissue observed in US images, larger amounts of training data are needed to allow for a robust determination of wound size and healing progress. While a prior study showed no significant inter-observer bias for annotating wound areas in US images [5], a study to better understand inter-observer variability from different institutes and to overcome the subjective perception of a single expert during the annotation process is needed. To facilitate this, a standardized measurement protocol and a detailed annotation process can help to make scans more comparable. As a result, we expect an improved performance for a machine-learning based analysis by either increasing label consistency or by being able to explicitly model annotation uncertainty during the training.

Along this path, we see the potential for automatic scoring and classification of wounds into different severity stages and a continuous non-invasive monitoring of therapy response by combining US imaging and machine learning, which can be implemented at the point-of-care for wound assessment. In this context, this monitoring can be integrated in eHealth applications, thus enabling improved personalized healthcare and therapy outcomes.

Acknowledgement. JVJ acknowledges NIH support under grant R21 AG065776.

References

1. Järbrink K, Ni G, Sönnergren H, Schmidtchen A, Pang C, Bajpai R et al. The humanistic and economic burden of chronic wounds: a protocol for a systematic review. Syst Rev. 2017;6(1):1–7.
2. Nelzén O, Bergqvist D, Lindhagen A. Long-term prognosis for patients with chronic leg ulcers: a prospective cohort study. Eur J Vasc Endovasc Surg. 1997;13(5):500–8.
3. Frykberg RG, Banks J. Challenges in the treatment of chronic wounds. Adv Wound Care (New Rochelle). 2015;4(9):560–82.
4. Medina A, Scott PG, Ghahary A, Tredget EE. Pathophysiology of chronic nonhealing wounds. J Burn Care Rehabil. 2005;26(4):306–19.
5. Mantri Y, Tsujimoto J, Penny WF, Garimella PS, Anderson CA, Jokerst JV. Point-of-care ultrasound as a tool to assess wound size and tissue regeneration after skin grafting. Ultrasound Med Biol. 2021;47(9):2550–9.
6. Wang C, Anisuzzaman DM, Williamson V, Dhar MK, Rostami B, Niezgoda J et al. Fully automatic wound segmentation with deep convolutional neural networks. Sci Rep. 2020;10(1):1–9.
7. Huang S, Dang J, Sheckter CC, Yenikomshian HA, Gillenwater J. A systematic review of machine learning and automation in burn wound evaluation: a promising but developing frontier. Burns. 2021.
8. Ronneberger O, Fischer P, Brox T. U-Net: Convolutional networks for biomedical image segmentation. Medical Image Computing and Computer-Assisted Intervention. Ed. by Navab N, Hornegger J, Wells WM, Frangi AF. 2015:234–41.
9. Shelhamer E, Long J, Darrell T. Fully convolutional networks for semantic segmentation. IEEE Trans Pattern Anal Mach Intell. 2017;39(4):640–51.
10. Chen S, Dorn S, Lell M, Kachelrieß M, Maier A. Manifold learning-based data sampling for model training. Proc BVM. 2018:269–74.
11. Perez L, Wang J. The effectiveness of data augmentation in image classification using deep learning. 2017.
12. Moghimi S, Miran Baygi MH, Torkaman G, Mahloojifar A. Quantitative assessment of pressure sore generation and healing through numerical analysis of high-frequency ultrasound images. J Rehabil Res Dev. 2010;47(2):99–108.

Classification of Vascular Malformations Based on T2 STIR Magnetic Resonance Imaging

Danilo W. Nunes[1], Michael Hammer[1], Simone Hammer[2], Wibke Uller[3], Christoph Palm[1,4]

[1]Regensburg Medical Image Computing (ReMIC), Ostbayerische Technische Hochschule Regensburg (OTH Regensburg), Regensburg, Germany
[2]Department of Radiology, University Hospital Regensburg, Regensburg, Germany
[3]Department of Diagnostic and Interventional Radiology, University Hospital Freiburg, Freiburg, Germany
[4]Regensburg Center of Biomedical Engineering (RCBE), OTH Regensburg and Regensburg University, Regensburg, Germany
christoph.palm@oth-regensburg.de

Abstract. Vascular malformations (VMs) are a rare condition. They can be categorized into high-flow and low-flow VMs, which is a challenging task for radiologists. In this work, a very heterogeneous set of MRI images with only rough annotations are used for classification with a convolutional neural network. The main focus is to describe the challenging data set and strategies to deal with such data in terms of preprocessing, annotation usage and choice of the network architecture. We achieved a classification result of 89.47 % F1-score with a 3D ResNet 18.

1 Introduction

Vascular malformations (VMs) are a rare and complex disease. VM can be categorized in high-flow (arterio-venous) and low-flow (venous, lymphatic, capillary or combined) malformations according to their hemodynamics [1]. Correct diagnosis and use of proper classification of VMs are mandatory since management of VMs is different depending on their subtype [2]. VM are congenital, therefore patients with VM are rather young and usually undergo magnetic resonance imaging (MRI) as first cross-sectional imaging for diagnosis. As VMs are very rare, most radiologists are not familiar with the distinctive features of high-flow and low-flow VM in MRI and correct classification is challenging.

In this work, we propose a pipeline for high or low-flow classification of MRI images of vascular malformations using three dimensional Convolutional Neural Networks (CNNs). Since the condition is rare we face a very inhomogeneous, unbalanced, and small 3D data set. On the other hand, the memory footprint of each volume is quite large. In this work, we describe approaches to handle such challenging data and use them for training CNNs with the goal of VM-subtype classification.

2 Materials and methods

In this section the data are described in more detail followed by a presentation of the CNN network architecture and the training procedures.

© Der/die Autor(en), exklusiv lizenziert durch
Springer Fachmedien Wiesbaden GmbH, ein Teil von Springer Nature 2022
K. Maier-Hein et al. (Hrsg.), *Bildverarbeitung für die Medizin 2022*,
Informatik aktuell, https://doi.org/10.1007/978-3-658-36932-3_57

Tab. 1. Minimum and maximum volume dimension [number of voxels] and voxel resolution [mm] in different planes over the used data.

Plane	Height [min,max]	Width [min,max]	Slices [min,max]	Row [min,max]	Column [min,max]	Thickness [min,max]
T	[210,576]	[320,640]	[20,140]	[0.51,1.34]	[0.51,1.34]	[3.0,8.0]
S	[320,512]	[320,512]	[20,28]	[0.40,0.62]	[0.40,0.62]	[2.0,4.5]
C	[320,704]	[320,704]	[20,256]	[0.60,1.34]	[0.60,1.34]	[0.8,6.0]
cC	[561,1756]	[321,685]	[19,51]	[0.66,1.34]	[0.66,1.34]	[4.4,6.6]

2.1 Data

The data for this work were provided by University Hospital Regensburg. This study is limited to regions of the leg and the foot. However, the pelvis may occur additionally in some of the images. 298 patients were examined several times resulting in 142 and 377 high-flow and low-flow MRI examinations, respectively. Each examination consists of several MRI T2 STIR sequences in different planes: coronal (C), sagittal (S), and transversal (T). Therefore, each resulting MRI image has the highest spatial resolution in this respective plane and a reasonably lower slice thickness. Regarding the whole data set, voxel resolutions and volume dimensions differ significantly especially due to the imaging plane. This is shown in Table 1, in which the minimum and maximum volume dimension and voxel resolution is listed for each plane. One slice of a high and a low-flow C volume is shown in Figure 1.

While T and S volumes consist of only one sequence per examination, C volumes may contain up to three different parts to cover the whole extremity. However, the field of view of each part is individual for each examination. The malformation can occur in just a small or nearly the whole extremity and in all or just one C data part. In case of more than one C data part, a composed sequence of all coronal data parts (cC) is given additionally.

The annotations of the physicians used twelve different descriptions of the extremity parts for examination and VM position. To condense this, these descriptions were grouped together into three parts: upper, lower, and whole extremity. Therefore, the following was annotated:

- the parts of the extremity examined,
- the rough position of the VM,
- and the label of the VM subtype.

However, it remained unclear which slices of which volume were affected exactly.

2.2 Network architectures

While in the medical domain three-dimensional (3D) data are mostly volumes like our MRI images, many recent developments in 3D neural networks have been driven by the growing interest in extracting information from video data.

The training of such networks was proven to be more challenging than training two-dimensional (2D) CNNs, as they contain three times more parameters and, thus, need even more data. The idea of transfer learning may help to reduce the number of training samples needed, which is frequently done for 2D CNNs using ImageNet data [3]. However, up to 2017, the lack of publicly available 3D data sets limited the development of 3D networks to shallower models compared to its 2D counterparts. This changed when DeepMind released its Kinects-400 video data set for human action classification [4]. It is considered to be equivalent to ImageNet [3] for training 3D networks, due to its variety and size [5].

The motivation of using 3D networks goes beyond just native 3D input support. Performing classification on video and MRI data, however, share some similarities. Videos do not encode only temporal but also spatial information throughout their frames. This latter can be exploited for MRI images, which encode only spatial information throughout their slices. Therefore, in this study, a 3D ResNet 18 [6] pretrained on the Kinetics-400 video data set is used.

2.3 Training and experimental setup

In order to define the optimal number of slices for classification of an MRI image and to analyze the behavior of the network when varying N as the number of slices used, four experiments were performed using variations of the same images containing 54, 28, 14, and 7 slices. The upper limit of 54 was set due to hardware limitations reached by the large memory footprint of the volumes. On a NVIDIA GeForce GTX 1080 Ti with 11 Gigabyte VRAM, a maximal batch size of 4 was applicable for training.

When partitioning the data into training, validation, and test, the multiple examinations for each patient have to be considered. Hence, the split has to occur on patient level resulting in 208, 60, and 30 training, validation and test patients, respectively. Additionally, it is important to have comparable distributions for the three data partitions in mind in terms of the sequence planes (C, S, T, cC), the position of the VM and the

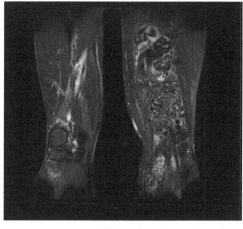 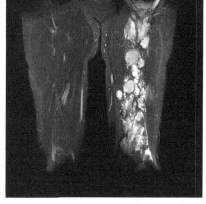

(a) High-flow   (b) Low-flow

Fig. 1. High-flow (left) and low-flow (right) vascular malformation.

label of the VM subtype. This ends up with 983 and 336 low-flow and high-flow VMs for training, 110 and 62 low-flow and high-flow VMs for validation, and 285 and 92 low-flow and high-flow VMs for testing, respectively.

In case of C, S and cC volumes having fewer slices than N, the first and the last slice, respectively, was repeated proportionally until reaching N. Similarly for volumes with more than N slices, the first and the last slices were removed symmetrically. This strategy also allowed the analysis of the importance of the middle slices and the minimum of information necessary to reach the optimal performance.

For the T volumes adjusting the number of slices means, in most cases, removing slices. However, due to the characteristics of the T plane, this can lead to the removal of the whole VM area (e.g. the lower leg). To avoid this, the radiologists annotations about the position of the VM was included in a preprocessing step for training, validation, and test volumes. This step is valid, because we can presume for classification, that the VM always has to be in the input field of view in a real world scenario. The description of the extremity part (upper, lower, whole) was used to determine, which slices of the T sequence were taken. If the VM is located in the upper extremity, the first N slices after a fixed offset were used. This holds true for the lower extremity annotation analogously for the last slices. The annotation whole extremity yielded to the extraction of the N middle slices. This procedure was applied to 519 T volumes.

Ultimately, all MRI slices were scaled to a resolution of 224x224. The only modification performed on the networks was the removal of the original fully connected (FC) layer at the end of the network and replacing it with two new neurons for the two output classes.

We used cross-entropy as loss function and optimized it using Adam [7] with an initial learning rate of 0.0001. The networks were trained during 300 epochs and the learning rate was reduced by 0.1 after 150 and 225 epochs. To minimize the bias of the unbalanced data set, resampling was employed during training by oversampling the low frequent class (high-flow) and by undersampling the high frequent one (low-flow).

Also during training, the augmentation techniques by TorchIO [8] were used, avoiding overfitting and increasing generalization, by performing random motion, random bias field and random flipping with a probability of 20 %, 30 % and 50 % respectively. Canonization and normalization were performed in all splits of the data. The models selected for evaluation were the ones that presented the highest F1-score in the validation set.

3 Results

The results of the performance for each $N \in \{54, 28, 14, 7\}$ are shown in Table 2. The best performance was obtained by the model with the highest N. However, the models trained with fewer slices (28 and 14 slices) performed only marginally worse, not proportional to the amount of slices being used.

Variations using 28 and 14 slices (45 % and 73 % fewer data, respectively) performed only marginally worse, with a significant drop in performance only seen on the model trained with only 7 slices, which uses only 14 % of the data used to train the model with 54 slices.

Tab. 2. Performance metrics of the 3D ResNet 18 network when varying N. The metrics are: receiver operator characteristic curve (ROC), precision recall curve (PR), and area under the curve (AUC).

N	Accuracy	F1 Score	ROC AUC	PR AUC
54	86.05 %	89.47 %	0.92	0.95
28	80.81 %	86.85 %	0.91	0.93
14	79.07 %	85.60 %	0.89	0.92
7	72.67 %	80.97 %	0.79	0.88

Figure 2 presents the precision recall (PR) curves of each model as well as its respective area under the curve (AUC) values, showing that despite the class unbalance, the models in general were not biased towards the higher frequency (low-flow), presenting PR AUC values above 0.9 for all classifiers, with the exception being the model trained with only 7 slices.

4 Discussion

This study shows a novel pipeline for the automatic classification of high-flow and low-flow VMs in the lower limb, using MRI images. To our knowledge, this is the first application of CNNs to perform such a task. We have shown that even with rough annotations and very heterogeneous data it was possible to train a good performing 3D Network.

The number of slices, varying from 14 to 54, had not impacted significantly the performance of the network. Only a reduction to 7 slices showed a significant lower

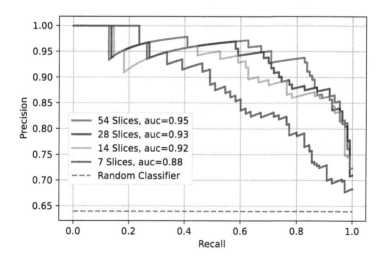

Fig. 2. Precision recall curves comparing 3D ResNets varying the number different number of slices.

performance, establishing a limit on how much information can be taken out until there is a negative impact. As addition or removal of slices were done at the first and the last slices, this result of similar performance also enhanced the importance of the information contained in the middle slices.

The preprocessing step for the T data described in Section 2.3 made our data set more robust regarding to the uncertainty about the VM position. Because of a total of 519 T sequences 325 contained VMs in the upper or lower leg, these regions could potentially be lost with a naive fixed slice area selection in the middle of the T volumes.

We have also indirectly validated the strategy used to select the regions of an MRI image, from which the slices should be extracted, as even with a reduced area, the network's performance was not drastically impacted, thus indicating that the selected section had the highest information density, i.e., with the VM present. In the future we plan to compare our results with physician diagnosis performance with focus on their experience level.

References

1. ISSVA classification of vascular anomalies. https://www.issva.org/classification. Accessed: 2021-10-24. International Society for the Study of Vascular Anomalies, 2018.
2. Sierre S, Teplisky D, Lipsich J. Vascular malformations: an update on imaging and management. Arch Argent Pediatr. 2016;114 2:167–76.
3. Jia Deng, Wei Dong, Socher R, Li-Jia Li, Kai Li, Li Fei-Fei. ImageNet: a large-scale hierarchical image database. Proc IEEE CVPR. IEEE, 2009:248–55.
4. Kay W, Carreira J, Simonyan K, Zhang B, Hillier C, Vijayanarasimhan S et al. The kinetics human action video dataset. 2017.
5. Hara K, Kataoka H, Satoh Y. Can Spatiotemporal 3D CNNs retrace the history of 2D CNNs and ImageNet? Proc IEEE CVPR. IEEE, 2018:6546–55.
6. Tran D, Wang H, Torresani L, Ray J, LeCun Y, Paluri M. A closer look at spatiotemporal convolutions for action recognition. Proc IEEE CVPR. IEEE, 2018:6450–9.
7. Kingma DP, Ba J. Adam: A method for stochastic optimization. Proc ICLR. 2014:1–15.
8. Pérez-García F, Sparks R, Ourselin S. TorchIO: a Python library for efficient loading, preprocessing, augmentation and patch-based sampling of medical images in deep learning. Comput Methods Programs Biomed. 2021;208:106236.

DICOM Whole Slide Imaging for Computational Pathology Research in Kaapana and the Joint Imaging Platform

Maximilian Fischer[1], Philipp Schader[1], Rickmer Braren[2], Michael Götz[1,3],
Alexander Muckenhuber[2], Wilko Weichert[2], Peter Schüffler[2], Jens Kleesiek[4],
Jonas Scherer[1,5], Klaus Kades[1], Klaus Maier-Hein[1], Marco Nolden[1]

[1]Division of Medical Image Computing, German Cancer Research Center (DKFZ), Heidelberg, Germany
[2]School of Medicine, Institute of Pathology, Technical University of Munich, Munich, Germany
[3]Clinic of Diagnostics and Interventional Radiology, Section Experimental Radiology, Ulm University Medical Centre, Ulm, Germany
[4]Institute for AI in Medicine (IKIM), University Medicine Essen, Essen, Germany
[5]Medical Faculty Heidelberg, University of Heidelberg, Heidelberg, Germany
`maximilian.fischer@dkfz-heidelberg.de`

Abstract. With the introduction of whole slide imaging (WSI) systems, several digital pathology applications have emerged. Despite all benefits, lacking appropriate infrastructure to process proprietary WSI file formats for remote diagnosis and annotation is a constraint for widespread application of digital pathology. The joint imaging platform (JIP) already includes a wide range of solutions for digital medical image processing, mainly focused on radiology. We extend the infrastructure in the JIP for accessing, storage, remote analysis and deep learning-based processing of pathological data. By converting proprietary WSI file formats into the DICOM standard, we enable the linkage of radiology and pathology on the JIP and show potential applications in current research studies.

1 Introduction

Clinical decision making for cancer diagnosis and treatment relies in major parts on radiological and pathological imaging. Even if both disciplines are located in the same institution, there is often no direct linkage between their case accession or reporting systems [1]. Recent research [2] has shown that combining both domains can improve clinical decision making. In [2] Jungmann et al. showed a strong association between regional Hounsfield Units and tumor cellularity for pancreatic ductal adenocarcinoma (PDAC). The authors suggest CT-based tumor cell estimates for non-invasive characterization of tumor cellularity in PDAC. Developing such approaches requires the linkage of radiological and pathological data. This connection is hard to establish because no common representation for radiological and pathological data is in wide use. The initial work of Herrmann et al. [3] showed that the Digital Imaging and Communications in Medicine[1] (DICOM®) standard, which is ubiquitously available in radiology, can be applied to pathology and requirements for digital pathology like "virtual microscopy",

---

[1]https://www.dicomstandard.org/

"telepathology" and "computational pathology" are satisfied in DICOM. Opposed to the lack of standardized digital tools for pathology, the advanced digitization of radiology has lead to the development of many software components to support workflows in this field. One example is the *(JIP)* [4], a software platform that combines several aspects of radiology research, designed to support imaging biomarker research in the german cancer consortium (DKTK). The platform provides storage for images, enables data exploration as well as cohort definition and the application of computational methods. By using containerized methods and workflows, method sharing across different JIP instances is enabled and building-blocks for standard tasks simplify the integration of own workflows. Most functionality is accessible via a web interface allowing for the simultaneous interaction with the imaging data stored on the platform by multiple users. The building blocks of the JIP are released as an open source toolkit under the name *Kaapana*, available on GitHub[2].

To better address studies like [2], we aim to extend the JIP and the underlying Kaapana toolkit to support digital pathology research in a standardized way. By extending it to support pathology data, new workflows like parallel viewing or application of computerized algorithms for error-prone tasks like cellulary count or mapping regions of interest on radiology and pathology data are enabled.

2 Materials and methods

The requirements for digital pathology infrastructures are already defined with "virtual microscopy", "telepathology", and "computational pathology" by [3]. Enabling these features on Kaapana requires that pathology data (i) can be stored and retrieved from the platform, (ii) can be viewed and annotated by users and (iii) can be processed in workflows. The following explains how these aspects are implemented in Kaapana.

2.1 Data standardization

To facilitate (i), we use the DICOM standard, first published in 1983 and since then continuously evolving, including support for WSI since 2010 [5, 6]. State of the art in the digital pathology landscape are WSI that are digitized at microscopic resolution and stored in vendor specific file formats with few meta data encoded [5]. Many formats are based on the Tagged Image File Format (TIFF[3]), and generate a multi-resolution image pyramid, which enables zooming and navigation on a slide in real time. In contrast to TIFF, DICOM defines standard protocols to transmit, store, retrieve, process and display medical imaging data, as well as a rich set of meta data elements.

Developed for radiology, Kaapana supports storing, viewing and processing of DICOM images. Choosing the DICOM representation of WSI data seems therefore evident and it was shown that the implementation of the DICOM standard for WSI can be achieved with reasonable effort [3]. Available WSI to DICOM converters[4,5] are

---

[2]https://github.com/kaapana/kaapana
[3]http://www.itu.int/itudoc/itu-t/com16/tiff-fx/docs/tiff6.pdf
[4]https://github.com/GoogleCloudPlatform/wsi-to-dicom-converter
[5]https://github.com/smujiang/WSI2DICOM

also based on [3]. Still, our aim is to provide a digital pathology environment that can easily be extended for individual use cases. Since not all requirements for the linkage of radiology and pathology data in Kaapana are yet fully known, we implement an own conversion to gain more flexibility for further use cases.

Our DICOM WSI conversion is based on [3] and the image pyramid is encoded as a series of image instances, as defined in [6]. This enables fast zooming through image levels for DICOM WSI files in appropriate viewers. To avoid size limitations in the standard (max. 64K columns and rows per frame), each pyramidal level is tiled into smaller pixel frames, compressed and capsulated as one or along with multiple frames to frame items. The maximum number of frames per file is limited to 4 gigabytes. Access patterns for multi-frame DICOM WSI are defined in [6]. Currently most of the available file formats from the OpenSlide[6] initiative are supported by our conversion. A set of mandatory tags is defined that are either extracted from the WSI file or can be provided in an additional YAML file. Linkage between radiology data and pathology data on Kaapana is established by existing DICOM tags like the mandatory StudyInstanceUID.

2.2 Viewing and annotating pathological imaging data

To enable virtual microscopy, viewing and annotating WSI data is a necessity. In the latest Kaapana implementation, the OHIF Viewer [7] is included and allows viewing of DICOM WSI data stored in the PACS. But it does currently not support the annotation of such data.

To overcome the missing annotation capabilities, the open-source Slide Microscopy (Slim) viewer [7] as an additional viewer with annotation capabilities for DICOM WSI is integrated. Like the OHIF Viewer, it is implemented as a web application and is suited to run inside the web interface of a Kaapana instance.

2.3 Computational pathology

To demonstrate a use case of computational pathology on Kaapana, a classification algorithm is implemented that classifies patches from lymph node images into tumor and non-tumor patches, based on the CAMELYON16 challenge [8]. The workflow system of the platform is used to monitor the generation of the DICOM WSI representation and the classification of the data. For classification of lymph node images, a VGG19 neural network architecture [9] is trained according to [10] on 270 lymph node WSI files from the challenge data set. On Kaapana, patches are sampled from the DICOM WSI image instance with the highest magnification. The predicted labels, 0 for no tumor and 1 for tumor, of each patch are stored in a 2-D Dask[7] dataframe with the shape of the original image. Dask is a Python library for parallel computing. Downsampling the dataframe and averaging the labels of several patches yields a heat map with probabilities for each region containing tumorous tissue or not. The heat map might be stored as parametric map or, if mapped to an image using a colormap as derived whole slide image, by the DICOM standard.

---

[6]https://openslide.org/
[7]https://dask.org/

3   Results

In the following, we first present the results of our implemented DICOM conversion algorithm. Then we present how telepathology is enabled in Kaapana and report the results of the computational pathology task.

3.1   Data conversion

As already been mentioned in section 2.1, we extract tiles from the WSI file and generate multi-frame DICOM WSI image instances. Our conversion is implemented with Pydicom[8] and tiles are compressed with lossy JPEG[9] compression and adjustable quality (default=95). Decreasing the quality factor results in smaller file sizes [3]. An example TIFF file with 97792 x 221184 pixels from [8] has a disk size of 2.2 gigabytes and with our conversion the resulting DICOM image instances have a disk size of 2.1 gigabytes. On the one hand using lossy jpeg compression decreases conversion time and relative data size but on the other hand due to data loss the performance of machine learning algorithms might be affected, which is not yet fully investigated [3].

Using DICOM to store WSI images and their annotations integrates well with existing services of the platform. Uploading a ZIP File with WSI data to the platform triggers automatically a workflow to execute the conversion. After the conversion is complete the resulting DICOM images are imported in the platform and the tags of the DICOM objects are also stored in the meta component of the platform. This allows exploration of stored data and also enables the definition of cohorts by allowing to query for certain DICOM tags. Metadata like the patient identifiers can be shared between the radiological and the pathological domain, thus combined processing of data from both areas is enabled. We implemented our own DICOM WSI converter for the JIP that can easily be extended for individual use cases. Our conversion is integrated into the modular concept of the JIP and can be replaced by another conversion if necessary.

3.2   Remote viewing and telepathology

For the integration in Kaapana, the Slim viewer is packaged in a Docker container and configured to retrieve images via the DICOMweb interface from the PACS component of the platform. Annotations generated in the viewer are again stored in the PACS of the platform as DICOM structured report. Before the annotations are stored their metadata are extracted and stored in the meta component of the platform. The viewer is fully integrated in the web interface of the platform as shown in figure 1. While in theory multiple categories of annotations are possible and supported by the Slim viewer, currently only a tissue and a tumor category is used.

3.3   Computational pathology

Figure 1 shows the result of the patch classification in the colorized heat map. The WSI file was transferred to Kaapana via our DICOM WSI conversion and patches were

---

[8]https://pydicom.github.io/
[9]https://jpeg.org/

extracted and classified. The resulting heat map is encoded as a new DICOM WSI image instance within the study of a DICOM WSI file. Both image instances can be visualized in the Slim viewer and a projection of the heat map into the original image is also possible.

4 Discussion

We demonstrated the potential of digital pathology in Kaapana and showed possible applications. An implementation of a common data format for radiology and pathology data and the integration of the Slim viewer on Kaapana was introduced. While we showed the principle capabilities of Kaapana to perform computational pathology, more elaborated tasks on the junction of radiology and pathology, e.g. the matching of pathological and radiological regions in approaches like [2], remain as further work.

Jungmann et al. reported in their study that the connection between radiological and pathological data was hard to establish and could only be realized during parallel viewing of the data by a radiologist and a pathologist. The digital infrastructure for pathology on Kaapana might not only provide computerized algorithms to support pathologists, but also allows for more flexibility in usage scenarios, e.g. through remote access.

Using DICOM as common representation for pathology and radiology reduces the gap between both domains. Cohort definition and sharing imaging data sets and their annotations as well as trained models is easily possible between different Kaapana instances and therefore different users. With this foundation, the first step was taken towards a federated learning infrastructure that is also accessible for WSI data. This

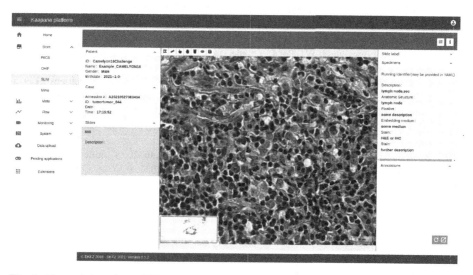

Fig. 1. The web interface of Kaapana with the integrated Slim viewer. The Viewer shows an example image from [8] together with its metadata. The tumor heat map created in section 2.3 is shown in the minimap of the viewer on its lower left corner.

enables the aggregation of distributed trained models across different clinics and incorporating knowledge of all training domains. During the integration of pathology into the JIP, we had an intensive exchange with experts from the pathology and DICOM community and became aware that the DICOM standard is currently still evolving very rapidly in pathology. We are happy to collaborate on this topic and combine knowledge in digital pathology infrastructure.

Acknowledgement. This work was partially supported by the DKTK Joint Funding UPGRADE, Project "Subtyping of pancreatic cancer based on radiographic and pathological features"(SUBPAN), and by the Deutsche Forschungsgemeinschaft (DFG, German Research Foundation) under the grant 410981386.

References

1. Soarce J, Aberle DR, Elimam D, Lawvere S, Tawfik O, Wallace DW. Integrating pathology and radiology disciplines: an emerging opportunity? BMC Med. 2012;10(100).
2. Jungmann F, Kaissis GA, Ziegelmayer S, Harder F, Schilling C, Yen HY et al. Prediction of tumor cellularity in resectable PDAC from preoperative computed tomography imaging. Cancers (Basel). 2021;13(9).
3. Herrmann MD, Clunie DA, Fedorov A, Doyle SW, Pieper S, Klepeis V et al. Implementing the DICOM standard for digital pathology. J Pathol Inform. 2018;9(1):37.
4. Scherer J, Nolden M, Kleesiek J, Metzger J, Kades K, Schneider V et al. Joint imaging platform for federated clinical data analytics. JCO Clin Cancer Inform. 2020;4:1027–38.
5. Clunie DA. DICOM format and protocol standardization: a core requirement for digital pathology success. Toxicol Pathol. 2021;49(4). PMID: 33063645:738–49.
6. DICOM standards committee wg2. DICOM supplement 145-whole slide microscopic image IOD and SOP classes.
7. Fedorov A, Longabaugh WJ, Pot D, Clunie DA, Pieper S, Aerts HJ et al. NCI imaging data commons. Cancer Res. 2021;81(16):4188–93.
8. Bejnordi BE, Veta M, Diest PJ van, Ginneken B van, Karssemeijer N, Litjens G et al. Diagnostic assessment of deep learning algorithms for detection of lymph node metastasis in women with breast cancer. JAMA. 2017;318(22):2199–210.
9. Simonyan K, Zisserman A. Very deep convolutional networks for large-scale image recognition. arXiv:1409.1556. 2015.
10. Berman AG, Orchard WR, Gehrung M, Markowetz F. PathML: a unified framework for whole-slide image analysis with deep learning. medRxiv. 2021.

Efficient DICOM Image Tagging and Cohort Curation Within Kaapana

Klaus Kades[1,2], Jonas Scherer[1,3], Jan Scholtyssek[1], Tobias Penzkofer[5,6],
Marco Nolden[1,4], Klaus Maier-Hein[1,4]

[1]Division of Medical Image Computing, German Cancer Research Center (DKFZ), Heidelberg, Germany
[2]Faculty of Mathematics and Computer Science, Heidelberg University, Heidelberg, Germany
[3]Medical Faculty, Heidelberg University, Heidelberg, Germany
[4]Pattern Analysis and Learning Group, Radio-oncology and Clinical Radiotherapy, Heidelberg University Hospital, Heidelberg, Germany
[5]Department of Radiology, Charité Universitätsmedizin Berlin, Berlin, Germany
[6]Berlin Institute of Health, Berlin, Germany
k.kades@dkfz-heidelberg.de

Abstract. The adaptation and application of medical image analysis algorithms inside a clinical environment comes with the challenge of defining, curating and annotating suitable training and testing cohorts from increasing numbers of available DICOM images. Systems for automated image retrieval and cohort selection have emerged in recent years. Commonly, however, a physician still needs to verify results and take a look at the images themselves to take a final decision. In this work, in order to assist this process and to provide functionalities for standard-conform tagging and adding of free-text to DICOM images, we combine two open source tools, namely Doccano and OHIF Medical Imaging Viewer. We integrate them into the Kaapana open source platform and imaging toolkit. We demonstrate how these functionalities can be leveraged to curate cohorts, add, adjust and enrich DICOM metadata and to tag images for image classification or image-text correlation tasks. Having these steps integrated in a DICOM-conform way also represents an important step towards adopting FAIR-principles in the scientific process.

1 Introduction

A key challenge in the medical image computing domain is to bridge the gap between novel algorithms and their application on routinely acquired imaging data in a clinical environment. In recent years, an increasing number of projects and toolkits focused on closing this gap by providing software and platform solutions which integrate themselves into the clinical landscape.

A proper cohort selection is a critical and often time-consuming step in many respective scenarios. In the best case, this cohort selection can be done automatically based on DICOM tags [1], but often a manual curation step taking into account the images themselves is necessary. On top of that, metadata in DICOM images might be inconsistently or wrongly labeled, not only complicating an automated cohort definition [2] but also hampering the re-use of the data for research purposes. Re-use of research data is one part of the FAIR[1] guiding principles for science, a topic of growing importance, nationally e.g. addressed by initiatives like the NFDI e.V.[2] or the Helmholtz Metadata Collaboration[3]. Curating and enriching data with high quality semantic metadata needs domain-specific tools to support this process in an efficient way, saving valuable domain expert time like in this case of a radiologist. Lastly, many supervised learning algorithm like image classification or image-text correlation algorithms depend on a tag or free-text based annotation. However, most of existing open-source annotation tools that provide the capability of tagging images are either limited to non-DICOM data or focus on the annotation of the image itself.

The introduction of the DICOM standard was a huge step towards standardization in medical imaging that simultaneously opened the door for a fast image retrieval based on metadata. Recent works analyzing the use of these metadata identify benefits but also determine challenges. While some studies argue that DICOM metadata from within one manufacturer is valuable for a cohort definition [1], others identified the cohort selection as a major challenge when assembling large medical imaging datasets, mostly because of inconsistent or missing metadata [2]. As a potential solution, it has been proposed to improve cohort definition by combining the information from Electronic Health Records and DICOM data [3]. In this work, we address the issues by allowing for dedicated, workflow-integrated and standard-conform steps of manual interaction during cohort curation. Moreover, our presented tool can also be used to adjust DICOM tags.

In addition to a proper cohort definition, detailed pixel-wise annotations of DICOM images are often required in the context of medical image computing projects, i.e. semantic segmentation or annotation as offered for example by the Medical Imaging Interaction Toolkit and others [4–7].

Complementary to these approaches, we are here focusing on the image-level fast and intuitive tagging of DICOM images. Technically, we leverage the annotation tool Doccano as well as the OHIF Medical Imaging Viewer, both integrated into Kaapana [4] [8, 9]. The proposed open source solution can be helpful in many scenarios that also go beyond cohort definition, i.e. for correcting wrong metadata of DICOM images, for adding free-text to a DICOM image, or for labeling DICOM images for later applications of machine and deep learning. We evaluate our tool with respect to the feasibility of these mentioned use cases.

2 Materials and methods

Instead of building a software solution from scratch, we make use of the following three open source tools in order to allow the tagging, editing and adding of free-text to DICOM metainformation.

Kaapana is an open-source toolkit to create state-of-the art platforms in the field of medical data analysis. The initial driving project, the Joint Imaging Platform (JIP) of

---

the German Cancer Consortium (DKTK), was realized using Kaapana [10]. Kaapana consists of multiple core components. All components are hosted on a Kubernetes cluster. For the storage of data it integrates the open source PACS system dcm4chee as well as the object store MinIO. For the management of metadata of the DICOM Images and datasets, the search engine Elasticsearch and the dashboard solution Kibana are available. In addition, Airflow is the central component for workflow management, which allows to create customized processing pipelines. Finally, the OHIF Medical Image Viewer serves to display the DICOM data within the platform [10].

The zero-footprint web-based OHIF Medical Imaging Viewer was created by the Open Health Imaging Foundation (OHIF). Besides viewing images it also supports a wide range of image manipulation and annotation tasks. Furthermore, through its support of DICOMweb it allows an direct access to image archives [9].

Doccano is an open-source text annotation tool with the support of various annotation feature, i.e. text classification, sequence labeling and sequence to sequence tasks [8]. The web-based tool offers the possibility to create projects, to upload text datasets in various formats and to add labels for the text classification tasks. The support of keyboard shortcuts allows a very efficient annotation of text data. Recently, Doccano started to support speech to text as well as image classification annotations. However, the image classification is limited to images provided in the Portable Network Graphics format, seldomly used for medical images, and not providing medical expert accustomed navigation and interaction tools.

To display DICOM images within Doccano, we used the straight forward approach of embedding an inline frame (iframe) of the OHIF Viewer into the Doccano user interface. Since the OHIF Viewer displays the images based on the Study Instance UID attribute (0020,000D), in this work, the image tagging is limited to the study level. Doccano's source code was modified to recognize a specially formatted text containing the DICOM-study ID which triggers the integration of the OHIF Viewer showing this study. This approach allows to tag and to add free-text data to a text sample that is referenced to the DICOM Images with the Study Instance UID.

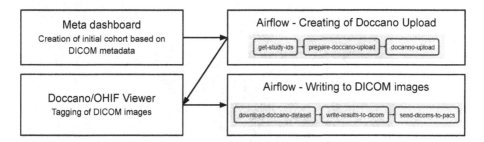

Fig. 1. Illustration of the interplay between the *meta dashboard*, *Airflow* and *Doccano* with the integrated *OHIF Viewer* within the Kaapana platform. On the meta dashboard a cohort is created based on the DICOM metadata. With the help of Airflow the request is processed and passed to Doccano, where a project is created. After finishing the annotation process the added information are written back to the DICOM images via another Airflow workflow.

The bridge to the Kaapana platform is established by making use of the Kibana meta dashboard and the Airflow component. Figure 1 illustrates the whole setup. The meta dashboard within Kaapana contains the extracted metadata of all DICOM images that were send to the internal image archive of the platform. Like [1], we first define a cohort which we want to work on as good as possible on the basis of the DICOM metadata. In a second step the Elasticsearch query of the cohort with the project information for Doccano is transferred to Airflow. In Airflow we implemented a directed acyclic graph (DAG) that uploads the collection of study IDs to Doccano. Once the annotation in Doccano is finished, we provided the possibility to trigger another workflow in Airflow. In its current form, this workflow downloads the annotated data from Doccano and writes the received data directly into the DICOM image. In detail, tags are added comma separated to the DICOM tag Clinical Trial Protocol ID Attribute (0012,0020). Within Kaapana this tag is used as a dataset identifier, because this is the DICOM tag into which the Application Entity Title (AE title) used during transmission is recorded. For classification tasks or when entering free-text the added information can be added to any suitable DICOM tag. For the correction of missing DICOM tags, one can specify, which DICOM tags should be examined when triggering the workflows. After the correction, the DICOM tags are overwritten inside the respective DICOM image.

3   Results

We evaluate our implementation based on the feasibility of three use case scenarios which we identified in cooperation with the projects that use Kaapana, like the Joint Imaging Platform [10]:

1. Curating a cohort selection which was created based on DICOM metadata for the application of a medical image analysis algorithm: For this scenario, the user of the

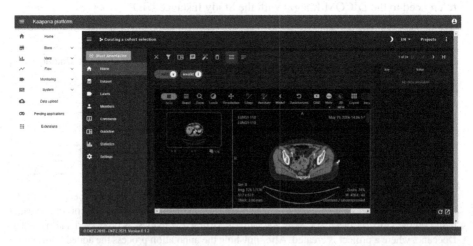

Fig. 2. Illustration of the tagging process for one sample, in which instead of a text sample, the OHIF Viewer with a corresponding study ID is displayed.

platform uses the meta dashboard of Kaapana to predefine the desired cohort based on the DICOM metadata. When sending the data to Doccano they are prompted with an input mask in which they can specify to create a classification project. In the next step, the user switches to Doccano, creates the necessary labels, e.g. a valid and invalid image label, and assigns the labels to the corresponding images. Due to the keyboard shortcuts only two clicks per image are necessary. Once the user went through all images he can send the results back to Airflow where the tags are added to the DICOM images. Figure 2 shows a screenshot of how the tagging of an image looks like inside the platform.

2. Editing the DICOM labels of a segmentation object since the labels given in the DICOM segmentation object are not in all cases correct: As in use case 1, the user can select images which they want to work on via the Kibana meta dashboard and can send the data to Doccano with the specification of which DICOM tags they want to edit. Inside Doccano a sequence to sequence project is created. At the top the user sees the image and at the bottom the specified DICOM tags that they can edit. Again due to the user-friendly implementation of Doccano these steps can be performed with only a few clicks per sample. After finishing the correction on all DICOM images they can save the corrections by triggering a workflow in Airflow which will modify the DICOM data as specified in Doccano.

3. A user wants to add a diagnosis to a DICOM image to use this for a text-image correlation task: Again, the user can define their cohort on the meta dashboard and send the data to Doccano. As in use case 2, a sequence to sequence project is created. The user can now add multiple diagnosis to the DICOM image. As before the number of clicks is negligible in comparison to the time needed to write the diagnosis. When finished, they can send the data back to Airflow where the diagnosis is written into a suitable DICOM tag.

4 Discussion

Overall, the approach of embedding an iframe of the OHIF Medical Image Viewer into Doccano and integrating this implementation into Kaapana unlocks the potential for a fast tagging and editing of DICOM tags as well as adding free-text to DICOM images. In this work, we proofed feasibility of the current version in multiple user scenarios, including the definition, curation and annotation of cohorts for subsequent medical image analysis workflows. In the future, the current iframe solution could be replaced or complemented by other web-based DICOM viewer tools like dcmjs, thus enabling more flexibility with respect to text-based annotations even on pixel-level. This could be achieved using the sequence labeling task of Doccano in combination with a bounding box that is linked to the text sequence. Finally, the dependency on the Study Instance UID Attribute could be resolved by allowing for a selection mechanism that is based on the Patient ID Attribute or the Series Instance UID Attribute. The presented workflow could in the future also be used to ensure high data quality by automatically sending images with missing metadata to Doccano for tagging. By following established or evolving metadata standards in the medical imaging research domain, this might improve the reusability and accessibility of data in the Kaapana platform.

Acknowledgement. This research was supported by the German Cancer Consortium (DKTK, Strategic Initiative *Joint Imaging Platform*), within *Hub Health* by Helmholtz Metadata Collaboration (HMC), and by the German Federal Ministry of Education and Research (BMBF) as part of the University Medicine Network (Project *RACOON*, 01KX2021).

References

1. Gauriau R, Bridge C, Chen L, Kitamura F, Tenenholtz NA, Kirsch JE et al. Using DICOM metadata for radiological image series categorization: a feasibility study on large clinical brain MRI datasets. J Digit Imaging. 2020;33(3):747–62.
2. Magudia K, Bridge CP, Andriole KP, Rosenthal MH. The trials and tribulations of assembling large medical imaging datasets for machine L learning applications. J Digit Imaging. 2021.
3. Almeida JR, Monteiro E, Oliveira JL. An architecture to define cohorts over medical imaging datasets. 2021 IEEE 34th International Symposium on Computer-Based Medical Systems (CBMS). ISSN: 2372-9198. 2021.
4. Nolden M, Zelzer S, Seitel A, Wald D, Müller M, Franz AM et al. The medical imaging interaction toolkit: challenges and advances : 10 years of open-source development. eng. Int J Comput Assist Radiol Surg. 2013;8(4):607–20.
5. Dong Q, Luo G, Haynor D, O'Reilly M, Linnau K, Yaniv Z et al. DicomAnnotator: a configurable open-source software program for efficient DICOM image annotation. J Digit Imaging. 2020;33(6):1514–26.
6. Rubin DL, Rodriguez C, Shah P, Beaulieu C. iPad: semantic annotation and markup of radiological images. AMIA Annual Symposium Proceedings. 2008;2008:626–30.
7. Stein T, Metzger J, Scherer J, Isensee F, Norajitra T, Kleesiek J et al. Efficient web-based review for automatic segmentation of volumetric DICOM images. Bildverarbeitung für die Medizin 2019. Ed. by Handels H, Deserno TM, Maier A, Maier-Hein KH, Palm C, Tolxdorff T. (Informatik aktuell). Wiesbaden: Springer Fachmedien, 2019:158–63.
8. Nakayama H, Kubo T, Kamura J, Taniguchi Y, Liang X. doccano: text annotation tool for human. Software available from https://github.com/doccano/doccano. 2018.
9. Ziegler E, Urban T, Brown D, Petts J, Pieper SD, Lewis R et al. Open health imaging foundation viewer: an extensible open-source framework for building web-based imaging applications to support cancer research. JCO Clin Cancer Inform. 2020;(4). PMID: 32324447:336–45.
10. Scherer J, Nolden M, Kleesiek J, Metzger J, Kades K, Schneider V et al. Joint imaging platform for federated clinical data analytics. JCO Clin Cancer Inform. 2020;(4). PMID: 33166197:1027–38.

Automatic Classification of Neuromuscular Diseases in Children Using Photoacoustic Imaging

Maja Schlereth[1,2], Daniel Stromer[2], Katharina Breininger[1], Alexandra Wagner[3], Lina Tan[3], Andreas Maier[2], Ferdinand Knieling[3]

[1]Department of Artificial Intelligence in Biomedical Engineering,
FAU Erlangen-Nürnberg, Erlangen
[2]Pattern Recognition Lab, FAU Erlangen-Nürnberg, Erlangen
[3]Department of Pediatrics and Adolescent Medicine, Universitätsklinik Erlangen, FAU
Erlangen-Nürnberg, Erlangen
maja.schlereth@fau.de

Abstract. Neuromuscular diseases (NMDs) cause a significant burden for both healthcare systems and society. They can lead to severe progressive muscle weakness, muscle degeneration, contracture, deformity and progressive disability. The NMDs evaluated in this study often manifest in early childhood. As subtypes of disease, e.g. Duchenne muscular dystropy (DMD) and spinal muscular atrophy (SMA), are difficult to differentiate at the beginning and worsen quickly, fast and reliable differential diagnosis is crucial. Photoacoustic and ultrasound imaging has shown great potential to visualize and quantify the extent of different diseases. The addition of automatic classification of such image data could further improve standard diagnostic procedures. We compare deep learning-based 2-class and 3-class classifiers based on VGG16 for differentiating healthy from diseased muscular tissue. This work shows promising results with high accuracies above 0.86 for the 3-class problem and can be used as a proof of concept for future approaches for earlier diagnosis and therapeutic monitoring of NMDs.

1 Introduction

DMD and SMA often manifest in early childhood and are hard to differentiate in early stages [1]. In severe cases, the muscles degenerate quickly, and reliable and fast diagnosis is necessary to start with the correct treatment as early as possible. Currently, confirmation of the diagnosis is typically done by genetic testing which takes up to several months [2]. To support an early assessment, imaging-based diagnosis has been proposed. Photoacoustic (PA) imaging has been investigated as an imaging modality for assessing neuromuscular diseases [3]. It comes with many advantages, as it is non-invasive, has a low acquisition time and is able to differentiate tissue composition based on their PA properties. While ultrasound (US) images depict the morphology of different tissue types, PA images contain functional information. For instance, the wavelength 800 nm helps to observe highly perfused and hemoglobin or myoglobin rich tissue, such as muscular or brain tissue [4, 5]. Regensburger et al. show that PA imaging can be successfully used to detect collagen tissue as a biomarker for DMD as muscular tissue degenerates in DMD and is replaced by collagen or fatty tissue [6]. The authors found significant differences between healthy and diseased tissue regarding signal intensity for

Springer Fachmedien Wiesbaden GmbH, ein Teil von Springer Nature 2022
K. Maier-Hein et al. (Hrsg.), *Bildverarbeitung für die Medizin 2022*,
Informatik aktuell, https://doi.org/10.1007/978-3-658-36932-3_60

collagen. To analyse the data, regions of interest were manually drawn and individually evaluated for each patient. To overcome these limitations, automatic image processing and classification can be used [7]. Zhang et al. propose a traditional machine learning (ML) and a deep learning (DL) method using AlexNet and GoogLeNet for classification of breast cancer for PA images with high accuracies [8], which motivates the use of DL for diagnosis of SMA and DMD.

Our main contributions are the development and evaluation of binary classifiers that differentiate between healthy volunteers and DMD or SMA patients as a proof-of-concept study as well as a three-class classifier (healthy control, DMD, SMA) for a differential diagnosis. As DMD and SMA are difficult to differentiate in early stages, an additional indicator could speed up the diagnostic process. We compare the use of US and PA images with different wavelengths and spectrally unmixed signals (SUS) as input to the network for classification. Furthermore, we analyse the performance of the classifiers across age groups/severity and identify next steps to provide clinicians with rapid diagnostic support for muscular diseases using PA imaging.

2 Materials and methods

In the following section, we will shortly describe the data sets, image preprocessing and the experimental setup for the two-class and three-class problem to differentiate between DMD, SMA and healthy volunteers.

2.1 Datasets

Image data from two studies considering both DMD and SMA were provided by the Department of Pediatrics and Adolescent Medicine at the University Hospital of Erlangen. In these studies PA raw data were generated from 10 patients with DMD, 10 patients with SMA and 20 age-matched controls using a handheld PA system (MSOT Acuity Echo, iThera Medical GmbH, Munich, Germany). In total, the dataset consists of 10 683 valid image frames per single-wavelength (WL) or per SUS. A WL or SUS is used for visualization of different tissue types. Each task was performed with four different input images, i.e., US images, two different WL images (800 nm, 920 nm) and a SUS image (Collagen). At this stage no raw data but only preprocessed data as provided by the vendor software were available, and combining different WL/SUS images did not provide a benefit within this setup.

For DMD, which usually worsens with age, the data is divided into age groups which correlate with the progress of the disease. Three patients aged 5–6, five patients aged 7–8 and two patients aged 9–10 were examined. For SMA, the data is divided by the type of SMA. Patients with type SMA 1 exhibit more obvious symptoms than patients with SMA 2 or 3. For SMA, two patients with SMA 1, four patients with SMA 2 and four patients with SMA 3 were considered. For each class, the data is split patient-wise into training, validation and test set with ratio 0.5, 0.2, 0.3 to represent each severity stage of DMD and SMA in the test set. As the selection of the input image and network architecture was highly exploratory, we opted not to use cross-validation.

2.2 Pre-processing

To obtain the required PA images, the provided raw data was processed with the vendor specific-software to obtain four images containing one WL/SUS each. Furthermore, they were resized to 224 × 224 pixel.

2.3 Experimental setup

A VGG16 network was trained for each classification task (control vs. DMD: 2-class DMD, control vs. SMA: 2-class SMA, control vs. DMD vs. SMA: 3-class) with each of the four different input image types separately. We then used the validation set to determine the best performing WL/SUS for each task for further investigation. For both the two-class and three-class classification tasks, a weighted cross entropy loss was used as loss function to counteract class imbalance. Stochastic gradient descent (SGD) with momentum was set as optimizer. VGG16 was pre-trained on the ImageNet dataset and all weights were frozen except for the last layer [9]. Here, random augmentation techniques were applied to improve the training process (random brightness, noise, saturation, rotation and left-right flipping). Finally, the data was normalized to match ImageNet statistics. For the three-class problem, gradient-weighted class activation mapping (Grad-CAM) was used to highlight regions relevant for the network predictions from VGG16 and further investigate the network prediction. The resulting images were evaluated jointly with a pediatrician (F.K.) experienced in working with US and PA images of muscular tissue.

3 Results

As discussed in the previous section, a separate neural network was trained for each input image type and each classification task. During validation, US showed the best accuracy across all tasks with 0.96 (2-class DMD), 0.83 (2-class SMA) and 0.91 (3-class). Out of the PA images, 920 nm provides the best validation accuracy for 2-class DMD (0.95) and the 3-class case (0.83), whereas the 800 nm image showed the best accuracy for 2-class SMA.

For the final evaluation on the test set, we use the VGG16 networks trained with US and best performing PA image on the validation set, i.e., the 920 nm WL for the 2-class DMD and the 3-class case, and the 800 nm WL for the 2-class SMA. Table 1 shows the final evaluation results on unseen images. All tasks show high accuracies ranging from 0.86 to 1.00 with better performance for the networks with US input, but also discriminative power from the networks with PA input.

Table 2 shows the true positive rate broken down by disease severity for all frames from the three DMD and SMA patients of the test set, respectively, using US and 920 nm input images. As expected, we mainly see errors in patients which are in an earlier stage of disease progression, i.e., DMD at age 5 and SMA type 3. While the error rates are similar for DMD across US and 920 nm, we see a considerably larger difference in errors for SMA between the input types. Table 3 shows the confusion matrix for the 3-class case using US and 920 nm images.

Tab. 1. Accuracy, recall, precision, AUC and F1 score for unseen test data for both 2-class and the 3-class tasks using US and the best PA WL/SUS as input and VGG16 as network architecture.

	Input	Accuracy	Recall	Precision	AUC	F1
2-class DMD	US	0.95	0.92	0.97	0.95	0.95
	920 nm	0.90	0.82	0.96	0.90	0.90
2-class SMA	US	1.00	1.00	0.99	0.99	0.99
	800 nm	0.86	0.97	0.69	0.89	0.86
3-class DMD	US	0.94	0.87	0.98	0.94	0.92
	920 nm	0.91	0.86	0.95	0.91	0.90
3-class SMA	US	0.94	1.00	0.99	0.94	0.99
	920 nm	0.91	0.59	0.93	0.91	0.72

Tab. 2. Percentage of frames classified correctly as DMD or SMA (true positive rate, 3-class case) for three DMD and three SMA patients broken down by different disease states using US and 920 nm images as input. Left: DMD, ages 5,7 and 10. Right: SMA type 1, 2 and 3.

	DMD			SMA		
	Age 10	Age 7	Age 5	Type 1	Type 2	Type 3
US	97 %	98 %	70 %	100 %	100 %	100 %
920 nm	90 %	99 %	69 %	100 %	49 %	31 %

Tab. 3. Relative confusion matrix for US and 920 nm of the 3-class case comparing network prediction and ground truth (GT) labels. Diagonal elements shows percentage of correctly classified frames.

GT	Predicted US			Predicted 920 nm		
	Healthy	DMD	SMA	Healthy	DMD	SMA
Healthy	98.6 %	1.3 %	0.1 %	97.3 %	2.3 %	0.4 %
DMD	12.5 %	87.5 %	0 %	14 %	86 %	0 %
SMA	0 %	0 %	100 %	33.6 %	7.1 %	59.3 %

Figure 1 shows the activated gradients for VGG16 in layer 29 of six different 920 nm WL images. One example each for SMA, DMD and healthy control which is correctly classified and one example each which is wrongly classified is exhibited. The visualization using Grad-CAM shows activated gradients for correctly classified SMA in the central muscle area. In the wrongly classified scan, no central activation is visible. For correctly classified DMD, strong activations are visible in more superficial muscular areas. For the correctly classified healthy scan, no central activations are present.

4 Discussion

In this paper, we show initial results for the classification of neuromuscular diseases based on US and PA images for pediatric patients suffering from DMD and SMA. These initial results on a small dataset are promising across the different settings and tasks. While US imaging provides slightly better quantitative classification results compared to PA input images in our study, clinical observations indicate the potential for an added value by PA images as it may offer finer gradation than US alone. Specifically, it is able to enrich the imaging data with functional information beyond the morphological structures visible in US. As we could not demonstrate a benefit in preliminary experiments yet, further research will have to investigate the potential of combining PA and US images and the limitations of this strategy under a more careful preprocessing scheme.

The dataset in the current study was acquired from a small study population with a comparatively simple network architecture and further evaluation has to be performed to validate our findings. In preliminary experiments, other architectures such as AlexNet, ResNet and EfficientNet-B0 were also considered and performed on par or slightly lower compared to VGG16. An evaluation of this performance difference will be interesting to discuss in future work. Due to the small dataset, we opted for a frame-wise evaluation of

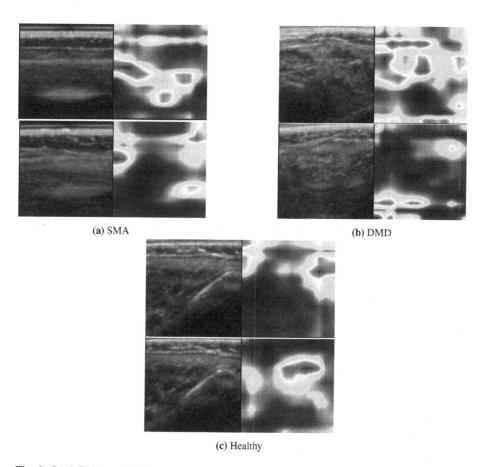

(a) SMA   (b) DMD

(c) Healthy

Fig. 1. Grad-CAM results for (a) SMA, (b) DMD and (c) healthy. Left: 920 nm image (yellow) overlayed on US image, right: heatmap of activated gradients. Highly activated regions are depicted in red and localize class discriminative features. Top row is correctly classified, bottom row is wrongly classified.

the classification. We expect that the classification performance can be increased further if multiple frames or scans of one patient are considered, e.g., via majority voting. On a larger dataset, we further see considerable potential for using multiple input images jointly for a classification to combine complementary information across US and PA, i.e., combining morphology and functional information. This also translates to other applications such as inflammatory diseases where increased blood circulation in the injured region may be identified in the PA images whereas morphological changes can be identified in US images.

Our analysis shows a connection between the number of correctly classified scans and age for DMD, and correctly classified frames and subtype for SMA. This matches well with the fact that older patients in the case of DMD also exhibit more distinct clinical symptoms [1] and that clinical symptoms vary in severeness in the different SMA subtypes [10]. It can therefore be postulated that the disease progression also has clear impact both on the measured US and PA signal. US and PA could potentially be used to monitor treatment process and medication response to support personalized treatment planning and assessment if further research confirms predictability of severity for each disease. Despite the slightly lower performance of PA compared to US, PA's inherent properties will make it an interesting choice for future applications.

References

1. Feldman EL. Atlas of neuromuscular diseases. Springer, 2005.
2. Stuberg WA. Muscular dystrophy and spinal muscular atrophy. Physical therapy for children. 2006:421–52.
3. Wagner AL, Danko V, Federle A, Klett D, Simon D, Heiss R et al. Precision of handheld multispectral optoacoustic tomography for muscle imaging. Photoacoustics. 2021;21:100220.
4. Phelps JE, Vishwanath K, Chang VTC, Ramanujam N. Rapid ratiometric determination of hemoglobin concentration using UV-VIS diffuse reflectance at isosbestic wavelengths. Opt Express. 2010;18(18):18779–92.
5. Kirchner T, Gröhl J, Holzwarth N, Herrera MA, Hernández-Aguilera A, Santos E et al. Photoacoustic monitoring of blood oxygenation during neurosurgical interventions. Photons Plus Ultrasound. Ed. by Oraevsky AA, Wang LV. Vol. 10878. International Society for Optics and Photonics. SPIE, 2019:14–8.
6. Regensburger AP, Fonteyne LM, Jüngert J, Wagner AL, Gerhalter T, Nagel AM et al. Detection of collagens by multispectral optoacoustic tomography as an imaging biomarker for Duchenne muscular dystrophy. Nat Med. 2019;25(12):1905–15.
7. Gröhl J, Schellenberg M, Dreher K, Maier-Hein L. Deep learning for biomedical photoacoustic imaging: a review. Photoacoustics. 2021;22:100241.
8. Zhang J, Chen B, Zhou M, Lan H, Gao F. Photoacoustic image classification and segmentation of breast cancer: a feasibility study. IEEE Access. 2019;7:5457–66.
9. Simonyan K, Zisserman A. Very deep convolutional networks for large-scale image recognition. https://arxiv.org/pdf/1409.1556. 2014.
10. Schara U, Schneider-Gold CJ, Schrank B. Klinik und Transition neuromuskulärer Erkrankungen. Berlin: Springer, 2015.

Realistic Evaluation of FixMatch on Imbalanced Medical Image Classification Tasks

Maximilian Zenk[1], David Zimmerer[1], Fabian Isensee[1], Paul F. Jäger[1],
Jakob Wasserthal[2], Klaus Maier-Hein[1]

[1]Division of Medical Image Computing, German Cancer Research Center (DKFZ)
[2]University Hospital Basel
m.zenk@dkfz-heidelberg.de

Abstract. Semi-supervised learning offers great potential for medical image analysis, as it reduces the annotation burden for clinicians. In this work, we apply the state-of-the-art method FixMatch to chest X-ray and retinal image datasets. Our comparison with the supervised-only method is based on a fair hyperparameter tuning budget and includes label imbalance in the labeled set, thus simulating a practical evaluation setup. We find that unlabeled data can be used effectively for the retinal images, especially when using additional methods to counteract label imbalance in the unsupervised loss. In experiments with CheXpert, however, FixMatch does not provide substantial gains.

1 Introduction

One big challenge biomedical image analysis with deep learning faces today is the small number of annotated training images available for model development. Although this problem also exists in the natural image domain, it is more severe for the medical field, as the annotation is usually time-consuming and requires medical expertise that crowdsourcing solutions usually cannot offer. Methods for semi-supervised learning (SSL) approach this topic by leveraging unlabeled data in addition to a small set of labeled data, in order to improve the performance on the learning objective. Recently, impressive results have been reported in natural image classification, reducing the number of labeled images down to 4 per class while still maintaining decent performance [1].

In the medical domain, several related works have demonstrated how to leverage unlabeled chest X-rays with SSL [2, 3]. However, we observe that two aspects are not always reported in sufficient detail: The supervised baseline model needs to be tuned with a fair budget, and further, label imbalance should be taken into account, which is ubiquitous in medical imaging.

Focusing on these two points, we study how FixMatch [1], a state-of-the-art SSL algorithm, performs on datasets for classifying chest X-rays [4] and fundus images [5] when a realistic evaluation protocol is applied. To the best of our knowledge, we are the first to apply FixMatch to these two datasets. We observe that the gain through FixMatch depends on the dataset as well as the number of labeled training samples, and show how to partially mitigate negative effects of label imbalance.

© Der/die Autor(en), exklusiv lizenziert durch
Springer Fachmedien Wiesbaden GmbH, ein Teil von Springer Nature 2022
K. Maier-Hein et al. (Hrsg.), *Bildverarbeitung für die Medizin 2022*,
Informatik aktuell, https://doi.org/10.1007/978-3-658-36932-3_61

2 Materials and methods

2.1 Datasets

2.1.1 Chest X-ray. The CheXpert [4] dataset contains 224,316 chest X-rays from 65,240 patients. In the publicly available official split, a training set with 64,540 patients and a validation set with 200 patients are included. Labels for 14 clinical observations have been extracted automatically for the training images from radiology reports, whereas radiologists manually labeled the validation samples. Note that every case has multiple (binary) labels, indicating which observations are present in it. The automatically generated labels take values in $\{nan, -1, 0, 1\}$, corresponding to "no mention", "uncertain", "absent", "present "; manual labels are in $\{0, 1\}$.

Following [4], we use 5 of the 14 observations for evaluation: atelectasis (AT), cardiomegaly (CM), consolidation (CS), edema (ED) and pleural effusion (PE). As is commonly done, we replaced nan-values with 0 for training. Moreover, all cases with uncertain labels and all lateral view images were excluded from the dataset. We do not use the official split due to the small validation set and the different annotation procedure. Instead, 80 % of the official training patients are used for model development and 20 % as a holdout test set. From our training set, 15 % are used for validation, resulting in 92,135/16,258/27,101 images in the training/validation/test set. Finally, varying numbers of labeled images (N_l) are randomly sampled from the training set. Images are resized to 224×224 pixels (preserving the aspect ratio through padding) and normalized with ImageNet statistics during preprocessing.

2.1.2 Retina images. Hosted on the kaggle platform, the Eyepacs dataset [5] contains retinal images acquired for diabetic retinopathy (DR) grading. The official split contains 35,126 images for training and 53,576 for testing; these include one image for the left and right eye for each case. Each image has been labeled by a clinician with a grade for the presence/severity of DR, ranging from 0 to 4.

Following [6], labels are binarized here into 0 (no or mild DR) and 1 (moderate or worse DR). We use the official split and additionally reserve 15% of the training data for validation purposes. To create a labeled-unlabeled split, we randomly sample image pairs (left and right eye) from the training set. We preprocess all images by cropping the optical disk and resizing the image (with padding) to 299×299 pixels, followed by normalization with ImageNet statistics.

2.2 Semi-supervised learning with FixMatch

In this study, we experiment with the FixMatch algorithm [1] for semi-supervised learning. FixMatch (FM) uses separate loss functions for the labeled batch of size B and the unlabeled batch of size μB. While the loss for labeled images l_s is regular cross entropy, the unsupervised loss is constructed using two differently augmented versions of an unlabeled image; one weakly augmented and one strongly augmented. Based on the weakly-augmented version, the classification network produces a pseudo-label for the image. The prediction on the strongly-augmented version is then evaluated against this pseudo-label using cross-entropy. Importantly, only pseudo-labels that exceed a certain confidence threshold τ are included in the unsupervised loss. Hence, given a model f and its prediction $q_b = f(\alpha(x_b))$ on an image x_b, weakly augmented with α, the unsupervised loss is $l_u = \frac{1}{\mu B} \sum_{b=1}^{\mu B} \mathbb{I}(\max q_b \geq \tau) H(\hat{q}_b, f(A(x_b)))$, where $\hat{q}_b = \arg\max q_b$ and the strong augmentation function is A. The total loss is then computed as the weighted sum $l = l_s + \lambda_u l_u$. Hyperparameters of FixMatch are λ_u, μ and τ.

2.3 Methods for imbalanced classification

Label imbalance refers to a situation where one class in the dataset is much more frequent than the other (assuming a binary classification task). To improve the performance on the minority class, we apply three methods: oversampling (OS), which uses weighted sampling of training images such that a batch is balanced on average [7]. Note that this is non-trivial for the multi-label samples of CheXpert. Here we simply divide the batch into five parts and ensure that in each, one of the five classes is present in about 1/5 of the samples, which only has a moderately balancing effect overall.

Alternatively, the supervised loss can be re-weighted such that misclassifications of the minority class incur higher cost (loss weighting, LW) [7]. For simplicity, we weight false positives in the supervised loss with 1 and false negatives with N_-/N_+, the overall ratio of negative and positive samples.

Our third approach is distribution alignment (DA) [1, 8], which acts on the unsupervised loss. Here, a "model class prior" $p_m(y)$ is estimated with a running average of the predictions on the weakly-augmented unlabeled samples. Then the model prediction q_b for pseudo-labeling is replaced with $\tilde{q}_b = \text{Normalize}(q_b \cdot p(y)/p_m(y))$, where $p(y)$ is estimated from the labeled data.

2.4 Model selection and evaluation

We attempt to make a fair comparison between FixMatch and the supervised baseline trained only on the labeled data by performing a random search with 60 hyperparameter tuning trials for each on both datasets and by using the same ResNet50 [9] architecture, pretrained on ImageNet. The tuning was performed with $N_l = 3000$ and 2000 labeled images for CheXpert and Eyepacs, respectively. For FixMatch, the learning rate of the Adam optimizer [10], weight decay and FixMatch-specific hyperparameters were tuned. We used rotation, translation, scaling and horizontal flipping as weak augmentation for CheXpert and additionally brightness, contrast and saturation adjustment for Eyepacs. Two transformations sampled from a pool of 14 geometric and intensity transforms (without color transform for chest X-ray data) were added on top of that for the strongly augmented version, following the RandAugment strategy in [1, 11]. For the supervised baseline, we tuned the learning rate, the weight decay and RandAugment's magnitude parameter m, using above strong augmentation method on labeled data. After identifying the best hyperparameters based on their best validation set score (details below), these were used for all experiments reported here.

The validation score for CheXpert is the area under the receiver operating curve (AUC) averaged over the 5 classes and for Eyepacs the AUC. The best model checkpoint according to this score was evaluated on the test set. If not noted otherwise, we report

Tab. 1. Comparison of FixMatch variants to supervised baseline on CheXpert. Mean and std. over 5 seeds are given. Baseline trained using *all* labels (3 seeds): AUC: 82.3 ± 0.1; AP: 53.8 ± 0.1.

CheXpert	AUC (mean over 5 classes)			AP (mean over 5 classes)		
$N_l =$	750	3000	12000	750	3000	12000
Supervised	72.5 ± 0.7	77.3 ± 0.4	79.2 ± 0.2	40.3 ± 0.6	46.0 ± 0.3	49.0 ± 0.3
FM	74.1 ± 0.2	$\mathbf{77.5} \pm 0.1$	$\mathbf{79.5} \pm 0.2$	41.7 ± 0.6	46.1 ± 0.2	$\mathbf{49.3} \pm 0.2$
FM + OS	73.0 ± 0.5	77.1 ± 0.2	79.2 ± 0.2	40.9 ± 0.3	45.7 ± 0.5	48.9 ± 0.2
FM + LW	73.6 ± 0.5	77.0 ± 0.2	79.4 ± 0.1	41.1 ± 0.7	45.6 ± 0.3	48.9 ± 0.2
FM + DA	$\mathbf{74.2} \pm 0.3$	$\mathbf{77.5} \pm 0.1$	79.4 ± 0.1	$\mathbf{41.8} \pm 0.7$	$\mathbf{46.3} \pm 0.2$	49.2 ± 0.1

Tab. 2. Comparison of FixMatch variants to supervised baseline on Eyepacs. Mean and std. over 5 seeds are given. Baseline trained using *all* labels (3 seeds): AUC: 90.9 ± 0.1; AP: 81.5 ± 0.1.

Eyepacs	AUC			AP		
$N_l =$	500	2000	8000	500	2000	8000
Supervised	75.2 ± 1.2	81.9 ± 0.5	87.0 ± 0.2	50.3 ± 3.1	63.8 ± 0.7	74.3 ± 0.1
FM	76.9 ± 2.0	83.7 ± 0.4	88.5 ± 0.2	55.2 ± 3.6	68.8 ± 0.7	$\mathbf{77.2} \pm 0.4$
FM + OS	77.7 ± 1.3	83.8 ± 0.4	88.3 ± 0.1	56.3 ± 2.5	68.3 ± 0.4	76.4 ± 0.2
FM + LW	79.2 ± 1.3	$\mathbf{84.9} \pm 0.4$	$\mathbf{88.7} \pm 0.2$	55.8 ± 4.4	69.1 ± 0.7	77.0 ± 0.5
FM + DA	$\mathbf{80.5} \pm 0.4$	84.5 ± 0.4	88.5 ± 0.2	$\mathbf{59.5} \pm 0.9$	$\mathbf{69.3} \pm 0.7$	77.1 ± 0.5

the performance of a model that is the exponential moving average (EMA; decay rate 0.9995) across all preceding training steps, as in [1].

3 Results

3.1 Out-of-the-box utility of FixMatch

To evaluate how much the FixMatch model can profit from unlabeled data, we perform experiments with various labeling budgets for both datasets, repeated with five different random seeds for the data split (labeled/unlabeled/validation). The correctness of our FixMatch implementation was validated in experiments with the CIFAR-10 dataset, on which we achieved similar performance as reported in [1].

Here we compare FixMatch to the supervised baseline trained on the same labeled set, using the AUC. In our CheXpert experiments, FixMatch only outperforms the baseline with 750 labeled images, indicating that the nearly 90k unlabeled images are not used optimally (Tab. 1, top two rows). For Eyepacs, however, it yields consistent performance gains, except for $N_l = 500$, where the improvement is not as clear due to the larger performance variance across random seeds (Tab. 2, top two rows).

3.2 Effect of label balancing methods

Both medical datasets feature class imbalance, with positive fractions of 42% (PE), 28% (ED), 18% (AT), 12% (CM), 7% (CS) for CheXpert and 20% for Eyepacs. We hypothesize that imbalance is one factor which degrades FixMatch performance and

Fig. 1. Training curves for Eyepacs with 500 labels. Lines and shaded areas are mean ± std. over 5 seeds. Left: Signs of overfitting for most FixMatch variants. Right: Except for distribution alignment, pseudo-labels are disproportionately biased. Dotted line represents the positive fraction in the dataset.

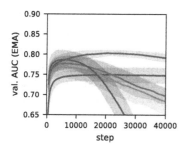 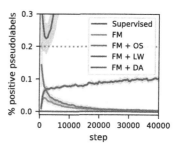

investigate how the methods from section 2.3 affect the learning outcome. This is motivated by the observation that pseudo-labels are biased towards the majority classes. For example, among the predictions on the CheXpert test set by the best model checkpoint (no EMA, $N_l = 3000$) from one training run, 84% are above threshold $\tau = 0.95$ for CM (60% for PE), but only 3% of these (44% for PE) are predicted positive.

To focus more on the performance of the positive classes, we report the average precision metric (AP) in tables 1 and 2 for all FixMatch variants, trained with the methods from section 2.3 (OS, LW, DA). While none of the extensions seem to help for CheXpert, AP values are clearly better for distribution alignment on the Eyepacs dataset. Gains through loss weighting and oversampling are less pronounced. The training curves for Eyepacs and $N_l = 500$ in figure 1 show the desired balancing effect with distribution alignment (purple). All other methods tend to collapse the pseudolabel predictions towards one class. Since the supervised baseline does not show signs of overfitting for Eyepacs, we suspect that those strong class biases originate from the unsupervised loss and are the main reason for the performance drop in the course of FixMatch training.

4 Discussion

In the previous section, we saw that FixMatch struggles to improve classification performance on the CheXpert dataset, while there are small but consistent benefits on Eyepacs. Tackling label imbalance is one option we investigated for improving the results and indeed we found a positive impact of distribution alignment for the Eyepacs dataset.

This improvement was most significant for the lowest N_l setting and did not transfer to CheXpert. It is still possible that other imbalance methods work better in these cases or that those we tried need additional tuning. In practice, hyperparameter tuning for SSL methods is difficult due to the need for labeled validation data. Our model selection used a large validation set, because we wanted to focus on the maximum achievable performance. We plan to evaluate how a realistically small validation set affects the tuning.

Another possible reason for our mixed results is label noise, caused by the automatic annotation for CheXpert and the presence of ungradable images in Eyepacs [6]. Moreover, some components of FixMatch are not dataset agnostic: The augmentation method was developed on RGB images and may not be optimal for X-rays. Further, the thresholding used for pseudo-labeling may not transfer to cases with multiple imbalanced labels per image.

FixMatch is of course only one recent SSL method and we plan to add more methods to our evaluation, to see if the problems encountered here are a general pattern. Results from related works in SSL for chest X-ray classification [2, 3] are unfortunately not directly comparable to ours due to the lack of a standardized data split and evaluation setup. This manuscript presents a first step towards adopting best practices for the evaluation of SSL methods and understanding success and failure modes.

Acknowledgement. This work is partially funded by the Helmholtz Association within the project "Trustworthy Federated Data Analytics "(TFDA) (funding number ZT-I-OO1 4).

References

1. Sohn K, Berthelot D, Li CL, Zhang Z, Carlini N, Cubuk ED et al. Fixmatch: simplifying semi-supervised learning with consistency and confidence. ArXiv. 2020.
2. Liu Q, Yu L, Luo L, Dou Q, Heng PA. Semi-supervised medical image classification with relation-driven self-ensembling model. IEEE Trans Med Imaging. 2020;39(11):3429–40.
3. Gyawali PK, Ghimire S, Bajracharya P, Li Z, Wang L. Semi-supervised medical image classification with global latent mixing. Med Image Comput Comput Assist Interv. Springer. 2020:604–13.
4. Irvin J, Rajpurkar P, Ko M, Yu Y, Ciurea-Ilcus S, Chute C et al. Chexpert: a large chest radiograph dataset with uncertainty labels and expert comparison. Proc Conf AAAI Artif Intell. Vol. 33. (01). 2019:590–7.
5. Kaggle. Diabetic retinopathy detection [online]. 2015.
6. Voets M, Møllersen K, Bongo LA. Reproduction study using public data of: development and validation of a deep learning algorithm for detection of diabetic retinopathy in retinal fundus photographs. PloS one. 2019;14(6):e0217541.
7. Johnson JM, Khoshgoftaar TM. Survey on deep learning with class imbalance. J Big Data. 2019;6(1):27.
8. Berthelot D, Carlini N, Cubuk ED, Kurakin A, Sohn K, Zhang H et al. Remixmatch: semi-supervised learning with distribution alignment and augmentation anchoring. ArXiv. 2019.
9. He K, Zhang X, Ren S, Sun J. Deep residual learning for image recognition. Proc IEEE Comput Soc Conf Comput Vis Pattern Recognit. 2016.
10. Kingma DP, Ba J. Adam: a method for stochastic optimization. ArXiv. 2014.
11. Cubuk ED, Zoph B, Shlens J, Le QV. RandAugment: practical automated data augmentation with a reduced search space. ArXiv. 2019.

Initialisation of Deep Brain Stimulation Parameters with Multi-objective Optimisation Using Imaging Data

Mehri Baniasadi[1,2], Andreas Husch[1], Daniele Proverbio[1], Isabel Fernandes Arroteia[2], Frank Hertel[2], Jorge Gonçalves[1]

[1]University of Luxembourg, Luxemburg Center for Systems Biomedicine, Campus Belval, 6 avenue du Swing, L-4367 Belvaux
[2]Centre Hospitalier de Luxembourg, National Department of Neurosurgery, 4 Rue Nicolas Ernest Barblé, L-1210 Luxembourg
mehri.baniasadi@uni.lu

Abstract. Following the deep brain stimulation (DBS) surgery, the stimulation parameters are manually tuned to reduce symptoms. This procedure can be time-consuming, especially with directional leads. We propose an automated methodology to initialise contact configurations using imaging techniques. The goal is to maximise the electric field on the target while minimising the spillover, and the electric field on regions of avoidance. By superposing pre-computed electric fields, we solve the optimisation problem in less than a minute, much more efficient compared to finite element methods. Our method offers a robust and rapid solution, and it is expected to considerably reduce the time required for manual parameter tuning.

1 Introduction

Deep brain stimulation (DBS) is a surgical treatment for a number of neurological disorders, including essential tremor (ET) and Parkinson's disease (PD). It reduces the symptoms of the disease by stimulating specific region of the brain (Target) via implanted electrodes.

After the electrode implantation, a parameter tuning session is performed. The goal is to cover the target region as much as possible with the effective electric field or the volume of tissue activated (VTA). Another goal of the parameter tuning session is to avoid stimulating the regions associated with side effects. Normally, the parameter tuning procedure is performed manually, until an improvement in symptoms is observed. Numerous possible combinations for contact configuration often cause the tuning procedure to be long and demanding for both patients and physicians. Moreover, it might not conclude with the maximal clinical benefits.

Several algorithms have been proposed to find the optimal parameters, including the simple scoring method [1], weighted metric method [2], fuzzy and probabilistic optimization [3], and constraint optimization [4].

We propose a novel method suggesting an initial contact configuration for the DBS parameter tuning session using the weighted sum method for the first time. The algorithm has three objectives: maximizing the electric field on the target, minimising the electric field outside of the target, and minimising the electric field on the region of avoidance

(ROA). We formulate our multi-objective problem by optimising over a weighted-sum cost function, which also includes priorities for each objective region to be defined by the user. We chose the weighted sum method, as it enables prioritization of the objective according to the subject's case. With two case studies, we demonstrate the importance of the user-defined weights enabling personalised medicine. Benefiting from FastField [5], an algorithm for electric field simulation, the optimisation algorithm solves in only 20-40 seconds. Thanks to its rapidity, the optimisation can also be solved for different amplitude values. Performing a trade-off between the evaluation metrics for different amplitude values, the optimal amplitude and its corresponding contact configuration can be chosen. The solution of this algorithm is robust and comprehensive and can be used for both cylindrical and directional leads.

2   Method

To maximise the effect of the DBS, a computational model of DBS-induced electric field in the patient's brain is necessary. We reconstruct the DBS target structures and the electrode using MRI and CT scan. Once the DBS case is reconstructed, our multi-objective approach is solved for the initial contact configuration.

2.1   Target and electrode reconstruction

The patient's MRI is registered to the Montreal Neurological Institute (MNI) space using Advanced Normalization Tool (ANTs)[1]. The location of the target is extracted using an atlas registered into the MNI space . For this study we use Distal and Thomas atlas. Patient's CT is registered to the MRI using FMRIB's Linear Image Registration Tool (FLIRT)[2]. We use the PaCER algorithm to extract the location of the electrode in the brain [6], and the DioDe algorithm to detect the rotation of the electrode [7].

2.2   Initialisation of DBS parameters

The procedure of finding the initial setting is divided into two parts. First, it identifies the contacts that are close to the target, in particular, the segmented contacts facing towards the target. Second, it solves the optimal contact configuration problem for the selected contacts, while fixing amplitude, pulse width and frequency to keep the energy consumed constant. The electric field $E(g)$ around the electrode is simulated using FastField [5] over a 3D grid G with constantly spaced points $\{g\}$. The points where the electric field value is higher than the threshold (200 V/mm) are considered as the VTA volume.

2.2.1   Ranking the contacts. We measure the Euclidean distance between the center gravity of each contact with the center gravity of the target. Contacts are ranked based on their proximity to the target (Fig. 1, left). For the segmented contacts, we measure

---

[1]http://stnava.github.io/ANTs/
[2]https://fsl.fmrib.ox.ac.uk/fsl/fslwiki/FLIRT

the angle between the center of the contact and the center of the target. Contacts facing towards the target are ranked higher (Fig. 1, right). Once all the contacts are ranked, the optimisation can be solved on the top 4 highly ranked contacts. This ranking step is optional and the optimisation can also be solved on all the contacts.

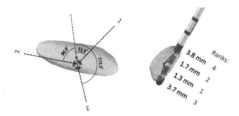

Fig. 1. A Boston Scientific Vercise directional lead is shown for the ranking. The 4 rings are ranked based on their distance to the target. The segmented contacts are ranked based on their angle to the target.

2.2.2   Optimisation problem. We solve a multi-objective optimisation for the weight of contacts (w_n). The objectives include maximizing the electric field on target, minimising the electric field outside of target and minimising the electric field on the region of avoidance (ROA). The latter is optional. We formulate this multi-objective problem with the weighted sum method as in (Eq. 2). Partition the simulation grid $\mathcal{G}$ into the three areas of interest: $\mathcal{K}$ (target), $\mathcal{O}$ (off-target), $\mathcal{R}$ (ROA), such that $\mathcal{G} = \{\mathcal{K}, \mathcal{O}, \mathcal{R}\}$. Solve

$$\min_{w_n} \left[\alpha \sum_{g \in \mathcal{G}} E(g, w_n) - \beta \sum_{g \in \mathcal{K}} E(g, w_n) + \gamma \sum_{g \in \mathcal{R}} E(g, w_n) \right] \tag{1}$$

$$\text{subject to } \sum_{n}^{N} w_n = 1, \text{ with } \forall_n \in N : w_n > 0 \tag{2}$$

where

$$E(g, w_n) = \sum_{n}^{N} E_n^0(g) \cdot \frac{w_n \cdot A}{A_0} \cdot \frac{\kappa_0}{\kappa} \tag{3}$$

is the electric field produced by each contact $n = [1 \ldots N]$ and computed at each point g of the 3D grid $\mathcal{G}$. α, β, γ are user-defined priority terms that can be used to prioritize one objective over another; their default values are 1, 2, and 1. $\alpha = 1$ and $\beta = 1$, and $\gamma = 0$ corresponds to minimising the electric field outside of the target. $\beta = 1, \alpha = 0$, and $\gamma = 0$ corresponds to maximizing the electric field on the target. $\gamma = 1, \alpha = 0$, and $\beta = 0$ corresponds to minimising the electric field on ROA.

N is the number of contacts of the electrode, w_n is the weight associated to each contact. E_n^0 is the pre-computed e-field for each contact. A is the amplitude and κ the brain conductivity value. A_0 and κ_0 are amplitude and conductivity values used to generate the pre-computed e-fields [5]. The brain conductivity value is 0.1 S/mm for all the calculations in this study. The optimisation problem is solved using MATLABs fmincon function with the interior point method.

2.3   Performance evaluation

To evaluate the performance, we measure the percentage of the target and the ROA covered by the VTA (Target coverage, and ROA coverage), and the percentage of the VTA outside of the target (VTA spillover).

2.4   Amplitude evaluation

The optimisation algorithm is solved for different amplitude values, ranging from 1 to 8 mA. A simple trade-off between the objectives is performed to initialise the amplitude value. The VTA spillover and the ROA coverage are deducted from the target coverage. The amplitude with the highest trade-off (TROFF) value is chosen as the initial stimulation amplitude.

3   Results

We use the imaging data from two de-identified patients to evaluate our optimisation approach.

3.1   Case study 1

Case 1 is an Essential tremor patient, with VIM as the target, VPL as the ROA, and a Boston Scientific Vercise directional lead implantation. The optimisation is solved for the contact configuration using amplitude values 1 to 8 mA. The target coverage, ROA coverage , and the VTA spillover for different amplitude values are shown in (Fig. 2). The amplitude with the highest TROFF value, and its corresponding contact configurations are chosen as the final setting, in this case, 5 mA with TROFF value of 16. The optimal Contact configuration for this case is shown in (Fig. 2). The Target coverage, ROA coverage, and the VTA spillover 62% , 2%, and 44%.

3.2   Case study 2

Case 2 is a Parkinson patient, with STN as the target, no ROA, and a Boston Scientific Vercise directional lead implantation. The optimisation is solved for the contact configuration using amplitude values 1 to 8 mA. The target coverage, and the VTA spillover for different amplitude values are shown in (Fig. 3). In this case, no ROA is considered. The amplitude with the highest TROFF value, and its corresponding contact configurations are chosen as the final setting, in this case, 2 mA with TROFF value of 23. The optimal Contact configuration for this case is shown in (Fig. 3). The Target coverage and the VTA spillover are 48% and 24%.

3.3 Evaluation of ranking and time efficiency

To evaluate the performance of the ranking method, the optimisation algorithm was run for both case 1 and 2 once on all contacts and once on the chosen contacts with the selected amplitudes values of 5 and 2 mA. The algorithm resulted in similar contact configuration in both cases.

Once extracting the location of the target, the time needed to run the optimisation algorithm was 41.7, and 20.0 seconds for case 1 and 2 respectively (MacBook Pro, 2.3 GHz Intel Cori5, 16 GB memory).

4   Discussion

In this paper, we propose an efficient method for optimising the contact configuration for DBS programming session. Our objective function is defined to satisfy three objectives

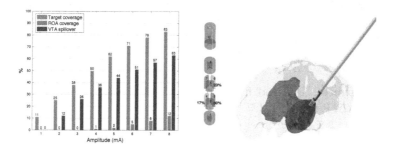

Fig. 2. Case study 1. The evaluation metrics when solving the optimisation with different amplitude values are plotted on the left. For this optimisation, the electrode is precisely inside the target; hence, we assign same priorities for the three objectives, $\alpha = 1$, $\beta = 2$, and $\gamma = 1$. On the right, the chosen contact configuration corresponding to amplitude 5 mA is plotted. VTA is plotted in red, VIM in green, VPL in yellow, and the whole Thalamus in gray.

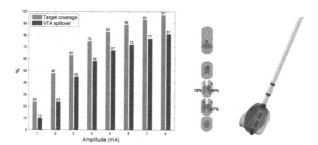

Fig. 3. Case study 2. The evaluation metrics when solving the optimisation with different amplitude values are plotted on the left. For this optimisation, the electrode is in the lateral part of the target, therefore, we assign a higher weight (β) to prioritize the maximisation of the electric field on the target. α, β, and γ values thus equal to 1, 4, and 0 were chosen. On the right, the chosen contact configuration corresponding to amplitude 2 mA is plotted. VTA is plotted in red, and STN in green.

while considering their corresponding weights, in contrast to other existing method that optimise the DBS settings on one of the objectives and maintain other objectives lower than a threshold. We leave the priority terms α, β, and γ as free parameters, to be chosen by practitioners depending on their needs. Examples of different priority values are shown in the case studies.

Like for other optimisation algorithms, the result depends on the correct image registrations, target segmentation, and electrode localization. Any uncertainty in the previous steps impacts the result of the optimisation. This work is evaluated on patients imaging data, but it has not been tested on patients. Future steps will involve testing the suggested contact configuration on patients and evaluate the symptoms response. We recall that this algorithm suggests plausible settings to initiate the tuning session, and not the final optimal setting. Thus, fine tuning from the practitioners' side might be necessary.

Overall, this study shows that the weighted sum method can be used to form the DBS multi-objective optimisation problem, to maximise the electric field on the target while reducing the electric field outside of the target and on the region of avoidance. The method is robust, efficient, and it is expected to considerably reduce the time needed for the DBS programming session. Furthermore, the method will be publicly available upon acceptance.

Acknowledgement. This work has been supported by Fonds National de la Recherché (FNR), grant AFR ref. 12548237.

References

1. McIntyre CC, Butson CR, Maks CB, Noecker AM. Optimizing deep brain stimulation parameter selection with detailed models of the electrode-tissue interface. Proc Annu Int Conf IEEE Eng Med Biol. 2006:893–5.
2. Xiao YZ, Peña E, Johnson MD. Theoretical optimization of stimulation strategies for a directionally segmented deep brain stimulation electrode array. IEEE Trans Biomed Eng. 2016;63(2):359–71.
3. Peña E, Zhang S, Deyo S, Xiao Y, Johnson MD. Particle swarm optimization for programming deep brain stimulation arrays. J Neural Eng. 2017;14(1).
4. Anderson DN, Osting B, Vorwerk J, Dorval AD, Butson CR. Optimized programming algorithm for cylindrical and directional deep brain stimulation electrodes. J Neural Eng. 2018;15(2).
5. Baniasadi M, Proverbio D, Gonçalves J, Hertel F, Husch A. FastField: an open-source toolbox for efficient approximation of deep brain stimulation electric fields. Neuroimage. 2020:1–12.
6. Husch A, V. Petersen M, Gemmar P, Goncalves J, Hertel F. PaCER - a fully automated method for electrode trajectory and contact reconstruction in deep brain stimulation. Neuroimage Clin. 2018;17(October 2017):80–9.
7. Hellerbach A, Dembek TA, Hoevels M, Holz JA, Gierich A, Luyken K et al. DiODe: directional orientation detection of segmented deep brain stimulation leads: a sequential algorithm based on CT imaging. Stereotact Funct Neurosurg. 2018;96(5):335–41.

Pathologiespezifische Behandlung von Labelunsicherheit bei der Klassifikation von Thorax-Röntgenbildern

Sebastian Steindl, Tatyana Ivanovska, Fabian Brunner

Fakultät Elektrotechnik, Medien und Informatik, OTH Amberg-Weiden
s.steindl@oth-aw.de

Zusammenfassung. Die Interpretation von Thorax-Röntgenbildern ist ein zentraler, nicht-trivialer Bestandteil der Diagnose von Lungen- oder Herzkrankheiten. Bei der Erzeugung der Label, die zum Einsatz von überwachten Deep Learning Methoden notwendig sind, herrscht eine gewisse Unsicherheit, die in den Labeln festgehalten werden kann. In dieser Arbeit soll die pathologiespezifische Behandlung dieser Labelunsicherheit im Vordergrund stehen. Es konnte gezeigt werden, dass dieses Vorgehen den durchschnittlichen ROC-AUC bei mehreren Modellarchitekturen verbessert.

1 Einleitung

Thorax-Röntgenbilder (CXR) stellen für Radiologen eine wichtige Grundlage zur Diagnose von Lungen- oder Herzkrankheiten dar [1]. Mit der Veröffentlichung von großen CXR-Datensätzen (z. B. ChestX-ray14 [2], PadChest [3], CheXpert [4]) in den letzten Jahren und durch die Covid-19 Pandemie ist das Forschungsinteresse an der automatisierten Diagnose mittels Deep Learning stark angestiegen.

Für die größeren Datensätze (mehr als 100.000 Bilder) ist es unpraktikabel, alle Label von Radiologen manuell erzeugen zu lassen. Daher wird für gewöhnlich ein NLP-Tool verwendet, das aus den textuellen Radiologieberichten automatisiert die Label extrahiert. CXR sind jedoch auch für erfahrene Radiologen nicht trivial zu interpretieren und in der Praxis werden für die Diagnose weitere Informationsquellen einbezogen. Auch eine „Inter-observer variability", also Abweichungen zwischen mehreren Radiologen, ist möglich [5].

Um die Unsicherheit in den Radiologieberichten im Datensatz widerzuspiegeln, existiert im CheXpert-Datensatz [4] neben der positiven (1) und negativen (0) Klasse auch eine „uncertain" (-1) Klasse. Für das ungeschulte Auge sind die Pathologien nicht zu erkennen (Abb. 1). In der Literatur wurden verschiedene Methoden, wie man mit solchen uncertain Labels umgeht, beschrieben. Irivin et al. [4] zeigte, dass bestimmte Strategien deutlich wirksamer für einige Diagnosen waren. Zum Beispiel wurde festgestellt, dass für Kardiomegalie das sogenannte U-MultiClass-Modell (AUC = 0.854) signifikant besser als das sogenannte U-Ignore-Modell funktionierte. Pham et al. [6] schlugen die sogenannte label smoothing regularization (LSR) vor. Dieses Verfahren erlaubte die

K. Maier-Hein et al. (Hrsg.), *Bildverarbeitung für die Medizin 2022*,
Informatik aktuell, https://doi.org/10.1007/978-3-658-36932-3_63

Leistung von Mehrklassen-Klassifizierungsmodellen durch Glätten des Label-Vektors jedes Sample zu steigern.

In dieser Arbeit werden die Verfahren mit Uncertain-Labels analysiert und eine effektive Erweiterung, nämlich das pathologiespezifische Smoothing, wird vorgeschlagen.

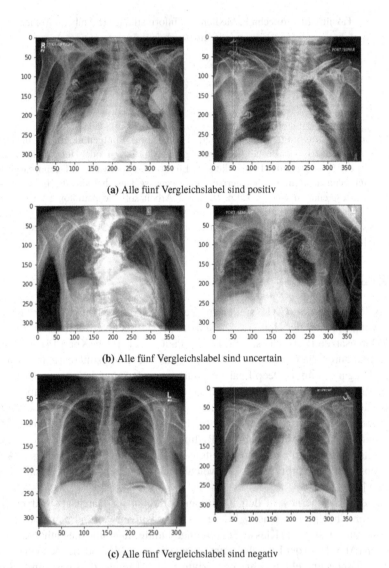

Abb. 1. Beispiel für CXR mit positiven, uncertain und negativen Klassen. In jeder Reihe werden zwei Beispiel gezeigt.

2 Material und Methoden

Im Folgenden wird der genutzte Datensatz, bisherige Ansätze sowie die Methode der pathologiespezifischen Behandlung der Labelunsicherheit vorgestellt.

2.1 Material

Der CheXpert-Datensatz [4] enthält 224.316 Bilder von 65.240 Patienten, die im Zeitraum zwischen Oktober 2002 und Juli 2017 am Standford Krankenhaus aufgenommen wurden. Der Datensatz enthält die folgenden 14 Label: No Finding, Support Devices, Fracture, Lung Opacity, Pneumothorax, Enlarged Cardiomegaly, Pneumonia, Lesion, Pleural Other, Atelectasis, Edema, Pleural Effusion, Consolidation und Cardiomegaly. Die Gütebewertung der Modelle findet allerdings nur anhand der letzten fünf Pathologien statt.

Bei etwa der Hälfte der Aufnahmen liegt die uncertain Klasse vor. Innerhalb der Vergleichspathologien ist der Anteil dieser unterschiedlich groß, und reicht bis zu knapp 15% bei dem Label Atelectasis und 12% bei Consolidation, womit -1 etwa genauso bzw. doppelt so häufig ist wie die positive Klasse 1. Dahingegen ist der Anteil bei Edema, Pleural Effusion und Cardiomegaly mit 6.17%, 5.02% und 3.52% deutlich geringer. Eine angemessene Behandlung dieser Label ist demnach von großer Bedeutung.

Der Validierungsdatensatz ist bei CheXpert standardisiert und enthält 234 CXR, die unabhängig voneinander durch drei Radiologen gelabelt wurden und deren Mehrheitsentscheid die finale Klasse festlegt [4].

2.2 Bisherige Ansätze

Irvin et al. [4] haben verschiedene Methoden vorgeschlagen, wie man mit den Uncertain Labels umgeht:

- U-Ignore: Ignorieren der Label bei der Loss-Berechnung.
- U-Zeros: Ersetzen von -1 durch 0.
- U-Ones: Ersetzen von -1 durch 1.
- U-SelfTrained: Zunächst wird mit U-Ignore ein Modell trainiert, das anschließend verwendet wird um die uncertain Label vorherzusagen.
- U-MultiClass: -1 wird neben 0 und 1 als weitere Klasse betrachtet.

Es wurde gezeigt, dass das U-Ignore Modell fast immer ineffektiv war, besonders für Kardiomegalie.

Pham et al. [6] nutzten eine andere Methode, die sogenannte Label Smoothing Regularization (LSR). Dabei wird -1 nicht durch einen festen Wert ersetzt, sondern durch einen zufällig aus einem Wertebereich gezogenen Wert. Die Autoren legen aufgrund empirischer Bewährtheit ein zu 0 tendierendes Intervall $[0, 0.3]$ und analog $[0.55, 0.85]$ fest. Diese Methoden wurden als U-Zeros+LSR und U-Ones+LSR bezeichnet. Dieses Label Smoothing soll verhindern, dass das Modell zu zuversichtlich ist auf Bildern, deren Label unsicher und eventuell falsch ist. Es wurde gezeigt, dass solche Regularisierung die Ergebnisse deutlich verbessert.

2.3   Pathologiespezifische Behandlung

Die bisher vorgestellten Methoden gehen indirekt davon aus, dass die tatsächliche Klasse eines uncertain Label unabhängig von der Pathologie ist. Allerdings ist durchaus denkbar, dass in Abhängigkeit von beispielsweise Symptomen, Dringlichkeit und weiteren Diagnostikmöglichkeiten die Radiologen ähnlich wie Modelle unterschiedliche Klassifikationsschwellwerte für einzelne Pathologien haben, und somit auch unterschiedlich starke Unsicherheiten in den Radiologieberichten entstehen.

Zudem ist die in dem Datensatz repräsentierte Auftrittshäufigkeit zwischen den Pathologien stark unterschiedlich. Während zum Beispiel Pleural Effusion bei 40% der Aufnahmen positiv ist, wurde Consolidation nur in rund 7% der Fälle festgestellt. Dies wird durch die Tatsache verstärkt, dass es sich bei der Problemstellung um eine Multilabel Klassifikation mit teilweise hierarchisch zusammenhängenden Krankheitsbildern handelt und einzelne Pathologien eine Art Überbegriff darstellen.

Demnach scheint es sinnvoll, die Behandlung der uncertain Label pathologiespezifisch zu gestalten. In dieser Arbeit wurde daher mit U-Mixed eine Kombination von U-Ones und U-Zeros aus der Arbeit von Irvin et al. [4] sowie als U-Mixed+LSR eine Erweiterung der LSR-Methode aus der Arbeit von Pham et al. [6] untersucht.

Im Paper von Irvin et al. [4] wurde präsentiert, für welche Pathologie der U-Ones bzw. U-Zeros Ansatz zu besseren ROC-AUC-Werten führte. Demnach war der U-Ones-Ansatz für Atelectasis, Edema und Pleural Effusion dem U-Zeros-Verfahren überlegen.

Somit wird mit der U-Mixed-Methode ein uncertain Label u bei den Pathologien Atelectasis, Edema und Pleural Effusion mit 1 und bei Consolidation und Cardiomegaly mit 0 ersetzt.

Analog definiert sich U-Mixed+LSR über das ersetzten von u durch o bei den Pathologien Atelectasis, Edema und Pleural Effusion sowie durch z bei Consolidation und Cardiomegaly, wobei o und z je gleichverteilt zufällig gezogen werden als $o \sim U(0.55, 0.85)$ und $z \sim U(0, 0.3)$. Die Gewichtungsintervalle wurden aus der originellen Arbeit von Pham et al. [6] übernommen.

2.4   Experimentaufbau

Für den Vergleich wurden drei Modellarchitekturen verwendet: Ein DenseNet-121, MobileNet-V2 und ein ResNet-50. Diese wurden mit den auf dem ImageNet-Datensatz vortrainierten Gewichten initialisiert und für 25 Epochen mit dem nach der Auftrittshäufigkeit der positiven Klasse gewichteten Binary Cross Entropy Loss und dem Adam Optimisierer trainiert. Die Lernrate betrug initial $1e-4$ und wurde bei einem Loss-Plateau um den Faktor 0.1 reduziert. Die Bilder wurden mit einer Batchgröße von 64 in die Netzwerke gegeben und für das Training auf die Auflösung 256×256 skaliert, bevor ein 224×224 Rechteck aus der Mitte ausgeschnitten wurde. Außerdem kam als Bildaugmentierung mit einer Wahrscheinlichkeit von $p = 0.5$ ein Links-Rechts-Spiegeln und eine zufällige Rotation um bis zu ± 10 Grad zum Einsatz. Die Bilder wurden mit Mittelwert und Standardabweichung des ImageNet-Datensatzes normalisiert. Nach Ende des Trainings wurde immer das Modell jener Epoche verwendet, in der der höchste ROC-AUC-Wert erzielt wurde.

Tab. 1. ROC-AUC-Werte der Modelle je nach uncertain Methode auf den Validierungsdaten. Die beste Methode je Modell ist kursiv hervorgehoben.

Methode	DenseNet-121	MobileNet V2	ResNet-50
U-Zeros	0.863	0.864	0.874
U-Ones	0.870	0.871	0.873
U-Mixed	0.880	0.878	0.874
U-Zeros+LSR	0.873	0.864	0.871
U-Ones+LSR	0.873	0.870	0.874
U-Mixed+LSR	*0.882*	*0.879*	*0.885*

Tab. 2. ROC-AUC-Werte des DenseNet-121 je nach uncertain Methode aufgeschlüsselt nach den Vergleichspathologien. Die beste Methode je Pathologie ist kursiv hervorgehoben.

Methode	Atelectasis	Edema	Pleural Effusion	Consolidation	Cardiomegaly
U-Zeros	0.792	0.916	0.926	0.909	0.775
U-Ones	0.845	0.918	0.913	0.877	*0.795*
U-Mixed	0.841	*0.925*	0.926	0.914	*0.795*
U-Zeros+LSR	0.797	0.923	0.910	*0.942*	*0.795*
U-Ones+LSR	0.817	0.923	0.909	0.933	0.783
U-Mixed+LSR	*0.852*	0.918	*0.932*	*0.942*	0.768

3 Ergebnisse

Der Vergleich der verschiedenen Methoden zeigt, dass der U-Mixed-Ansatz für alle verglichenen Architekturen bessere Resultate liefert als U-Zeros und U-Ones (Tab. 1). Des Weiteren wurden mit U-Mixed+LSR höhere ROC-AUC-Werte erzielt als mit U-Ones+LSR oder U-Zeros+LSR und diese Methode führte auch insgesamt zu den besten Ergebnissen. Diese Resultate zeigen, dass eine auf die jeweilige Pathologie angepasste Behandlung der Labelunsicherheit zu Verbesserungen der Modelle führen kann.

Bei der Betrachtung der ROC-AUC-Werte der einzelnen Pathologien, die mit dem DenseNet-121 erreicht wurden (Tab. 2) ist ersichtlich, dass die pathologiespezifische Behandlung (U-Mixed oder U-Mixed+LSR) bei vier von fünf Labeln den besten ROC-AUC-Wert erzielt. Einzig die Kardiomegaly sticht heraus, bei der mit der U-Mixed+LSR-Methode der geringsten ROC-AUC-Wert erreicht wurde. Da bei dieser der Anteil der uncertain Klasse am geringsten ist, sind die Unterschiede zwischen den einzelnen Methoden aber auch kleiner.

Bei den beiden Pathologien für die der uncertain Anteil am höchsten ist (Atelectasis und Consolidation) erzielte der U-Mixed+LSR-Ansatz die besten Ergebnisse.

4 Diskussion

Die Einschätzungen, ob die Unsicherheit bei einer Pathologie tendenziell eher mit der positiven oder negativen Klasse ausgeglichen werden soll, stützt sich in dieser Arbeit auf die empirischen Ergebnisse von Irvin et al. [4]. Durch medizinisches Fachwissen und mit einer genaueren Untersuchung des Verhaltens des Labeling-Tools bezüglich der Radiologieberichte könnte diese Einschätzung verfeinert und abgesichert werden.

Außerdem wurden die Grenzwerte für die LSR ohne weitere Untersuchungen von der Arbeit von Pham et al. [6] übernommen. Diese wurden jedoch für den Einsatz auf allen fünf Labeln gewählt. Daher ist davon auszugehen, dass in der Feinabstimmung dieser Grenzen auf die einzelnen Pathologien weiteres Optimierungspotenzial liegt. Dies sollte in einer zukünftigen Arbeit untersucht werden. Da die Testdaten nicht öffentlich sind, werden in Anlehnung an Pham et al. [6] die Resultate auf dem Validierungsdatensatz gezeigt.

Insgesamt zeigen die Ergebnisse, dass eine pathologiespezifische Behandlung der Labelunsicherheit die Klassifikationsresultate verbessern kann.

References

1. De Lacey G, Morley S, Berman L. The chest x-ray: a survival guide e-book. Elsevier Health Sciences, 2012.
2. Wang X, Peng Y, Lu L, Lu Z, Bagheri M, Summers RM. Chestx-ray8: hospital-scale chest x-ray database and benchmarks on weakly-supervised classification and localization of common thorax diseases. Proc IEEE Comput Soc Conf Comput Vis Pattern Recognit. 2017:2097–106.
3. Bustos A, Pertusa A, Salinas JM, Iglesia-Vayá M de la. Padchest: a large chest x-ray image dataset with multi-label annotated reports. Med Image Anal. 2020;66:101797.
4. Irvin J, Rajpurkar P, Ko M, Yu Y, Ciurea-Ilcus S, Chute C et al. Chexpert: a large chest radiograph dataset with uncertainty labels and expert comparison. Proc Conf AAAI Artif Intell. Vol. 33. 2019:590–7.
5. Çallı E, Sogancioglu E, Ginneken B van, Leeuwen KG van, Murphy K. Deep learning for chest x-ray analysis: a survey. Med Image Anal. 2021:102125.
6. Pham HH, Le TT, Tran DQ, Ngo DT, Nguyen HQ. Interpreting chest X-rays via CNNs that exploit hierarchical disease dependencies and uncertainty labels. Neurocomputing. 2021;437:186–94.

3D CNN-based Identification of Hyperdensities in Cranial Non-contrast CT After Thrombectomy

Alexandra Ertl[1,2], Alfred Franz[3], Bernd Schmitz[4], Michael Braun[4]

[1]Faculty of Medical Engineering and Mechatronics, Ulm University of Applied Sciences
[2]mbits imaging GmbH
[3]Institute of Computer Science, Ulm University of Applied Sciences
[4]Department of Neuroradiology, District Hospital Günzburg
ertl@mbits.info

Abstract. To restore blood flow after an ischemic stroke due to large vessel occlusion, thrombectomy is a common treatment method. The postoperative non-contrast computed tomography (CT) often shows hyperdense regions which are due to hemorrhagic transformation or contrast staining. Since further treatment decisions depend on the presence of hyperdensities, their reliable detection is necessary. The Deep Learning based approach presented in this study can support radiologists in this task. The dataset consists of 241 postoperative volumetric non-contrast CTs. They are labeled by a binary classification regarding the presence or absence of a hyperdensity. A shallow 3D CNN architecture and a preprocessing pipeline were proposed. A part of the preprocessing is windowing the CTs to enhance contrast. Different windowing thresholds were defined based on knowledge regarding the CT values of brain tissue and hyperdensities. Using the proposed window with a level of 50 HU and a width of 60 HU, the network achieved an accuracy of 89 % on the test data. Without windowing, an accuracy of only 46 % was achieved. The present study demonstrates the importance of appropriate preprocessing and how domain knowledge can be included to optimize it. The results indicate that reducing the input information in a meaningful way accentuates relevant features in the images and enhances the network performance.

1 Introduction

Worldwide, approximately one in four people will suffer a stroke during their lifetime [1]. Ischemic strokes account for the majority of those. They are caused by a vascular occlusion in the brain arteries. Thereupon the subsequent brain tissue is no longer adequately supplied and damaged irreversibly. To restore blood flow, the thrombus can be removed by thrombolysis or thrombectomy. During thrombectomy, the thrombus is located by performing an angiography with the use of a contrast agent. It is then removed by a catheter, which is inserted into the occluded vessel. On the postoperative non-contrast computed tomography (CT), hyperdensities can be found in many cases. They are caused by hemorrhagic transformation or contrast staining [2, 3]. While contrast staining usually disappears within 48 h, hemorrhagic transformation requires appropriate treatment depending on the extent of the bleeding. Accordingly, if hyperdensities are found, further investigation is necessary to identify the cause.

© Der/die Autor(en), exklusiv lizenziert durch
Springer Fachmedien Wiesbaden GmbH, ein Teil von Springer Nature 2022
K. Maier-Hein et al. (Hrsg.), *Bildverarbeitung für die Medizin 2022*,
Informatik aktuell, https://doi.org/10.1007/978-3-658-36932-3_64

The goal of this study was to develop a deep learning (DL) network for detecting hyperdensities in postoperative cranial non-contrast CT of thrombectomy patients. The CTs should be labeled per volume by performing a binary classification. The two classes are defined as "positive" and "negative" regarding the presence or absence of a hyperdensity. The network could assist physicians in reviewing postoperative CTs to accelerate the diagnosis, reduce the chances of missing hyperdensities and thus improve patient treatment.

The authors are not aware of any work on DL-based detection of hyperdensities in postoperative non-contrast CT of thrombectomy patients. Therefore, the literature review focused on DL-based approaches for the detection and classification of intracranial hemorrhage.

Arbabshirani et al. [4] developed a five layers deep 3D convolutional neural network (CNN) to identify intracranial hemorrhages on non-contrast CT. The dataset consisted of about 40,000 CT volumes. The "bleeding window" with a level of 40 Hounsfield Units (HU) and a width of 80 HU was applied to increase the contrast in the images. The network achieved an area under the curve (AUC) of 84.6 %.

Ker et al. [5] designed a 3D CNN to classify four different types of brain hemorrhage and normal cases using 399 non-contrast CT volumes. The three layers deep network achieved F1-scores of 71 % to 90 % for binary classification (normal versus hemorrhage), depending on the type of hemorrhage. The authors also investigated a thresholding procedure, which is applied to the images. This further improved the F1-scores to 92 % to 95 %.

In a study building on the work of Ker et al., Singh et al. [6] investigated the same 3D CNN for the identification of four different types of brain hemorrhages and normal cases in non-contrast CT images using 491 CT volumes. They tested an intensity normalization method similar to the thresholding method of Ker et al. The network was compared with a 3D ResNet and two different 3D VggNets. Their shallow 3D CNN achieved F1-scores of 93 % to 99 % for binary classification (normal vs hemorrhage), depending on the type of hemorrhage, and provided the best results of the study.

In the present study, a 3D CNN was evaluated for a new use case, the identification of hyperdensities in post-thrombectomy non-contrast CT. CNNs often rely on large datasets, as in the study of Arbabshirani et al., whereas the present study uses a comparably small dataset. A shallow CNN architecture was developed since Singh et al. discovered that these networks might give better results than very deep and complex architectures. Following the ideas behind windowing and thresholding the CTs in the mentioned studies, a windowing procedure was investigated. In the present study, the thresholds of the window were defined by including prior knowledge about the intensity values of brain tissue and hyperdensities and optimized by evaluating different thresholds.

2 Materials and methods

2.1 Data

The dataset was provided by the department of neuroradiology of the District Hospital Günzburg. It consists of postoperative non-contrast CTs of 241 different patients. The

CTs were acquired immediately after thrombectomy. The resolution of each axial slice is 512 x 512. Each CT consists of approximately 200 to 230 slices with a slice thickness of 1.5 mm. Each CT volume was labeled under supervision of an experienced radiologist. A CT volume was assigned to the positive class if a hyperdensity was found in any of the slices or to the negative class if no hyperdensity was found in the entire CT. The dataset was randomly separated into training and test data. The class distribution is shown in Table 1. Figure 1 shows slices of four different patients with hyperdensities.

	Tositive	Negative	Total
Training data	116	88	204
Test data	21	16	37
Total	137	104	241

Tab. 1. Class distribution and total number of cases in the training data, test data and the entire dataset.

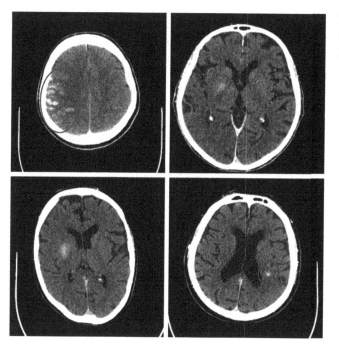

Fig. 1. Hyperdensities in slices of four different postoperative CTs.

2.2 Preprocessing

The preprocessing of the CTs consists of two steps, segmenting the brain and applying different image preprocessing operations.

1. The brain segmentation was automated by using the image computing software package 3D Slicer. First, the cranial bone is selected using the thresholding operation

with an threshold of 300 HU. Next, the largest cavity within the skull, which corresponds to the brain, is segmented by using the "Wrap Solidify" [7] extension.

2. The segmented volumes were resized to 256 x 256 x 128 using spline interpolation. Since the voxel values in a cranial CT typically range from -1024 HU to more than 1000 HU, windowing is applied to limit the values to the dynamic range of interest and enhance contrast. The intensity values of healthy brain tissue range from about 25 HU to 35 HU, while those of hyperdensities range from about 60 HU to 100 HU. Considering these values, different windows were defined and evaluated. The best results on the validation data were achieved by using a window with a level of 50 HU and a width of 60 HU.

2.3 Proposed network

The proposed network architecture is shown in Figure 2. The network consists of five convolutional layers, each followed by a max-pooling layer. The number of filter kernels for the convolutional layers are 32, 64, 128, 256, and 512. The kernel size is 3 x 3 x 3. After the final max-pooling layer, a batch normalization layer and a flatten layer are added to normalize the values and reshape the feature maps to a 1D feature vector. A dense layer consisting of 1024 neurons follows to classify the vector. For the convolutional layers and the dense layer Rectified Linear Unit (ReLU) activation and L2 regularization are used. The output layer contains two neurons which are activated by a softmax function and represent the two classes "positive" and "negative".

The network is trained for 75 epochs while evaluating the loss on the validation data to identify the best epoch. The respective weights are stored in the final model. The network was trained using five-fold cross-validation. Adam optimizer and categorical cross-entropy loss were used. A grid search was used to optimize batch size, learning

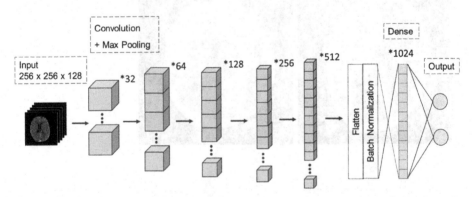

Fig. 2. Architecture of the proposed network. The input has a shape of 256 x 256 x 128. The network consists of five convolutional layers, each followed by a max-pooling layer. The blue boxes represent the respective feature maps. The number of filter kernels for each layer is shown next to the feature maps. A batch normalization layer and a dense layer consisting of 1024 neurons follow. The output layer contains two neurons.

Tab. 2. Performance on the test data without windowing and using the proposed windowing with level = 50 HU and width = 60 HU.

Windowing	Precision	Recall	F1-Score	Accuracy
None	0.52	0.57	0.55	0.46
L: 50 HU, W: 60 HU	0.95	0.86	0.90	0.89

rate, and learning decay. The best results on the validation data were achieved by using a batch size of 2, a learning rate of 0.0001, a decay rate of 0.1, and 10000 decay steps.

The network was implemented using Tensorflow and trained using a Nvidia RTX Titan GPU with 24 GB dedicated storage.

Five-fold cross-validation results in five trained models. A majority vote is used to aggregate the classification of the test data of all five models to a final consent. The following test results are based on the calculated majority vote. To assess the effect of windowing, the proposed network was trained and tested using the original full dynamic range of the image values as well as using the proposed window.

3 Results

The first row in Table 2 shows the results of the test data without using windowing. All statistical parameters have values of about 50 %.

The second row in Table 2 shows the classification results of the test data using the proposed window with a level of 50 HU and a width of 60 HU. It is noticeable that the precision of 95 % is higher than the recall of 86 %. All statistical parameters have values of about 90 %.

4 Discussion

A 3D CNN based architecture was chosen to process spatial information along all axes of the input. 3D filter kernels enable the network to efficiently recognize 3D patterns in the data. Therefore interrelationships between the slices of CTs can be taken into account. In this case, 3D filters might help detect hyperdensities that are visible in multiple slices.

Since 3D filter kernels have an additional dimension compared to the more common 2D kernels, the amount of parameters grows and with it the amount of required data. A large number of parameters makes training the network more difficult. Parameter optimization becomes more complex and the network might be more susceptible to overfitting [8, 9]. To keep the number of parameters low despite the use of a 3D model and to be able to learn from a small dataset, a shallow architecture was developed. Studies show that such shallow 3D CNNs can outperform deeper and more complex networks [6, 10].

The results in Table 2 show that without windowing, the network only achieved an accuracy of 46 % and therefore was not able to distinguish between the postive and negative class. Only by using the proposed window, the test data was classified reliably with an accuracy of 89 %. The enhancement of the performance by windowing can be attributed to shifting the network's focus on the relevant information in the data. The contrast in the images is improved and the difference in the intensity values between healthy brain tissue and hyperdensities is enhanced. The patterns to recognize hyperdensities are thereby accentuated which makes them easier to detect. This allows the use of a more simple network architecture that contains fewer parameters and requires less training data. Similar performance enhancements by using thresholding methods were observed in other studies as well [5].

In this work, promising results were only achieved by the use of appropriate pre-processing methods. For this purpose, simple image processing techniques performed in an automated way can be sufficient. The work demonstrates that preprocessing based on domain knowledge can enable the network to learn meaningful patterns even from a small dataset. The results further indicate that reducing the information in the input data to accentuate relevant features can improve the network output significantly.

To improve the accuracy of the network and the significance of the results, it is recommended to use the approach with a larger dataset. Furthermore, transfer learning could help overcome the challenges of a small data set. In future work, the proposed approach could be applied to other similar use cases.

References

1. Virani SS, Alonso A, Benjamin EJ, Bittencourt MS, Callaway CW, Carson AP et al. Heart disease and stroke statistics-2020 update: a report from the American heart association. Circulation. 2020;141(9):e139–e596.
2. Ng FC, Campbell BCV. Imaging after thrombolysis and thrombectomy: Rationale, modalities and management implications. Curr Neurol Neurosci Rep. 2019;19(8):57.
3. Puntonet J, Richard ME, Edjlali M, Ben Hassen W, Legrand L, Benzakoun J et al. Imaging findings after mechanical thrombectomy in acute ischemic stroke. Stroke. 2019;50(6):1618–25.
4. Arbabshirani MR, Fornwalt BK, Mongelluzzo GJ, Suever JD, Geise BD, Patel AA et al. Advanced machine learning in action: identification of intracranial hemorrhage on computed tomography scans of the head with clinical workflow integration. NPJ Digit Med. 2018;1(1):9.
5. Ker J, Singh SP, Bai Y, Rao J, Lim T, Wang L. Image thresholding improves 3-dimensional convolutional neural network diagnosis of different acute brain hemorrhages on computed tomography scans. Sensors (Basel). 2019;19(9).
6. Singh SP, Wang L, Gupta S, Gulyas B, Padmanabhan P. Shallow 3D CNN for detecting acute brain hemorrhage from medical imaging sensors. IEEE Sens J. 2020:1.
7. Weidert S, Andress S, Linhart C, Suero EM, Greiner A, Böcker W et al. 3D printing method for next-day acetabular fracture surgery using a surface filtering pipeline: feasibility and 1-year clinical results. Int J Comput Assist Radiol Surg. 2020.
8. Singh SP, Wang L, Gupta S, Goli H, Padmanabhan P, Gulyás B. 3D deep learning on medical images: a review. Sensors (Basel). 2020;20(18).
9. Yeo M, Tahayori B, Kok HK, Maingard J, Kutaiba N, Russell J et al. Review of deep learning algorithms for the automatic detection of intracranial hemorrhages on computed tomography head imaging. J Neurointerv Surg. 2021;13(4):369–78.
10. Polat H, Danaei Mehr H. Classification of pulmonary CT images by using hybrid 3D-deep convolutional neural network architecture. Appl Sci (Basel). 2019;9(5):940.

Predicting Aneurysm Rupture with Deep Learning on 3D Models

Annika Niemann[1,2], Bernhard Preim[1], Oliver Beuing[3], Sylvia Saalfeld[1,2]

[1]Institut für Simulation und Graphik, Otto-von-Guericke Universität Magdeburg,
[2]Forschungscampus STIMULATE,
[3]AMEOS Hospital Bernburg
annika.niemann@ovgu.de

Abstract. Rupture risk analysis of intracranial aneurysms is important for treatment decisions. Morphological parameters like size, diameter or aspect ratio are used to capture the relevant aspects of the aneurysm shape and predict the rupture of intracranial aneurysms. Automatic calculation of these parameters is cumbersome, whereas manual measurements are time-consuming, error-prone and subject to inter-observer variance. Instead of classification based on morphological parameters, here, deep learning on aneurysm surface meshes is used to classify 3D surface meshes of intracranial aneurysm into ruptured and unruptured. We compared several deep learning approaches on surfaces meshes and point clouds showing patient-specific aneurysm geometries. Using 150 aneurysms for training and 40 for testing, a test accuracy of 82,5% was achieved.

1 Introduction

Intracranial aneurysms are a pathological vessel deformation with a prevalence between 2% and 4% [1]. They bear the risk of rupture yielding stroke and/or fatal consequences for the patient. The risk of aneurysm rupture is estimated between 0.3% and 15% and highly differs between patients. On the contrary, treatment of unruptured intracranial aneurysms exposes a risk of 1% mortality and around 5% morbidity [1, 2].

For intracranial aneurysm treatment with minimal risk to the patient, evaluation of the rupture risk of an aneurysm is important. An established tool for this is the PHASES Score [2] and the UIATS score [3]. The risk factors included in the PHASES score are population, hypertension, age, aneurysm size, earlier subarachnoid hemorrhage (SAH) and site of aneurysm. Depending on these factors a PHASES score between 0 and 22 is determined, where aneurysms with a score >5 are at high risk to rupture within five years.

The unruptured intracranial aneurysm treatment score (UIATS) uses patient specific risk factors (for example age, previous SAH, smoking, ethnicity, hypertension, kidney disease, drug/alcohol abuse), aneurysm features (diameter, irregularity, location, changes in serial imaging) and also evaluates treatment risk. Depending on the score the UIATS suggest "treatment", "conservative management", or "not definitive" [3].

© Der/die Autor(en), exklusiv lizenziert durch
Springer Fachmedien Wiesbaden GmbH, ein Teil von Springer Nature 2022
K. Maier-Hein et al. (Hrsg.), *Bildverarbeitung für die Medizin 2022*,
Informatik aktuell, https://doi.org/10.1007/978-3-658-36932-3_65

Feghali et al. [4] calculated the PHASES and UIATS values for 992 ruptured aneurysms. Of these, 54% had a low rupture risk according to the PHASES score. The UIATS would have recommend conservative treatment for 26% and "not definitive"for 38%, indicating the weakness of these metrics.

Several studies explored suitable parameters for reliable aneurysm rupture prediction. A wide variation of morphological parameters were introduced, for example diameter, aspect ratio, aneurysm height, volume, ellipticity index, non-spherical index, undulation index [5].

The PHASES score is popular, as it is simple to use. More advanced methods often require significant effort or time, for example complex calculation of morphological parameters or manual measuring the aneurysm. Additionally, these parameters can be measured slightly different. For example can the aneurysm height be defined as maximal or as orthogonal distance between dome and neck. This has an impact on the rupture prediction [6].

To use the aneurysm shape without the need for morphological parameters, deep learning directly on 3D models of intracranial aneurysm could be utilized. In this paper, several architectures for deep learning on 3D models are used to classify aneurysms in ruptured and unruptured aneurysms.

2   Materials and methods

In this study, 3D meshes of intracranial aneurysms from the public available aneurisk dataset [7] and meshes derived from aneurysm data collected at the University Hospital Magdeburg were used.

Each mesh comprises at least one aneurysm and various surrounding vessels. The meshes are cut such that each mesh only shows the aneurysm and the parent vessel. Two different mesh cutting approaches are used: manual mesh cutting using MeshLab and a semi-automatic mesh cutting. For the semi-automatic approach, the meshes were first automatically segmented into parts based on convexity [8]. The next step is the manual identification of sections belonging to the aneurysm and the vessel sections directly at the aneurysm (parent vessel). Figure 1 shows the result of the automatic part segmentation (coloured segments) in the user interface for the semi-automatic mesh cutting. From these parts the user selects the aneurysm and the parent vessel. Figure 2 shows an example of the mesh after semi-automatic mesh cutting. Next, the meshes are remeshed to a similar number of faces. The semi-automatic approach offers an reproducible way to cut the meshes and minimizes the user-depends. The length of the included parent vessel in the semi-automatic approach depends on the shape, especially the presence or absence of bifurcating vessels and the bend of the parent vessel. While this indirectly encodes additional information, it also leads to higher variance in the inclusion of the parent vessel compared to manual segmentation.

Several algorithms were used: MeshNet [9] and MedMeshCNN [10] for classification of meshes and Pointnet++ [11] for point cloud classification. Each algorithm has a different focus. Pointnet++ only uses the vertices of the mesh. MeshNet calculates several features for each face of the mesh, while MedMeshCNN calculates features per edge.

Pointnet++ is the extension of Pointnet [12]. It adds hierarchical point set feature learning. Pointnet++ can be used for classification and segmentation.

MeshNet uses the face centers as a spatial descriptor. The mesh structure is captured using the face corners and normals. In mesh convolution blocks these features are aggregated with neighboring information.

MedMeshCNN, which is an extension of MeshCNN [13], uses five features per edge: dihedral angle, inner angles of the two adjacent faces and edge-length ratio for each face. Then an edge collapse process is used for mesh pooling.

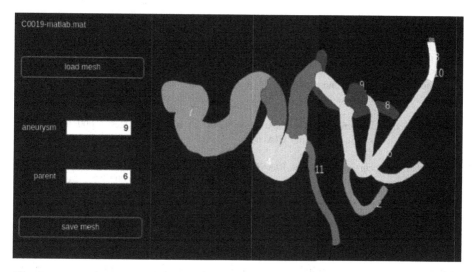

Fig. 1. User interface for semi-automatic mesh cutting: after automatic part segmentation the aneurysm and parent vessel are selected. Each automatic segmented section is shown in a different colour.

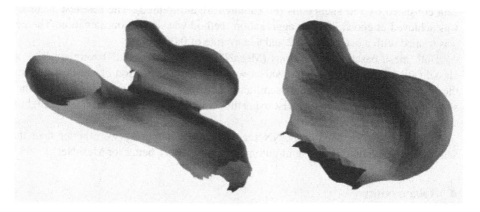

Fig. 2. Example result of semi-automatic mesh cutting: right: mesh showing only the aneurysm and left: mesh of aneurysm with parent vessel.

Tab. 1. Selected results of deep learning aneurysm classification (RIA: ruptured intracranial aneurysm, UIA: unruptured intracranial aneurysm).

Algorithm	Dataset	Training data	Test data	Parameters	Accuracy
MeshNet	aneurysm and parent, based on convex split	RIA: 89 UIA: 61	RIA: 20 UIA: 20	max number faces: 1025 learn rate: 0.0001 batch size: 2	test: 82,5% train: 99,33% at epoch 73
MeshNet	only aneurysm	RIA: 42 UIA: 42	RIA: 20 UIA: 20	max number faces: 5000 learn rate: 0.0001 batch size: 2	test: 80% train: 100% at epoch 95
MeshNet	manual cut, only bifurcation aneurysms	RIA: 34 UIA: 26	RIA: 10 UIA: 10	max number faces: 5000 learn rate: 0.0004 batch size: 2	test: 80% train: 85% at epoch 92
MeshNet	aneurysm and parent, based on convex split	RIA: 61 UIA: 61	RIA: 20 UIA: 20	max number faces: 5000 learn rate: 0.0004 batch size: 2	test: 72,5% train: 90,98% at epoch 138
MedMeshCNN	aneurysm and parent, manual cut	RIA: 108 UIA: 198	RIA: 10 UIA: 10	max input edges: 17000 learn rate: 0.0002 batch size: 8	test: 70% at epoch 21
MedMeshCNN	aneurysm and parent, based on convex split	RIA: 62 UIA: 62	RIA: 20 UIA: 20	max input edges: 17000 learn rate: 0.0001 batch size: 2	test: 65.0% at epoch 4
PointNet++	aneurysm and parent, manual cut	RIA: 73 UIA: 73	RIA: 20 UIA: 20	number of points: 5000 learn rate: 0.002 batch size: 4	test: 67,5% epoch: 197

3   Results

Table 1 shows selected results of deep learning classification for intracranial aneurysms.

The best classification was achieved with MeshNet on meshes showing the aneurysm and parent vessel according to the semi-automatic, convexity-based mesh cutting. The test accuracy on 20 ruptured and 20 unruptured aneurysms was 82.5%. The training data consisted of 150 aneurysms (89 ruptured/61 unruptured). The best test accuracy was achieved at epoch 73. The aggregation method was set as concatenation. The net was trained with a batch size of 2 and a learn rate of 0.0001.

Both mesh-based classifications (MeshNet and MedMeshCNN) were superior to classification on point clouds. MeshNet was best in classification of meshes showing the aneurysm and parent based on semi-automatic cutting. The performance on meshes showing only the aneurysm, likewise using the semi-automatic mesh cutting, was slightly worse.

In this study, for MedMeshCNN the manually cut meshes were better than the semi-automatic, contrary the semi-automatic meshes were better for MeshNet.

4   Discussion

While the results suggest that deep learning on 3D data might be useful for aneurysm rupture prediction, there are several limitations. The number of training data is small, especially as there is a high variance in intracranial aneurysm shape.

Each algorithm has a large number of parameters. Additionally, several choices of data preprocessing are possible. The possibility cannot be ruled out that other parameter choices lead to different results. Some parameter combinations are limited by current hardware capacity. Due to technical limitations batch size, mesh size and neural net size cannot be independently changed.

The semi-automatic cutting based on the automatic, convexity based part segmentation encourages consistent mesh cutting between users. While the variation between users is minimized compared to the manual cutting, the variation between aneurysms increases. The length of the included parent vessel changes, as the automatic part segmentation can split up the parent vessel into a few large or several smaller parts, depending on the curvature. In contrast, the manual cutting includes similar roughly large portions of the parent vessel. Therefore, this splitting could add some useful attributes, as it indirectly encodes the curvature of the vessel, or hinder the deep learning with unnecessary information and larger variation between data.

Compared to other mesh classification tasks, like classification of furniture, aneurysm classification is not easily solvable for a human. Risk factors like female gender, age and smoking might be not visible in the aneurysm shape. Currently, the available data is too small to evaluate whether shape as sole basis for rupture prediction is feasible or not. Very similar shapes might have a different outcome depending on other patient attributes. Including patient features might improve the results.

In conclusion, deep learning on surface meshes can be used to predict aneurysm rupture. With 150 meshes of intracranial aneurysms MeshNet was trained to classify aneurysms in ruptured or unruptured. Based on 40 test aneurysms it achieved an accuracy of 82.5%. For the optimal result MeshNet and semi-automatic mesh cutting was used. Here, mesh-based deep learning architectures were better than classification on point clouds.

Acknowledgement. This work is partly funded by the German Research Foundation (SA 3461/2-1) and the Ministry of Economics, Science and Digitization of Saxony-Anhalt within the Forschungscampus STIMULATE (grant number 13GW0473A).

References

1. Bijlenga P, Gondar R, Schilling S, Morel S, Hirsch S, Cuony J et al. PHASES score for the management of intracranial aneurysm. Stroke. 2017;48(8):2105–12.
2. Greving JP, Wermer MJH, Brown RD, Morita A, Juvela S, Yonekura M et al. Development of the PHASES score for prediction of risk of rupture of intracranial aneurysms: a pooled analysis of six prospective cohort studies. The Lancet Neurology. 2014;13(1):59–66.
3. Etminan N, Brown RD, Beseoglu K, Juvela S, Raymond J, Morita A et al. The unruptured intracranial aneurysm treatment score. Neurology. 2015;85(10):881–9.
4. Feghali J, Gami A, Xu R, Jackson CM, Tamargo RJ, McDougall CG et al. Application of unruptured aneurysm scoring systems to a cohort of ruptured aneurysms: are we underestimating rupture risk? Neurosurg Rev. 2021.
5. Saalfeld S, Berg P, Niemann A, Luz M, Preim B, Beuing O. Semiautomatic neck curve reconstruction for intracranial aneurysm rupture risk assessment based on morphological parameters. Int J Comput Assist Radiol Surg. 2018;13(11):1781–93.

6. Lauric A, Baharoglu MI, Malek AM. Ruptured status discrimination performance of aspect ratio, height/width, and bottleneck factor is highly dependent on aneurysm sizing methodology. Neurosurgery. 2012;71(1):38–46.

7. Aneurisk-Team. AneuriskWeb project website. Web Site. 2012.

8. Kaick O van, Fish N, Kleiman Y, Asafi S, Cohen-Or D. Shape segmentation by approximate convexity analysis. ACM Trans. on Graphics. 2014;34(1).

9. Feng Y, Feng Y, You H, Zhao X, Gao Y. MeshNet: mesh neural network for 3D shape representation. AAAI 2019. 2018.

10. Schneider L, Niemann A, Beuing O, Preim B, Saalfeld S. MedMeshCNN - enabling MeshCNN for medical surface models. CoRR. 2020;abs/2009.04893.

11. Qi CR, Yi L, Su H, Guibas LJ. PointNet++: deep hierarchical feature learning on point sets in a metric space. CoRR. 2017;abs/1706.02413.

12. Qi CR, Su H, Mo K, Guibas LJ. PointNet: deep learning on point sets for 3D classification and segmentation. CoRR. 2016;abs/1612.00593.

13. Hanocka R, Hertz A, Fish N, Giryes R, Fleishman S, Cohen-Or D. MeshCNN: a network with an edge. ACM Transactions on Graphics (TOG). 2019;38(4):90:1–90:12.

GAN-based Augmentation of Mammograms to Improve Breast Lesion Detection

Amir El-Ghoussani, Dalia Rodríguez-Salas, Mathias Seuret, Andreas Maier

Fakultät für Pattern Recognition, FAU Erlangen-Nürnberg
amir.el-ghoussani@fau.de

Abstract. Mammography is an important part of breast cancer diagnostics, as it allows to inspect the inner breast structure without physically penetrating breast tissue. Commonly, mammograms tend to vary in their visual appearance based on the specific device and the circumstances under which the mammogram is acquired. Such images could cause artificial intelligence algorithms to fail as they can introduce an undesired variation into the data. This study intends to put these images to use by utilizing a cycle-consistent Generative Adversarial Network (GAN) in order to augment the training data by diversifying instances of each visual domain into all the available ones. A publicly available dataset was augmented to train a detection network; the GANs used for the augmentation were trained with an in-house dataset with three visually different domains. Results show that using our augmentation technique consistently increases the detection performance by reaching a mean average precision of up to 0.82 against 0.77 without augmenting the data.

1 Introduction

Despite many medical breakthroughs breast cancer is still one of the main causes of death caused by malignant disease among women. In Germany, 67297 women were diagnosed in the period of 2015 and 2016. In 18396 cases, this led to death ($\approx$ 27%) [1]. The high mortality rate is associated with the fact, that cancer, and especially breast cancer, tends to evolve in silent and often unrecognized ways. If the cancer remains unrecognized in the body, mortality rate increases significantly. X-ray mammography is the current gold standard for early detection of breast cancer. This imaging method along with annual screening has proven to be the most effective tool to decrease the associated mortality rate [2]. Recent developments in the field of artificial intelligence (AI) have made possible, to support or even replace manual assessment of mammograms. In particular, the field of deep learning (DL) has given rise to multiple ways of engineering computer-aided detection (CAD) systems in order to aid and automate the diagnosing process in mammography [3, 4]. However, early detection of suspicious structures, facilitated by DL, remains a challenging task for various reasons. Most publicly available datasets either lack annotations or the dataset is biased. Additionally, default image properties, such as brightness, contrast, saturation, etc. may differ, because of different acquisition devices or manufacturers. Large variations of these properties could introduce noise, thereby harming the performance of a DL based detection system.

Several approaches to overcome both issues have been made. Jendele et al. [5] proposed increasing the amount of training samples by adversarial augmentation. They used a cycle-consistent geneerative adversarial network (cycleGAN), to balance benign and malignant mammography samples. Their approach was tested on lesion detection. They achieved a slight improvement in the classification performance when compared to classification without augmentation; F1-score is 0.638 with augmentation and 0.625 without augmentation. Sun et al. [6] used cycleGAN in a similar way to augment brain and liver MRI scans. In contrast to Jendele et al., their method considerably improves the F1-score on a brain tumor classification task; 0.644 without augmentation and 0.776 with augmentation.

In this paper, we propose exploiting the variation in the input data by first, visually identifying different domains and second, translating each domain samples into all other domains. This involves training and testing a cycleGAN. During the GAN training phase the cycleGAN is trained on translation of different domains. In our in-house dataset, 3 levels of brightness were visually identified; consequently, the samples were subdivided into "bright", "normal" and "dark" domains. At test time the cycleGAN generators are extracted and used to augment training data on a breast detection task. In contrast to Jendele et al. [5], we propose to balance the training data based on the visual domain of training samples rather than the ratio of benign and malignant samples.

The rest of this paper is organized as follows: the next section gives an overview of all materials and methods by describing the datasets and models used. It follows a section presenting the results obtained in all experiments. Finally, a discussion section which shortly discusses and summarizes results.

2 Materials and methods

During the GAN training phase, cycleGANs were trained with an in-house dataset containing 3 different visual domains. Thus, in total 2 cycleGANs were trained. During the GAN testing phase relevant cycleGAN generators were extracted in order to augment training samples during YOLO training phase, in which a YOLO convolutional neural network (CNN) was trained on the detection of breast lesions in mammograms. To account for inter-device variations, YOLO training was performed on a publicly available dataset acquired with a different scanner.

2.1 UKE dataset

This in-house dataset was acquired by various institutions of the University Clinic Erlangen (UKE) in and around Erlangen. It consists of mammography screenings of 279 patients. The full field digital mammography (FFDM) images were acquired in cranio-caudal (CC) and medio-lateral oblique (MLO) view; additionally, 92 Region of Interest (RoI) annotations were provided.

The visual inspection of the images shows an apparent variation in image brightness. This variation is caused by different mammography devices. According to the respective acquisition device, the dataset was subdivided into "dark", "bright" and "normal" domain samples, indicating the contrast and brightness of a mammogram (Fig. 1). In total, it contains 120 "dark", 844 "normal" and 152 "bright" domain samples.

2.2   INbreast dataset

The studied approach utilizes the INbreast dataset [7] to train and evaluate the augmentation technique at YOLO training and test time. INbreast contains a total of 410 breast cancer screening samples, provided in both CC and MLO view with RoI annotations. In this paper only samples labeled "Mass " were used, summing up to a total of 89 samples, as masses were found in both UKE and INbreast datasets. INbreast samples showed resemblance to UKE "normal" domain samples. Consequently G_{nb} and G_{nd}, previously trained on UKE data, were utilized to augment INbreast samples during YOLO training phase.

2.3   Cycle-consistent GAN

A total of two separate cycleGANs were trained (Fig. 2), and the particular generators extracted. G_{nb} for training the translation "normal" to "bright " UKE samples, and G_{nd} for translating "normal" to "dark" samples, respectively. A U-Net generator was tested in this study, inspired by the U-Net architecture introduced by Ronneberger et al. [8]. In total, it consists of four up- and downsampling stages, containing double convolutional blocks. Feature maps are compressed to a shape of 1×1 at the saddle point of the architecture. The discriminator architecture used, was based on PatchGAN [9].

2.3.1   Loss functions. Two kinds of loss constraints were applied in two architectural modifications. First a geometric loss was implemented, inspired by Huan et al. [10]. The core idea is to enforce consistency between the geometric transformation $T(x)$ of the prediction y and the ground truth $\hat{y}$ such that $T(y) \approx T(\hat{y})$.

Additionally, a feature loss inspired by the perceptual losses introduced by Johnson et al. [11] was included. Only feature loss was utilized since the style loss was found to introduce artefacts into the data. The objective was obtaining a feature map consistency $F_l(x)$ between the feature map of the predicted output $F_l(y)$ and the feature map of the ground truth $F_l(\hat{y})$ at layer l. All feature maps were computed using VGG-16 architecture

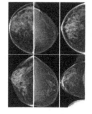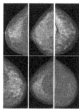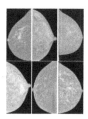

Fig. 1. UKE samples in craniocaudal (CC) view; left stack represents "dark", middle represents "normal" and right represents "bright" domain samples.

[12] pretrained on ImageNet. The loss was computed based on the consistency between layers 5, 9, 16. Both loss functions were applied in a cyclic and an acyclic manner. In case of cyclic loss, the Mean square error (MSE) between an initial "normal" sample x_n and the reconstructed "normal" sample $\hat{x}_n = G_{nd}(G_{dn}(x_n))$ is minimized. In case of an acyclic loss the MSE between an initial bright sample x_b and the generated normal sample $y_n = G_{bn}(x_b)$ is minimized. Cyclic and acyclic loss schemes are illustrated in Figure 2.

Finally, identity loss was used to constrain the feature recognition of generators. Classical cycleGAN generators often fail to identify the specific transformation domain leading to transformation of arbitrary features from one into another domain [13].

2.4 Breast lesion detection

For breast lesion detection, we used a YOLO-based architecture; specifically, the YOLOv5 implementation found in [14] and all hyperparameters were kept on default. It was trained with 72 INbreast samples on identifying masses on a test set of 17 INbreast and 12 UKE mammography samples. All samples contained lesions. The input image size was set to 512×512 pixels.

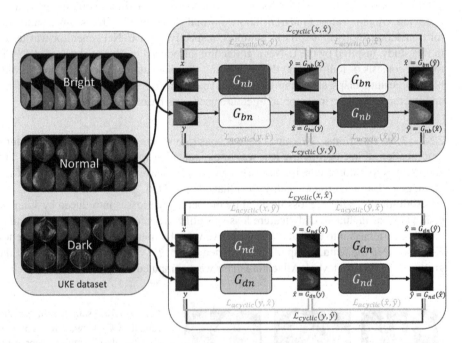

Fig. 2. During the GAN training phase, instances are sampled from the corresponding UKE data domains in order to train "normal" to "bright" translation (top right box), and "normal" to "dark" translation (bottom right box) respectively. After GAN training G_{nb} and G_{nd} were extracted and utilized for the augmentation of YOLO training data.

Tab. 1. Detection results with the augmented samples. The second column "Losses" lists the combination of loss functions used for the particular experiment. Bold entries indicate the two best performing models that were obtained with the particular architecture.

ID	Loss	Precision	Recall	$mAP@0.5$	$mAP@0.5:0.95$
Baseline	-	0.83	**0.81**	0.77	0.41
U-Net$_{adv}$	Adversarial	1.00	**0.77**	**0.79**	**0.45**
U-Net$_{cyc-geo}$	Adversarial, geometry, cycle	0.96	0.71	0.78	**0.45**
U-Net$_{acyc-geo}$	Adversarial, geometry, acycle	0.96	0.71	**0.82**	0.44
U-Net$_{cyc-feat}$	Adversarial, feature, cycle	1.00	0.71	0.77	0.44
U-Net$_{acyc-feat}$	Adversarial, feature, acycle	1.00	0.64	0.76	0.41

3 Results

CycleGANs were tested with all of the mentioned modifications. Cyclic loss functions were compared to acyclic ones and geometric loss was compared to feature loss. In total, this consists of five separate experiments including the default adversarial architecture: U-Net$_{cyc-geo}$, U-Net$_{acyc-geo}$, U-Net$_{cyc-feat}$, U-Net$_{acyc-feat}$, U-Net$_{adv}$. All experiments were compared to the baseline approach in which the training data was not augmented. In the augmented case, the INbreast images were augmented to the UKE domains "bright" and "dark" . Therefore, the amount of training samples increased to 228.

CycleGANs were trained using an Adam optimizer with a learning rate of 0.0002, batch size of 2 for 50 epochs. The performance of all augmentation approaches was evaluated based on the quantitative measurements of the highest recall and the associated precision at an Intersection over Union (IoU) of 0.7. Additionally, the average precision at IoU of 0.5 ($mAP@0.5$) and the mean value of average precision at IoUs ranging from 0.5 to 0.95 with an increment of 0.05 ($mAP@0.5:0.95$). These results can be seen in Table 1.

4 Discussion

Inspection of the precision and the recall indicates, that all augmentation models improve the precision significantly, while recall decreases only slightly. This suggests that the proposed augmentation can significantly improve the detector precision, while only trading a slight amount of recall. This interpretation is backed when investigating $mAP@0.5$ or $mAP@0.5:0.95$. It can be observed that all augmentation models improve the mAP, when compared to the baseline model.

Overall, cycleGAN generators performed well when transforming from the "bright" to the "normal" UKE domain and vice versa. However, when samples were translated from "dark" to "normal" domain only marginal difference was obtained in the visual appearance. This was attributed to the low variation between the "normal" and "dark" UKE samples. Due to this, in YOLO training phase INbreast samples were given to G_{bn}, in order to generate "dark" domain samples. In conclusion, GANs can be successfully used for augmenting mammograms. The presented approach seems to consistently improve the performance of breast lesion detection. In future work, our augmentation technique could be extended to different medical domains and/or tested on different tasks such as classification and segmentation.

Acknowledgement. We would like to thank the Women's Hospital of the UKE for providing us the dataset.

References

1. Robert Koch Institute (RKI). Krebs in Deutschland. `https://www.krebsdaten.de/Krebs/DE/Content/Krebsarten/Brustkrebs/brustkrebs_node.html`. Accessed: October 25th, 2021. 2021.
2. Misra S, Solomon NL, Moffat FL, Koniaris LG. Screening criteria for breast cancer. Adv Surg. 2010;44(1):87–100.
3. Jiménez-Gaona Y, Rodríguez-Álvarez MJ, Lakshminarayanan V. Deep-learning-based computer-aided systems for breast cancer imaging: a critical review. Appl Sci. 2020;10(22):8298.
4. Al-antari MA, Al-masni MA, Choi MT, Han SM, Kim TS. A fully integrated computer-aided diagnosis system for digital x-ray mammograms via deep learning detection, segmentation, and classification. Int J Med Inform. 2018;117:44–54.
5. Jendele L, Skopek O, Becker AS, Konukoglu E. Adversarial augmentation for enhancing classification of mammography images. CoRR. 2019;abs/1902.07762.
6. Sun L, Wang J, Ding X, Huang Y, Paisley JW. An adversarial learning approach to medical image synthesis for lesion removal. CoRR. 2018;abs/1810.10850.
7. Moreira IC, Amaral I, Domingues I, Cardoso A, Cardoso MJ, Cardoso JS. INbreast: toward a full-field digital mammographic database. Acad Radiol. 2012;19(2):236–48.
8. Ronneberger O, Fischer P, Brox T. U-Net: convolutional networks for biomedical image segmentation. Vol. 9351. 2015:234–41.
9. Liu MY, Breuel T, Kautz J. Unsupervised image-to-image translation networks. CoRR. 2017;abs/1703.00848.
10. Fu H, Gong M, Wang C, Batmanghelich K, Zhang K, Tao D. Geometry-consistent generative adversarial networks for one-sided unsupervised domain mapping. Proceedings of the IEEE/CVF Conference on Computer Vision and Pattern Recognition. 2019:2427–36.
11. Johnson J, Alahi A, Fei-Fei L. Perceptual losses for real-time style transfer and super-resolution. Computer Vision – ECCV. 2016:694–711.
12. Simonyan K, Zisserman A. Very deep convolutional networks for large-scale image recognition. arXiv. 2014.
13. Taigman Y, Polyak A, Wolf L. Unsupervised cross-domain image generation. arXiv. 2016.
14. Jocher G, Stoken A, Borovec J, NanoCode012, ChristopherSTAN, Changyu L et al. ultralytics/yolov5: v3.1 - Bug fixes and performance improvements. Version v3.1. Zenodo. 2020.

Multiscale Softmax Cross Entropy for Fovea Localization on Color Fundus Photography

Yuli Wu[1], Peter Walter[2], Dorit Merhof[1]

[1]Institute of Imaging and Computer Vision, RWTH Aachen, Germany
[2]Department of Ophthalmology, RWTH Aachen, Germany
yuli.wu@lfb.rwth-aachen.de

Abstract. Fovea localization is one of the most popular tasks in ophthalmic medical image analysis, where the coordinates of the center point of the *macula lutea*, i.e. *fovea centralis*, should be calculated based on color fundus images. In this work, we treat the localization problem as a classification task, where the coordinates of the x- and y-axis are considered as the target classes. Moreover, the combination of the softmax activation function and the cross entropy loss function is modified to its multiscale variation to encourage the predicted coordinates to be located closely to the ground-truths. Based on color fundus photography images, we empirically show that the proposed multiscale softmax cross entropy yields better performance than the vanilla version and than the mean squared error loss with sigmoid activation, which provides a novel approach for coordinate regression.

1 Introduction

Outputting coordinates is common in computer vision tasks, such as in bounding-box regression for object detection and in keypoint localization for facial recognition. Regression losses are typically selected to calculate the error between the ground-truth and the prediction, e.g. mean squared error (MSE) loss and mean absolute error (MAE) loss, which measure L2 and L1 distances between the ground-truth and the prediction, respectively. In contrast, probabilistic losses are usually used in classification tasks, which includes cross entropy (CE) loss as one of the most popular choices (categorical cross entropy in the case of multi-class). One significant difference between these two categories is that MSE or MAE punishes incorrect predictions less, which are however close to the ground-truth, while categorical CE combined with softmax activation function treats all incorrect predictions equally to the maximum.

An accurate localization of the fovea, an important anatomical landmark in the retina, can be beneficial to the computer aided diagnosis of retinal diseases. Huang et al. [1] take advantage of the geometrical relationship between optic disc and fovea to achieve a more accurate localization and Xie et al. [2] utilize a three-stage network with coarse-fine fusion. MSE loss is used in both approaches. Kopaczka et al. [3] combine soft-argmax loss [4] and L1 distance loss to localize and track rodents, which shows the

© Der/die Autor(en), exklusiv lizenziert durch
Springer Fachmedien Wiesbaden GmbH, ein Teil von Springer Nature 2022
K. Maier-Hein et al. (Hrsg.), *Bildverarbeitung für die Medizin 2022*,
Informatik aktuell, https://doi.org/10.1007/978-3-658-36932-3_67

feasibility of probabilistic loss functions in classification tasks. In this work, we consider the localization task as two classification tasks, referring to the x- and y-axis, by using a combination of the softmax activation function and the cross entropy loss function. Trying to bridge the functional gap between the regression and probabilistic losses, we propose multiscale softmax cross entropy (MSCE), which takes the last feature map learned from the backbone convolutional neural network and combines multiple downsampled feature maps with independent softmax cross entropy.

2 Materials and methods

2.1 Dataset

The dataset of color fundus images, REFUGE2 [5], contains 1200 images with and 400 images without ground-truth annotations for training and testing, respectively. The metrics used to evaluate the predicted localization coordinates is taken from the latest Gamma Challenge (https://gamma.grand-challenge.org), namely the reciprocal of the average Euclidean distance (R-AED) value, which is defined as

$$\text{R-AED} = \frac{1}{d(\mathbf{p}, \mathbf{q}) + 0.1} \tag{1}$$

where the Euclidean distance is used between the normalized coordinates of ground-truth $\mathbf{p}$ and prediction $\mathbf{q}$ as $d(\mathbf{p}, \mathbf{q}) = \|\mathbf{p} - \mathbf{q}\|_2$

2.2 Network architecture

We adopt the neural network architecture from cellpose [6], which is a modified U-Net [7] with residual connections inside each convolutional block and a style vector fused to the upsampling pathway. The original image is first resized and fed into the cellpose network, which outputs the feature map of identical size. The learned feature map is pooled multiple times to generate the multiscale branches, each of which is first reduced per axis (via e.g. sum or mean). The multiscale loss is then calculated with independent softmax cross entropy for each branch. Finally, the final loss is aggregated with weighted sum, which we denote as MSCE. The detailed introduction of MSCE is presented in Section 2.3. The implementation of hyperparameters during the experiments can be found in Section 2.4.

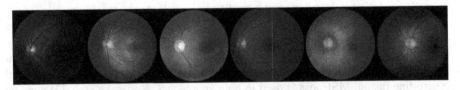

Fig. 1. Examples of color fundus images from REFUGE2 [5].

2.3 Loss

We present MSCE, which takes two logit vectors of different sizes and calculates a weighted summation of softmax cross entropy from them

$$SCE = -\sum_{i=1}^{C} t_i \log(\frac{e^{s_i}}{\sum_{j=1}^{C} e^{s_j}}) \qquad (2)$$

$$MSCE = \sum_{m=1}^{M} \lambda_m \cdot \left(-\sum_{i=1}^{C_m} t_i \log(\frac{e^{s_i}}{\sum_{j=1}^{C_m} e^{s_j}}) \right) \qquad (3)$$

Based on the original softmax cross entropy (SCE) in Equation 2, the multiscale version can be defined as shown in Equation 3. In both equations, s denotes the predicted logit and t_i indicates whether the i-th of total C class labels is the correct classification. In Equation 3, M denotes the number of multiscales (or the number of the branches in Figure 2) and λ_m denotes the weights for the SCE term of each scale. In this work, we set all $\lambda_m = 1$. In Figure 3, different loss functions are compared with a toy example, where we assume the 70th class, $i.e.$ coordinate, of a 256 dimensional vector is the ground-truth and the normalized loss values are calculated for each possible prediction. Figure 3a illustrates MSE, an example from the category of regression loss, which progressively attracts the wrong predictions to the ground-truth. In the case of SCE (Fig. 3b), however, the incorrect coordinates have been opposed expressly and unanimously, no matter where they are located rather than the ground-truth. The proposed MSCE is expected to neutralize the characteristics of MSE and SCE, which not only distinguishes the predictions in a stepwise regressive manner but also drastically encourages the prediction to converge towards the single actual ground-truth without decreasing the reward ratio. The desired feature can be better approached, if the number of the multiscales M is set to the maximum ($M = 8$ in case of 256 classes) comparing Figure 3c and Figure 3d.

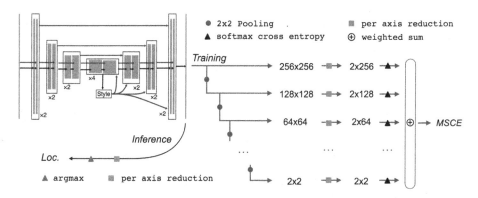

Fig. 2. Network architecture for training and inference. The network backbone is adopted from the cellpose network [6] and the corresponding figure is adapted from it.

2.4   Hyperparameters

The *style* mechanism from the cellpose network [6] has been preserved, as it is assumed to play a role when combining the disease grading task and the fovea localization task in future work. The images are first resized to 256 by 256 and no augmentation techniques have been then applied. We use `MaxPooling` when downsampling the feature map to generate multiscales ones (blue dots in Figure 2) and `sum` as the reduction operator to obtain the per axis logit vectors (orange squares in Figure 2). It has been empirically shown that `MaxPooling` and `sum` yield better results than `AveragePooling` and `mean` reduction. The training process is optimized by stochastic gradient descent that uses an exponential decay schedule with an initial learning rate of 0.01, decay steps of 400 and a decay rate of 0.9. The maximal number of epochs is set to 1000 and the `EarlyStopping` mechanism has been applied with a patience of 100 epochs in terms of overall loss values.

3   Results

Experimental results are shown in Table 1 *w.r.t.* the reciprocal of the average Euclidean distance (R-AED, Equation 1). It is found that `MaxPooling` with `sum` reduction plays a significant role to boost the performance with SCE and MSCE, in which case MSCE

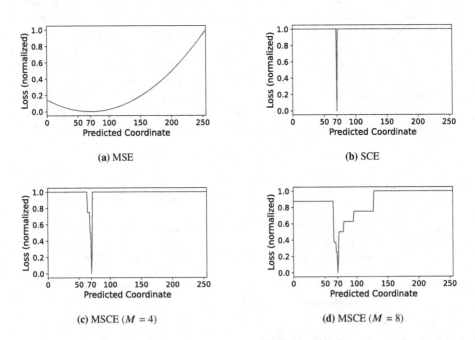

Fig. 3. Toy experiments in 1D coordinate: loss values of different loss functions. Predicted coordinates are presented in x-axis and the normalized loss values in y-axis, with the assumption that the 70th coordinate of total 256 is the ground-truth. MSE: mean squared error; SCE: softmax cross entropy; MSCE: multiscale softmax cross entropy. M denotes the number of the multiscales (Eq. 3).

Tab. 1. Results from ablation experiments with different loss functions and network settings *w.r.t.* the reciprocal of the average Euclidean distance (R-AED). `Ave/mean` denotes `AveragePooling` with `mean` reduction and `Max/sum` denotes `MaxPooling` with `sum` reduction. Best results from each experimental group are marked in bold face.

Loss	Network	Batch Size	R-AED ($\uparrow$)
Mean squared error (baseline)	`Ave/mean`	8	**5.69**
Softmax cross entropy	`Ave/mean`	8	3.45
Multiscale softmax cross entropy	`Ave/mean`	8	4.36
Mean squared error (baseline)	`Max/sum`	16	5.18
Softmax cross entropy	`Max/sum`	16	4.16
Multiscale softmax cross entropy	`Max/sum`	16	**5.31**
Mean squared error (baseline)	`Max/sum`	8	5.53
Softmax cross entropy	`Max/sum`	8	4.99
Multiscale softmax cross entropy	`Max/sum`	8	**6.12**

outperforms MSE loss. Generally, the modified MSCE yields better results than the vanilla SCE, which empirically demonstrates the feasibility of probabilistic losses in the regression tasks. Predicted fovea locations are illustrated in Figure 4, where the final coordinate vectors are illustrated on the original fundus images with MSE, vanilla SCE and MSCE in Figures 4a-4c, respectively. From Figure 4d, it can be noted that MSE (blue) and SCE (green) result in a larger offset than MSCE (white). A typical failed prediction happens if the fovea is located far away from the central region and blends into the dark marginal area, as shown in Figure 4e.

4   Discussion

Although the proposed MSCE loss has surpassed the commonly used MSE loss and the vanilla SCE loss based on the ablation experiments, some unstable predictions haven been noticed during the experiments. We assume that finetuned hyperparameters, including the weights λ_m in Equation 3, could mitigate this issue. In practice, the fovea is usually localized with the help of the relative position of the optic disc by surgeons. Therefore, it is expected that fusing the relative spatial information via optic disc segmentation would achieve better results for fovea localization. Additionally, the segmentation-based feature map of our approach could further strengthen the advantages by combining different ophthalmic tasks with fovea localization based on fundus images, such as vessel segmentation, optic disc and optic cup segmentation, and disease (e.g. glaucoma) grading.

5   Conclusion

This work addresses the fovea localization task based on the feature map that is initially tailored for segmentation. Furthermore, the task of coordinate regression from logits is performed based on a probabilistic loss, which usually contributes to classification tasks. The modified multiscale version of softmax cross entropy (MSCE) has empirically

Fig. 4. Examples of predicted fovea locations with different losses. (a)-(c) illustrate the final coordinate vectors on the original images. (d) compares the predicted locations with crosses (blue, green, white denote MSE, SCE, MSCE, respectively). (e) shows a failed prediction, if the optic disc instead of the fovea is located in the center.

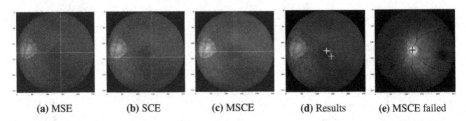

| (a) MSE | (b) SCE | (c) MSCE | (d) Results | (e) MSCE failed |

shown the capability for localization tasks. The performance of MSCE surpasses both the vanilla SCE and the mean squared error loss with the identical network backbone and hyperparameter setups, which offers a novel loss alternative for fovea localization and is promising for other general coordinate regression tasks like bounding boxes in object detection.

Acknowledgement. This work was funded by the Deutsche Forschungsgemeinschaft (DFG, German Research Foundation) – grant 424556709/GRK2610.

References

1. Huang Y, Zhong Z, Yuan J, Tang X. Efficient and robust optic disc detection and fovea localization using region proposal network and cascaded network. Biomed Signal Process Control. 2020;60:101939.
2. Xie R, Liu J, Cao R, Qiu CS, Duan J, Garibaldi J et al. End-to-end fovea localisation in colour fundus images with a hierarchical deep regression network. IEEE Trans Med Imaging. 2021;40(1):116–28.
3. Kopaczka M, Jacob T, Ernst L, Schulz M, Tolba R, Merhof D. Robust open field rodent tracking using a fully convolutional network and a softargmax distance loss. Proc BVM. 2020:242–7.
4. Honari S, Molchanov P, Tyree S, Vincent P, Pal C, Kautz J. Improving landmark localization with semi-supervised learning. Proc IEEE CVVR. 2018:1546–55.
5. Orlando JI, Fu H, Barbosa Breda J, van Keer K, Bathula DR, Diaz-Pinto A et al. REFUGE challenge: a unified framework for evaluating automated methods for glaucoma assessment from fundus photographs. Med Image Anal. 2020;59:101570.
6. Stringer C, Wang T, Michaelos M, Pachitariu M. Cellpose: a generalist algorithm for cellular segmentation. Nat Methods. 2021;18(1):100–6.
7. Ronneberger O, Fischer P, Brox T. U-Net: convolutional networks for biomedical image segmentation. Proc MICCAI. 2015:234–41.

Tibia Cortical Bone Segmentation in Micro-CT and X-ray Microscopy Data Using a Single Neural Network

Oliver Aust[1], Mareike Thies[2], Daniela Weidner[3], Fabian Wagner[2], Sabrina Pechmann[4], Leonid Mill[2], Darja Andreev[3], Ippei Miyagawa[3], Gerhard Krönke[3], Silke Christiansen[4], Stefan Uderhardt[3], Andreas Maier[2], Anika Grüneboom[1]

[1]Leibniz Institute for Analytical Sciences ISAS, Dortmund
[2]Pattern Recognition Lab, FAU Erlangen-Nürnberg
[3]Department of Internal Medicine 3 - Rheumatology and Immunology and Deutsches Zentrum für Immuntherapie (DZI), FAU Erlangen-Nürnberg and Universitätsklinikum Erlangen
[4]Fraunhofer Institute for Ceramic Technologies and Systems IKTS, Forchheim
oliver.aust@isas.de

Abstract. X-ray microscopy (XRM) allows the investigation of osteocyte lacunae and recently discovered trans-cortical vessels in murine tibia bones due to higher resolution than conventional micro-CT (μCT) approaches. However, segmentation methods for XRM data are not yet established. Here, we propose a deep learning approach utilizing a U-Net-based neural network trained on a similar modality – μCT – that is capable of segmenting in both domains. We altered the XRM data to more closely resemble the μCT data to allow segmentation in the shifted XRM domain. Segmentation error on μCT data was evaluated by the F1 score (0.954) and IoU (0.913), whereas the segmentation on XRM data was verified visually. We conclude that the obtained model indeed allows the segmentation of cortical bone in both XRM and μCT data, although it was only trained on μCT images.

1 Introduction

The recent discovery of trans-cortical vessels (TCVs) in the tibae of mice and humans has opened up many new possibilities to investigate the effects of aging and diseases in bone [1]. Due to their size of approximately 8-15 μm it is difficult to observe the channels in which they reside with traditional X-ray techniques such as μCT. However, recent XRM devices achieve resolutions down to 500 nm and thus allow resolving TCV channels [1]. Additionally, the technique allows to image lacunae – even smaller cavities in the bone where osteocytes reside [1, 2]. Osteocytes play a role in bone turnover [3] and form connections with TCVs interacting with them [1].

Both murine and human tibia consist of two main compartments: cortical bone, a tubular solid outer bone (Fig. 1 (a, b) orange), and trabecular bone, a supportive sponge-like bone structure inside the cortical bone located at the epiphysis (Fig. 1 (a, b) white). As the name implies, TCVs are only found in the cortical part of the bone. This means it is required to segment the cortical bone from trabecular bone to be able to calculate several parameters such as TCV density in the cortical bone or the effects of decomposed TCVs to the cortical bone density. Further, to compare cortical bone osteocytes or osteocytes that are in proximity of TCVs to trabecular bone osteocytes requires the segmentation of cortical bone from trabecular bone. Additionally, the age-related loss of trabecular bone in tibae is a well-known effect [4]. Segmentation of the cortical bone at the same time yields the trabecular bone and thus, the ratio of them can be calculated.

The segmentation of tibia cortical bone has already been tackled. However, traditional segmentation methods usually deal with the more commonly spread CT systems [5]. There are also many different disease models commonly investigated that have strong effects on the structure of the bone, such as osteophyte growth (arthritis) [6], loss of bone density (osteoporosis) [7] or increase in bone density (osteopetrosis) [8] that changes the way the data needs to be handled. For example, samples with osteoporosis will have a thinner cortical bone due to erosion which means segmentation based on thickness is no longer possible. Previous works have shown the capability of deep learning for segmentation in CT data [9].

Here, we demonstrate that it is possible to use a single model trained with μCT data from different disease models to segment the cortical bone from the trabecular bone in

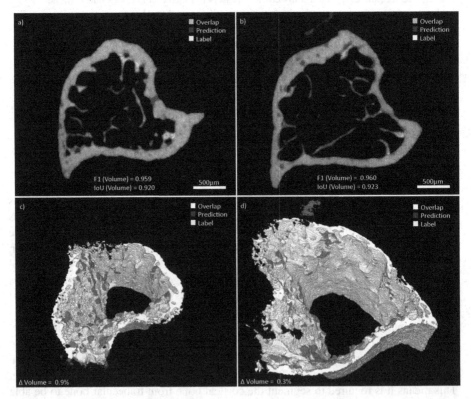

Fig. 1. Examples of the predictions obtained by the model with μCT data. (a) and (b) show exemplary slices from different datasets. (c) and (d) are the 3D views of the volumes obtained from segmenting with the label (yellow) and the prediction (purple) with the overlap colored white on the datasets (a) and (b) respectively.

both diverse μCT data and in XRM data despite the difference in domains. By utilizing a neural network we are able to segment more diverse datasets than traditional methods would allow. We use the nnU-Net for neural network training as it not only provides state-of-the-art performance but also allows model to be easily made ready to use for biologists and medical staff via pretrained models [10].

2 Materials and methods

2.1 Sample preparation

Sample preparation was carried out in compliance with all ethical regulations for organ removals at the University of Erlangen and carried out as approved by the local animal ethic committees of the Regierung für Mittelfranken. For μCT measurements, tibiae from four different mouse models were retrieved. Twelve week old C57BL/6 Twinkle Runx2 transgenic mice without bone phenotype were taken as control mice (license TS-10/2021). Collagen-induced arthritis (CIA) was used as a model for rheumatoid arthritis (license 55.2.2-2532-2-424). To cover osteoporosis, tibia samples from ovariectomized mice (license 55.2.2-2532.2-1058-10) were used. Tibia samples from mice that showed an osteopetrosis phenotype were also included (license 55.2.2-2532.2-933-21). The total distribution of the 22 samples was: 8 control mice, 5 osteoporosis, 7 rheumatoid arthritis and 2 ostepetrosis samples. For XRM, tibia samples were retrieved from 56-93 weeks old C57BL/6 mice (license TS-10/2021).

2.2 μCT and XRM measurements

All μCT imaging was performed using the cone-beam desktop micro computer tomograph "μCT 40" by SCANCO Medical AG, Bruettisellen, Switzerland. An isotropic voxel size of 8.4 μm (field of view: 16.38 mm) and fixed thresholds (Hounsfield Units) were chosen for the visualization of calcified bone tissue. The volume of interest was determined as starting 0.42 mm from the middle of the tibia growth plate (near the knee) and extending 1680 mm (200 tomograms) distally.

XRM scans were acquired by a Zeiss Xradia Versa 620 (Carl Zeiss X-ray Microscopy Inc., Pleasanton, CA, USA) with a high framerate CMOS detector. Per tomography, 1401 projection X-ray radiographs (field of view: 2.85 mm) were recorded at sample rotation angles between 100 ° and −100 °. Magnification was achieved by geometric magnification with subsequent optical magnification by an 4x objective. The single projections were reconstructed by proprietary software (Zeiss XMReconstructor, Carl Zeiss X-ray Microscopy Inc., Pleasanton, CA, USA) with a filtered back-projection algorithm. The resulting volumetric images have a three-dimensional isotropic voxel size of 1.4 μm.

2.3 Neural network training and prediction

Cortical bone segmentation is performed using the nnU-Net framework [10]. A total of 22 μCT datasets each consisting of 200 images were used. Labels were manually created.

Every second slice was labelled while the intermediate slices were automatically interpolated by the SCANCO software. The datasets were converted to 16-bit images and the pixel size information was removed to ensure compatibility with XRM datasets. From the total of 22 datasets, 3 datasets were conserved as test datasets. The nnU-Net configuration 3D full resolution was used with 15 training and 4 validation datasets. All μCT predictions were carried out using the resulting model. The model is publicly available with documentation under https://github.com/OliverAust/Tib-Cort-Seg.

To be able to utilize the same model for XRM data, the images were downscaled from 1997×2038 pixels to 350×357 resulting in a downsampling factor of approximately 6 to account for the lower resolution of μCT data (8.4 μm) in comparison to XRM data (1.4 μm). No downscaling in Z-dimension was carried out to ensure all slices are predicted. The pixel size information was removed during downsampling. The μCT model was then used to predict on the downsampled XRM images. In the obtained predictions, all 3D objects except for the largest were removed. Since the cortical bone is by far the largest object in the predictions, falsely predicted segmented trabecular structures are removed leaving only the cortical bone and any non-segmented trabecular structures. The predictions were then scaled to 1997×2038 again and enlarged by 5 pixels to ensure the entirety of the cortical bone is captured. A total of 7 XRM mice tibia datasets were predicted and evaluated.

3   Results

To assess the quality of the predictions obtained by the neural network, the F1 score and Intersection-Over-Union (IoU) were calculated from the obtained predictions and the manual labels. For the three test datasets the average F1 score is 0.954 and the average IoU is 0.913 (Fig. 1 (a, b)). The average volume error is 4.2 %. Manual labels were drawn conservatively, i.e., labels are slightly larger on the outer side of the cortical bone to ensure the entire bone is included. The labels are then used to segment the cortical bone which is usually followed by a threshold to obtain the final cortical bone volume. This means that the difference in label on the outer side of the cortical bone will not make any difference in the final analysis of the cortical bone. Thus, to calculate the final error of the desired cortical bone volume itself, both the manual annotations and the predictions from the model were applied to the original raw data as a segmentation mask and the resulting volumes were compared. This reduced the average volume error of the three test data sets to 0.6 % (Fig. 1 (c, d)).

Since no XRM data was labelled manually, the quality of the cortical bone segmentation needed to be evaluated qualitatively. Firstly, to obtain the total bone volume a hand-picked threshold was applied to separate background from bone. Then, the processed prediction was used to separate cortical bone from trabecular bone (Fig. 2 (a, b)). Qualitative evaluation was performed on the resulting volumes (Fig. 2 (c, d)). We recognized that the resulting segmentations include more misclassifications of trabecular bone as cortical bone than in the predictions of μCT data but still found the results satisfactory.

4   Discussion

The major factor that allows the use of XRM data with the μCT model is that the structure that we extract is large, in return meaning downsampling effects are minimized. Cortical bone is the largest compartment in tibia XRM data. This also means that it is a better strategy to segment cortical bone to obtain the trabecular bone as a negative, i.e., subtracting the cortical bone from the entire image yields the trabecular bone, than the other way around, as trabecular bone structures are smaller and hence more error prone. We also tried several preprocessing options, such as contrast enhancement or adjustment of the histogram so that the XRM data better resembles the μCT training data, but the predictions were not consistently improved.

Downsampling XRM data for prediction also adds, aside from shorter computing times, the major benefit of greater context in predictions. For an image with a resolution of 1997×2038 and over 1500 slices to fit into the VRAM, exceptionally strong hardware

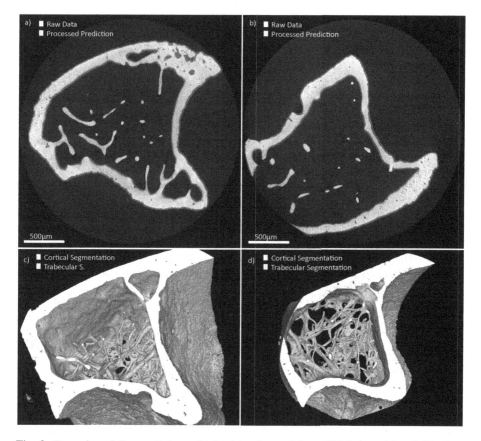

Fig. 2. Examples of the predictions obtained by the model on XRM data. (a) and (b) show exemplary slices from different datasets. (c) and (d) show 3d views of the segmented volumes from (a) and (b) respectively with the trabecular bone (yellow) and the cortical bone (white).

is required which is often not available. While smaller patch sizes would still allow to load the image, it would also most likely decrease segmentation quality as the patch size will contain less context [10]. To further improve segmentation quality of the cortical bone in XRM images, it would be possible to utilize the obtained labels as a basis to retrain on XRM data only. For example, manual adjustments to the obtained labels can accelerate manual labelling of XRM data.

In conclusion, the trained nnU-Net showed high segmentation accuracy on µCT tibia data from both healthy and diseased mice. The same model was also able to correctly segment cortical bone on XRM data of mouse tibia after downsampling, although more trabecular bone was included. The obtained cortical and trabecular bone segmentations are sufficient to be used for follow-up analysis of TCV channels and osteocyte lacunae in mice.

Acknowledgement. We thank the Leibniz-Institut für Analytische Wissenschaften - ISAS and European Research Council (ERC) (Grant agreement No. 810316) for funding. We also thank Brenda Krishnacoumar for additional sample preparation.

References

1. Grüneboom A, Hawwari I, Weidner D, Culemann S, Müller S, Henneberg S et al. A network of trans-cortical capillaries as mainstay for blood circulation in long bones. Nat Metab. 2019;1(2):236–50.
2. Kegelman CD, Coulombe JC, Jordan KM, Horan DJ, Qin L, Robling AG et al. YAP and TAZ mediate osteocyte perilacunar/canalicular remodeling. J Bone Miner Res. 2020;35(1):196–210.
3. Aarden EM, Nijweide PJ, Burger EH. Function of osteocytes in bone. J Cell Biochem. 1994;55(3):287–99.
4. Chen H, Washimi Y, Kubo Ky, Onozuka M. Gender-related changes in three-dimensional microstructure of trabecular bone at the human proximal tibia with aging. Histol Histopathol. 2011;26(5).
5. Buie HR, Campbell GM, Klinck RJ, MacNeil JA, Boyd SK. Automatic segmentation of cortical and trabecular compartments based on a dual threshold technique for in vivo micro-CT bone analysis. Bone. 2007;41(4):505–15.
6. Ruiz-Heiland G, Horn A, Zerr P, Hofstetter W, Baum W, Stock M et al. Blockade of the hedge-hog pathway inhibits osteophyte formation in arthritis. Ann Rheum Dis. 2012;71(3):400–7.
7. Bonucci E, Ballanti P. Osteoporosis—bone remodeling and animal models. Toxicol Pathol. 2014;42(6):957–69.
8. Stark Z, Savarirayan R. Osteopetrosis. Orphanet J Rare Dis. 2009;4(1):1–12.
9. Folle L, Meinderink T, Simon D, Liphardt AM, Krönke G, Schett G et al. Deep learning methods allow fully automated segmentation of metacarpal bones to quantify volumetric bone mineral density. Sci Rep. 2021;11(1):1–9.
10. Isensee F, Jaeger PF, Kohl SA, Petersen J, Maier-Hein KH. nnU-Net: a self-configuring method for deep learning-based biomedical image segmentation. Nat Methods. 2021;18(2):203–11.

Reinforcement learning-basierte Patchpriorisierung zur beschleunigten Segmentierung von hochauflösenden Endoskopievideodaten

Samuel Schüttler[1], Frederic Madesta[1], Thomas Rösch[2], René Werner[1],
Rüdiger Schmitz[3]

[1]Institut für Computational Neuroscience,
[2]Klinik und Poliklinik für Interdisziplinäre Endoskopie,
[3]I. Medizinischen Klinik und Poliklinik, Universitätsklinikum Hamburg-Eppendorf, Hamburg
r.schmitz@uke.de

Zusammenfassung. Bei endoskopischen Computer-Vision-Anwendungen sind Echtzeitverarbeitung der Videodaten sowie geringe Latenzen für einen praktischen klinischen Einsatz maßgeblich. Gleichzeitig führt die kontinuierliche Hardwareweiterentwicklung zu einer stetigen Verbesserung der Bildauflösung. Eingangsbilddaten hoher Auflösung erfordern i. d. R. eine patchweise Verarbeitung, wobei durch Patch-Priorisierungsstrategien die Verarbeitung der Daten beschleunigt und Latenzen reduziert werden können. Mit der Bildsegmentierung als Beispielaufgabe wird im vorliegenden Beitrag untersucht, wie das Patch-Sampling zur Inferenzzeit als Reinforcement Learning (RL)-Problem formuliert werden kann. Anhand von synthetischen und realen Daten wird gezeigt, dass durch das entwickelte RL-basierte Patch-Priorisierungsmodell (PPM) eine beschleunigte Segmentierung relevanter Bildregionen realisiert werden kann.

1 Einleitung

Neuronale Netze und maschinelles Sehen sind in der klinischen Endoskopie angekommen [1]. Die automatische Detektion und Delineation von Polypen wurde in klinischen Studien erfolgreich evaluiert, z. B. [2], und in mehreren, kommerziell erhältlichen Systemen umgesetzt. Eine schnelle Verarbeitung und geringe Latenz sind für den Praxiseinsatz maßgebend. Die Auflösung der erzeugten Bilddaten hat sich von Gerätegeneration zu Gerätegeneration jedoch erhöht [3]. Die Einführung von 4K-Systemen im viszeralchirurgischen Bereich sowie die Entwicklung von Weitwinkeloptiken lassen eine Fortsetzung dieser Entwicklung erwarten.

Die Verarbeitung hochauflösender Bilddaten erfolgt in der Regel patch-basiert. Gegenstand der vorliegenden Arbeit ist die Entwicklung von Strategien zum effizienten Aufteilen der Bilddaten in Teilbilder (Patch-Sampling) zur beschleunigten Weiterverarbeitung semantisch relevanter Bildbereiche mit neuronalen Netzwerken. Bei typischen Netzwerk- und Hardwarekonfigurationen rangieren Patchgrößen in Bereichen von ca. 224×224 bis selten über 512×512 Pixel [4, 5]. In der Regel wird das Patch-Sampling als systematisches Abrastern des Ursprungsbildes von z. B. oben links nach unten rechts umgesetzt, was hinsichtlich einer möglichst schnellen Abdeckung des semantisch relevanten Areals selten optimal ist [6].

Zur Priorisierung und Auswahl der zu analysierenden Patches schlagen wir die Nutzung eines vorgeschalteten Modells (Patchpriorisierungsmodell, PPM) vor, welches aus einer geringer aufgelösten Version des Ursprungsbildes die prioritär zu verarbeitenden Patches auswählt. Es wird gezeigt, dass und wie diese Aufgabe als Reinforcement Learning (RL)-Problem aufgefasst werden kann. Geeignete Methoden werden anhand synthetischer Daten evaluiert und die Übertragbarkeit des Ansatzes auf reale endoskopische Bilddaten demonstriert.

2 Material und Methoden

Das RL-PPM soll anhand von downgesampelten Inputbildern die priorisiert zu segmentierenden Bildbereiche (Patches) auswählen. In dieser Arbeit wurde der Input des RL-PPM als 500×500 px Bild gewählt, aus dem anhand eines 5×5- bis 10×10-Gitter gesampelt wird. In der praktischen Anwendung würden Anzahl und Größe der vom RL-PPM zu verarbeitenden Patches durch die Auflösung des Originalinputs und die nachgeschaltete Segmentierungspipeline vorgegeben. Beispielsweise erforderte ein Bild der Auflösung von 3840×2160 px (4K) mit einer Segmentierungspipeline für 512×512 px große Patches das Sampling von 60 Patches (10×6-Gitter bei 25% Überlappung).

2.1 Synthetische Koloskopiebilder

Zur Exploration verschiedener methodischer Ansätze und RL-Strategien wurden zunächst synthetische Daten generiert, die grob dem gestellten Problem entsprechen (Abb. 1). Das endoskopische Lumen wurde durch einen konzentrischen Verlauf von Graustufen approximiert, demgegenüber sich ein bis vier Ellipsen verschiedener Größe, Position und Orientierung als „Polypen" abheben, und zudem ein additives Rauschen hinzugefügt wurde. Parallel wurde eine binäre Maske als Grundwahrheit (Ground Truth, GT) entsprechend der eingefügten „Polypen" erzeugt. Dabei wurden für jede Episode des Trainings und der Evaluierung jeweils neue Bilder generiert.

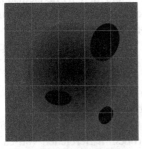 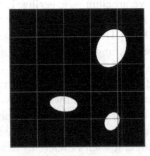 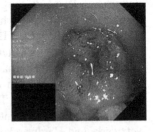

(a) Synthetisches Bild   (b) Ground Truth zu (a)   (c) Beispiel Realdaten

Abb. 1. Beispielbild für die synthetisch erzeugten Daten mit angedeutetem 5×5 Raster zur Illustration verwendeter Patchgrößen, sowie Beispielbild aus Kvasir-SEG.

2.2 Realdaten

Zur Demonstration der Übertragbarkeit des entwickelten Ansatzes auf endoskopischen Realdaten wurde der Kvasir-SEG-Datensatz [7] genutzt. Alle Daten wurden durch proportionale Skalierung und Padding auf eine Größe von 500×500 px transformiert und per „ITU-R 601-2 luma transform" in Graustufen umgewandelt. Der Datensatz, bestehend aus N=1000 Einzelbildern und zugehörigen Polypensegmentierungen von je unterschiedlichen Patienten, wurde randomisiert zu 80%/20% in Trainings- und Testdatensatz aufgeteilt.

2.3 RL-Environment

Auf Basis des OpenAI-Gym-Toolkits (https://gym.openai.com/) wurden problemspezifische RL-Environments wie folgt definiert: Eine Observation ist ein zweikanaliges Eingabebild mit einer Auflösung von 500×500 px, mit dem zu segmentierenden Bild als erstem und einer Maske der schon bearbeiteten Pixel als zweitem Kanal. Zu Beginn jeder Episode wird die optimale Schrittzahl s_{opt} für das Environment aus der Ground-Truth (GT) berechnet als Anzahl der Patches, die mindestens ein Polypenpixel enthalten. Mit einer aktuellen Schrittzahl (Anzahl gewählter Patches) s definieren wir den RL-Reward als

$$R_s = \begin{cases} R_{patch,raw} & \text{wenn } s \leq s_{opt} \\ R_{patch,raw} \cdot \gamma_{rew}^{s-s_{opt}} & \text{wenn } s > s_{opt} \\ 0 & \text{wenn Patch bereits gewählt worden ist} \end{cases} \qquad (1)$$

wobei

$$R_{patch,raw} = \begin{cases} \frac{1}{\text{Anzahl Patches mit Polypenpixel}} & \text{wenn Polypenpixel in Patch} \\ 0 & \text{sonst} \end{cases} \qquad (2)$$

und γ_{rew} als Discounting-Faktor $\gamma_{rew} = 0.5$. Der zu erreichende Reward je Episode ist folglich auf 1.0 normiert. Eine Episode des Environments wird abgeschlossen, wenn alle Patches mit Polypenpixeln augewählt wurden oder die Schritt- die Patch-Anzahl übersteigt.

2.4 Training

Zum Training wurden folgende Algorithmen in der Implementation von Stable-Baselines3 (https://github.com/DLR-RM/stable-baselines3) genutzt: (Synchronous) Advantage Actor-Critic (A2C) [8], Deep-Q-Network (DQN) [9] und Proximal Policy Optimization (PPO) [10], jeweils mit dem in [9] dargestellten CNN als zugrundeliegende Netzarchitektur. Als Hyperparameter der Algorithmen wurden die Standardwerte gewählt (Ausnahme Replay-Buffer DQN: 100.000 Schritte). Für die synthetischen Daten umfasste das Training in jedem Versuch 1 Million, für die Realdaten 3 Millionen Zeitschritte.

2.5 Evaluierung

Zentraler Gegenstand der Arbeit ist der Verlauf des Dice-Koeffizienten mit der Anzahl der ausgewerteten Bildpatches in Abhängigkeit der Sampling-Strategie bzw. eine
möglichst schnelle Konvergenz dieser Kurve. Es wurden trainierte PPMs mit dem zufälligen Sampeln von Patches („Random Policy") sowie systematischem zeilenweisen
Rastern („Strided Policy") verglichen. Für die gesampelten Patches nahmen wir durch
ein weiterverarbeitendes Netz, das nicht Gegenstand dieser Studie war, eine perfekte
Segmentierung an, die der GT-Maske des ausgewählten Patches entsprach.

Die Konvergenz des Lernprozesses wurde anhand von über 500 Episoden geglätteten
Reward-Kurven beurteilt. Die auf synthetischen Daten trainierten Policies wurden für
1000 Episoden evaluiert. Auf Realdaten wurde per PPO gegenüber den synthetischen
Daten *ohne* Anpassung jeglicher Hyperparameter und bis zur Konvergenz des Rewards
auf den Trainingsdaten evaluiert; die Evaluation fand auf den Testdaten statt.

Alle Versuche wurden auf einer Workstation mit Intel Xeon E-2186G @3.8GHz
sowie Geforce GTX 1080Ti mit 11 GB GPU-RAM durchgeführt.

3 Ergebnisse

Auf synthetischen Daten zeigte sich PPO unter den untersuchten Algorithmen am ge-
eignetsten hinsichtlich Konvergenzeigenschaften sowie Lerngeschwindigkeit (Abb. 2a).
Anhand von PPO wurde dann die Skalierbarkeit des Ansatzes bei steigender Gitterauf-
lösung untersucht. Bei einer Auflösung von 8×8 Patches zeigte sich eine verringerte
Performanz, die bei weiterer Reduktion der Patchgröße weiter abnahm (Abb. 2b).

Für Auflösungen bis zu einem 5×5-Gitter konnten durch Sampling entsprechend des
RL-PPMs bis zu fünf mal schneller alle relevanten Teile des Bildes für eine nachfolgende
Segmentierung ausgewählt werden, verglichen mit zufälliger Patchauswahl oder dem
zeilenweisen Abrastern des Bildes als Baseline-Ansätze.

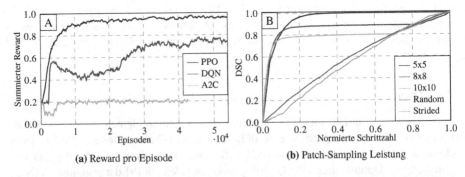

Abb. 2. Patch-Priorisierung auf RL-Environment für synthetische Daten: (A) Reward je Episode
für Daten wie in Abbildung 1 dargestellt, mit unterschiedlichen Algorithmen bearbeitet. (B)
Dice-Koeffizient (DSC) gemäß gesampelten Patches, normiert auf die maximal zu sampelnde
Anzahl an Patches bis zur Bildbedeckung, für PPO bei unterschiedlichen Gitter-Auflösungen
sowie zufälligem (random) und systematischem (strided) Sampling.

Anhand des Kvasir-SEG-Datensatzes wurde die Übertragbarkeit des Ansatzes auf reale Endoskopiedaten analysiert. Trotz begrenztem Umfang des Datensatzes lernt die Policy, Patches derart zu priorisieren, dass eine deutlich beschleunigte Konvergenz der Abdeckung der semantisch relevanten Bildbereiche (hier: Polypen) durch die ausgewählten Patches erreicht wird (5×5 Patch-Gitter; Abb. 3). Die Inferenzzeit für die Auswahl eines Patches liegt bei 2,566 ms (95%-CI: [2,563; 2,568] ms); die Trainingszeit betrug ca. 48 h.

4 Diskussion

Zur Beschleunigung zeitkritischer Evaluationen hochauflösender endoskopischer Daten wurde das Teilproblem des Patch-Sampling als Reinforcement Learning-Problem aufgefasst. Anhand synthetischer Daten wurden Güte und Grenzen gängiger RL-Algorithmen untersucht und Proximal Policy Optimization (PPO) als besonders geeignet für das Training eines Patch Prioritisation Models (PPM) identifiziert. Anhand der Segmentierung von Polypen als Beispielaufgabe wurde die Übertragbarkeit des Ansatzes auf Realdaten demonstriert und die Überlegenheit des RL-PPM gegenüber Baseline-Ansätzen wie dem zeilenweisen Abrastern des Bildes oder der zufälligen Priorisierung von Patches gezeigt. Die Patchpriorisieurng im Rahmen von PPO wird durch eine vergleichsweise flache Architektur mit lediglich drei Convolutional Layern erreicht. Die Übersetzung der beschleunigten Konvergenz in reale Geschwindigkeitsvorteile hängt von der Komplexität des nachgeschalteten Modells ab.

Alternativ könnte ein Modell zur Patchpriorisierung auch als konventionell supervidiertes Segmentierungsmodell implementiert werden, nach dessen grob aufgelöstem Output hochauflösende Patches für die Weiterverarbeitung gesampelt würden. Ferner können Patches anhand händisch definierter Merkmale priorisiert werden, z. B. im Sinne des Vorziehens von Bereichen hoher Entropie [6]. Beidem gegenüber bietet die Formulierung als RL-Problem folgende Vorteile. *Erstens* erlaubt die Konstruktion der

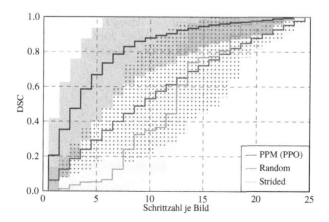

Abb. 3. Durchschnittliche Patch-Sampling-Leistung über alle Bilder der realen Testdaten. (Schattierung: eine Standardabweichung).

Observations auf native Weise die Integration von Feedback vom weiterverarbeitenden Modell durch das PPM. Zweitens ermöglicht die Fassung als RL-Strategie die Integration zusätzlicher Kriterien für die Priorisierung, sei es z. B. das Vorziehen kleiner oder randständiger Läsionen, die mutmaßlich schwerer zu entdecken bzw. kürzer sichtbar sind, beispielsweise bei Weitwinkeloptiken und Einsatz mehrerer Displays.

References

1. Schmitz R, Werner R, Repici A, Bisschops R, Meining A, Zornow M et al. Artificial intelligence in GI endoscopy: stumbling blocks, gold standards and the role of endoscopy societies. Gut. 2021:gutjnl–2020–323115.

2. Repici A, Badalamenti M, Maselli R, Correale L, Radaelli F, Rondonotti E et al. Efficacy of real-time computer-aided detection of colorectal neoplasia in a randomized trial. en. Gastroenterology. 2020;159(2):512–520.e7.

3. Zimmermann-Fraedrich K, Groth S, Sehner S, Schubert S, Aschenbeck J, Mayr M et al. Effects of two instrument-generation changes on adenoma detection rate during screening colonoscopy: results from a prospective randomized comparative study. en. Endoscopy. 2018;50(09):878–85.

4. Mendel R, Ebigbo A, Probst A, Messmann H, Palm C. Barrett's esophagus analysis using convolutional neural networks. Proc BVM. 2017:80–5.

5. Groof AJ de, Struyvenberg MR, Putten J van der, Sommen F van der, Fockens KN, Curvers WL et al. Deep-learning system detects neoplasia in patients with barrett's esophagus with higher accuracy than endoscopists in a multistep training and validation study with benchmarking. en. Gastroenterology. 2020;158(4):915–929.e4.

6. Madesta F, Schmitz R, Rösch T, Werner R. Widening the focus: biomedical image segmentation challenges and the underestimated role of patch sampling and inference strategies. MICCAI. 2020;12264:289–98.

7. Jha D, Smedsrud PH, Riegler MA, Halvorsen P, Lange T de, Johansen D et al. Kvasir-seg: a segmented polyp dataset. International Conference on Multimedia Modeling. Springer. 2020:451–62.

8. Mnih V, Badia AP, Mirza M, Graves A, Lillicrap T, Harley T et al. Asynchronous methods for deep reinforcement learning. Proc Int Conf Mach Learn. 2016;48:1928–37.

9. Mnih V, Kavukcuoglu K, Silver D, Rusu AA, Veness J, Bellemare MG et al. Human-level control through deep reinforcement learning. Nature. 2015;518(7540):529–33.

10. Schulman J, Wolski F, Dhariwal P, Radford A, Klimov O. Proximal policy optimization algorithms. 2017.

Offer Proprietary Algorithms Still Protection of Intellectual Property in the Age of Machine Learning?
A Case Study Using Dual Energy CT Data

Andreas Maier[1], Seung Hee Yang[2], Farhad Maleki[3], Nikesh Muthukrishnan[3], Reza Forghani[3]

[1]Pattern Recognition Lab, FAU Erlangen-Nürnberg
[2]Department Artificial Intelligence in Medical Engineering, FAU Erlangen-Nürnberg
[3]McGill University Hospital, McGill University
andreas.maier@fau.de

Abstract. In the domain of medical image processing, medical device manufacturers protect their intellectual property in many cases by shipping only compiled software, i.e. binary code which can be executed but is difficult to be understood by a potential attacker. In this paper, we investigate how well this procedure is able to protect image processing algorithms. In particular, we investigate whether the computation of mono-energetic images and iodine maps from dual energy CT data can be reverse-engineered by machine learning methods. Our results indicate that both can be approximated using only one single slice image as training data at a very high accuracy with structural similarity greater than 0.98 in all investigated cases.

1 Introduction

Medical image processing and analysis is heavily relying on device manufacturers as any treatment to patients has to follow medical device legislation [1]. As such vendors have great interest to protect their intellectual property such that it cannot be easily reproduced by their competition. This often results in monolithic software packages which are shipped in binary software only such that analyses can be performed while the underlying algorithm is not accessible to third parties.

As reverse engineering attacks are very expensive and require in depth knowledge [2], image processing algorithms are generally assumed to be robust against these attacks by companies in the healthcare sector. Yet, in the age of machine and deep learning [3, 4], this may no longer hold since very complex processing systems can be approximated by such techniques.

In this paper, we investigate how well image processing algorithms can be approximated using standard open source software. In particular, we will use the learning module provided in CONRAD [5], which is based on the WEKA machine learning toolbox [6], to learn algorithms related to dual energy imaging. In the first attack case, we look into computation of mono-energetic images from dual energy data given the same sampling grid. In the second case, we look into non-linear material decomposition estimated from manually pre-processed images as commonly found in clinical practice.

© Der/die Autor(en), exklusiv lizenziert durch
Springer Fachmedien Wiesbaden GmbH, ein Teil von Springer Nature 2022
K. Maier-Hein et al. (Hrsg.), *Bildverarbeitung für die Medizin 2022*,
Informatik aktuell, https://doi.org/10.1007/978-3-658-36932-3_70

2   Methods

Dual energy CT is based on the acquisition of X-ray images acquired at different kilovoltage peaks (kVp) [7]. Due to the differences in physical absorption, the materials in the imaged volume can be analysed in a quantitative way based on their physical spectral properties allowing advantages with respect to medical image analysis [8]. In particular, reconstruction of virtual monochromatic images and iodine maps are very common in this framework. The acquisition using already two photon energies (I_{low} and I_{high}) allows to estimate a wide spectrum of other acquisition energies virtually I_{virt} as described in [9]:

$$I_{virt} = \alpha \cdot I_{high} + (1 - \alpha)I_{low} \tag{1}$$

Above approximation is quite common in the world of medical physics and offers the straight forward hypothesis that also commercial algorithms should be explainable using a linear model.

Dual energy imaging also allows to perform material decomposition such as the extraction of water and iodine maps [10]. The relation between the actual energies and the materials is generally non-linear and is typically estimated using polynomial estimators. Several authors [11–13] suggested that a general machine learning model f is also suited to perform the decomposition into material maps I_{mat}:

$$I_{mat} = f(I_{high}, I_{low}) \tag{2}$$

As such, we are to expect general non-linear computations in material decomposition algorithms.

3   Experiments and results

In order to investigate above dual energy algorithms, we explored the dual energy data from a clinical scan of the neck (which includes part of the skull base and brain superiorly and part of the lungs inferiorly) using machine learning algorithms. For the training, one axial slice of the brain was selected. For testing one axial slice through the skull base and one axial slice through the lung were chosen in order to demonstrate that the learned parameters generalize over different anatomical regions as displayed in figure 1. The acquisition protocol used fast kVp-switching between 140 and 80 kV.

The original raw DICOM data only contained one of the acquisition energies in the respective DICOM field. Yet, the DICOM header offered four additional proprietary DICOM fields which stored additional pixel data in 16-bit encoding which was extracted using a custom DICOM reader supplied within the CONRAD software framework [5]. Amongst the extracted data, we found the second energy image as well as additional correction factors which are apparently used by the vendor to compute the resulting mono-energetic and material decomposition images.

All machine learning methods were trained with pixel-wise correspondences, as one would expect for single energy computation or material decomposition. None of the approaches considered a local neighborhood which implies that changes in resolution and operations such as noise reduction cannot be modelled by the learning approach.

All experiments used the default parameter setting of WEKA. No additional parameter tuning was applied. The created software was added to the CONRAD [5] repository[1].

3.1 Single energy estimation

In order to explore how well the computation of mono-energetic images is protected, single energy slices from 40 to 140 keV in steps of 20 keV were created. As observed in equation 1, we assume a linear relation between the dual energy raw data and the produced results.

The results summarized in Table 1 indicate that the linear model is able to recover all parameters of the mono-energetic image computation correctly. Correlation coefficient r and structural similarity (SSIM) lie above 0.999 in all cases indicating that the computation is identical up to 16-bit precision.

Mono-energetic Image Estimation	r	SSIM	Slice
40 kV	0.999	0.999	Skull
40 kV	0.999	0.999	Lung
60 kV	0.999	0.999	Skull
60 kV	0.999	0.999	Lung
80 kV	0.999	0.999	Skull
80 kV	0.999	0.999	Lung
100 kV	0.999	0.999	Skull
100 kV	0.999	0.999	Lung
120 kV	0.999	0.999	Skull
120 kV	0.999	0.999	Lung
140 kV	0.999	0.999	Skull
140 kV	0.999	0.999	Lung

Tab. 1. All mono-energetic slices could be reproduced with correlations and SSIMs greater than 0.999 which essentially shows that the ground truth algorithm could be extracted.

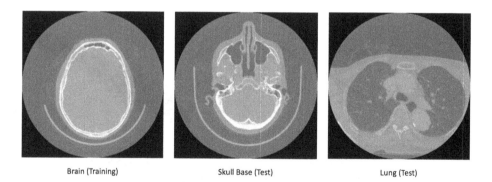

Brain (Training)   Skull Base (Test)   Lung (Test)

Fig. 1. All machine learning models were only estimated using a single slice through the brain in this paper. Evaluations were performed on a section through the skull base and the lung.

---

[1]The trained models are available at https://github.com/akmaier/CONRAD/tree/master/data/KEVS_models

3.2 Iodine map prediction

For the reliability analysis of the material decomposition, we created an Iodine map using the software on the clinical work station. In order the make the attack task even more realistic, the image resolution was and dimensions were changed from 512×512 to 1200×1024. To estimate the correct slice orientation, images were manually registered and re-sampled to match the raw data orientation. Based on the alignment, a linear and a non-linear machine learning estimator was trained. For the non-linear model WEKA's Reduced Error Pruning (REP) Tree [6] was chosen as it is faster than random forests while being more robust than the classical tree learners.

The results shown in Table 2 indicate that a linear model is not able to describe the material decomposition entirely yielding correlation and SSIM values of only 0.88 even in the case of the training slice in the brain area. The non-linear model performs much better with consistent correlation and SSIM values of over 0.98. Visual analysis of the predicted Iodine image and the ground truth indicated that the mismatch mainly comprised in changes of noise patterns, image resolution, and image alignment. Hence, the REP Tree model delivers a very close approximation of the ground truth algorithm of the vendor.

Tab. 2. The linear model only creates a coarse estimation of the material decomposition. The non-linear REP Tree, however, consistently achieves correlation and SSIM values greater than 0.98. The main difference between the produced images in this case is the change of orientation and resolution.

Mono-energetic Image Estimation	r	SSIM	Slice
Iodine (linear)	0.894	0.888	Brain
Iodine (linear)	0.825	0.808	Skull
Iodine (linear)	0.766	0.475	Lung
Iodine (REP Tree)	0.997	0.997	Brain
Iodine (REP Tree)	0.993	0.993	Skull
Iodine (REP Tree)	0.985	0.985	Lung

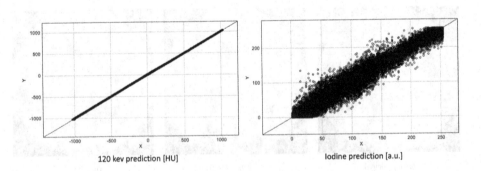

120 kev prediction [HU]   Iodine prediction [a.u.]

Fig. 2. Regression analysis on the lung slice data set: The left image shows the strong correlation between ground truth values and the machine learning estimates for the prediction of 120 kV images. The right side shows a scatter analysis between the ground truth iodine maps and the predictions by the tree model with an SSIM of more than 0.98.

4 Discussion

The presented results indicate that linear prediction algorithms can be approximated by pixel-wise machine learning methods very well. Furthermore, even in adverse conditions in a non-linear setting with changes in resolution and slice alignment, very high correlation values and structural similarity could be obtained using a tree learning. We assume that advanced machine learning models [4] would be able to capture such differences as well. Yet, they would probably require more than a single slice image as training data.

Generally, it is surprising to see how common open source tools already are able to approximate vendor algorithms. As such one might wonder whether closed source software still offers sufficient protection of algorithms and their intellectual property. In the machine learning world, even industrial players started to publish source code and trained models. One reason for this is of course that doing so allows them to incorporate contributors outside their payroll. Open-sourcing such software with appropriate licenses that protect the vendor's intellectual property might be a more promising approach in comparison to closed-source software that can be easily reverse-engineered.

Given the results in this paper, the advantage of closed source in terms of algorithm protection might not be as strong as one might expect. Hence, even industrial players in field field of medical image processing may want to reconsider the disadvantages of open source with respect to software and intellectual security. Given enough data, we expect many other algorithms could fall to the presented attack scheme.

Developing in open source domain may be even of advantage in the future for many medical device manufacturers as they would be able to harness the ingenuity of the entire academic community. The authors of this paper strongly believe that this direction would be beneficial for the entire medical image processing community.

5 Conclusion

Closed source software is no longer a sufficient protection strategy for many image processing algorithms as demonstrated by the results in this paper. Even non-linear material decomposition algorithms can be estimated by rather simple means in adverse conditions using only a single slice image. Generally, results yielded correlation and structural similarity of 0.98 or higher which indicates that the machine learning methods were able to precisely estimate the closed source algorithms correctly.

References

1. Sorenson C, Drummond M. Improving medical device regulation: the united states and europe in perspective. Milbank Q. 2014;92(1):114–50.
2. Canfora G, Di Penta M, Cerulo L. Achievements and challenges in software reverse engineering. Communications of the ACM. 2011;54(4):142–51.
3. LeCun Y, Bengio Y, Hinton G. Deep learning. nature. 2015;521(7553):436–44.
4. Maier A, Syben C, Lasser T, Riess C. A gentle introduction to deep learning in medical image processing. Z Med Phys. 2019;29(2):86–101.
5. Maier A, Hofmann HG, Berger M, Fischer P, Schwemmer C, Wu H et al. CONRAD: a software framework for cone-beam imaging in radiology. Med Phys. 2013;40(11):111914.

6. Hall M, Frank E, Holmes G, Pfahringer B, Reutemann P, Witten IH. The WEKA data mining software: an update. ACM SIGKDD explorations newsletter. 2009;11(1):10–18.

7. Maier A, Steidl S, Christlein V, Hornegger J. Medical imaging systems: an introductory guide. Springer, 2018.

8. Chen S, Zhong X, Hu S, Dorn S, Kachelrieß M, Lell M et al. Automatic multi-organ segmentation in dual-energy CT (DECT) with dedicated 3D fully convolutional DECT networks. Med Phys. 2020;47(2):552–62.

9. Krauss B, Schmidt B, Flohr TG. Dual energy CT in clinical practice. Medical Radiology, Berlin, Heidelberg: Springer Berlin Heidelberg. 2011.

10. Liu X, Yu L, Primak AN, McCollough CH. Quantitative imaging of element composition and mass fraction using dual-energy CT: three-material decomposition. Med Phys. 2009;36(5):1602–9.

11. Lu Y, Geret J, Unberath M, Manhart M, Ren Q, Fahrig R et al. Projection-based material decomposition by machine learning using image-based features for computed tomography. The 13th International Meeting on Fully Three-Dimensional Image Reconstruction in Radiology and Nuclear Medicine. 2015:448–51.

12. Lu Y, Kowarschik M, Huang X, Xia Y, Choi JH, Chen S et al. A learning-based material decomposition pipeline for multi-energy x-ray imaging. Med Phys. 2019;46(2):689–703.

13. Geng M, Tian Z, Jiang Z, You Y, Feng X, Xia Y et al. PMS-GAN: parallel multi-stream generative adversarial network for multi-material decomposition in spectral computed omography. IEEE Trans Med Imaging. 2020;40(2):571–84.

Abstract: Face Detection From In-car Video for Continuous Health Monitoring

Vinothini Selvaraju[1,2], Nicolai Spicher[2], Ramakrishnan Swaminathan[1],
Thomas M. Deserno[2]

[1]Department of Applied Mechanics, Indian Institute of Technology Madras, Chennai, India
[2]Peter L. Reichertz Institute for Medical Informatics of TU Braunschweig and Hannover
Medical School, Braunschweig, Germany
vinothini.selvaraju@plri.de

Face detection in videos from smart cars or homes is becoming increasingly important
in human-computer interaction, emotion recognition, gender and age identification,
driving assistance, and vital sign measurements, as heart rate and respiratory rate is
derived from the video. However, face detection suffers from variations in illumination,
subject motion, different skin colors, or camera distances. In this work [1], we compare
three algorithms for in-car application: Haar cascade classifier (HCC), histogram of
oriented gradients (HoG), and a deep neural network (DNN). For evaluation, we consider
the freely available "driver monitoring dataset" (DMD) multimodal database and self-
collected videos recorded in a research car. We analyze run-time, accuracy, and F1-score.
HoG has highest computational time as compared to HCC and DNN with 2.99 frames
per second (FPS), 7.00 FPS, and 18.25 FPS, respectively. For DMD, the F1-scores
are 91.75%, 95.91%, and 99.48% for HCC, HoG, and DNN respectively, and 88.05%,
83.68%, and 99.66% for our dataset, respectively. All in all, DNN is fastest and most
accurate. Moreover, we observed that DNN handles occlusions and varying illumination
better than the other approaches. In conclusion, DNN can be applied successfully for
in-car face detection as a first step towards real-time continuous health monitoring.

References

1. Selvaraju V, Spicher N, Swaminathan R, Deserno TM. Face Detection From In-car Video
   for Continuous Health Monitoring. Proc SPIE. 2022:(*accepted*).

Autorenverzeichnis

Printed in the United States
by Baker & Taylor Publisher Services